ROSS & WILSON PHARMACOLOGY

ROSS & WILSON PHARMACOLOGY

Allison Grant, BSc, PhD, FHEA

Lecturer, School of Health and Life Sciences
Glasgow Caledonian University
Glasgow
UK

ELSEVIER

Notices

ISBN: 978-0-7020-8098-2

Content Strategist: Andrae Akeh
Content Project Manager: Fariha Nadeem
Design: Margaret M. Reid
Illustration Manager: Muthukumaran Thangaraj
Marketing Manager: Deborah Watkins

Printed in India

Last digit is the print number: 9 8 7 6 5 4 3 2 1

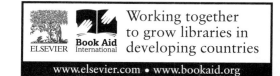

Contents

Preface

Records dating from ancient civilisations in Sumeria, Egypt, India, and China show the origins of medicine and mankind's attempts to understand and treat disease. Healing practices in antiquity often relied on the intervention of gods, the wearing of talismans to ward off disease, a strong belief in magic, and the use of ceremonial rituals to increase the patient's chance of recovery; however, the concept that external substances swallowed, applied topically, or inhaled could influence outcomes was also very familiar to the earliest physicians. These early medicines were derived from the natural world and included plant, animal, and mineral extracts; most were useless, and many were actively harmful.

Fast forward to the 21st century, and the use of drugs to prevent, cure, or manage diseases has become a cornerstone of therapeutics. Very few human diseases or disorders are managed without the use of drugs, and all healthcare professionals require a thorough, evidence-based understanding of clinical pharmacology to prescribe safely, to monitor the effectiveness of treatment, and to competently advise and inform patients from a solid, evidence-based knowledge base. This text has been written with this role in mind. It goes beyond the simple listing of drugs, their actions, and side-effects and explains the science underpinning the mechanisms of action of drugs, but without being bogged down with excessive detail. Understanding what a drug does to a living system and how it exerts its biological effects explains the rationale behind its use in the disease for which it is being used and the reason why it may have apparently unconnected side-effects. Understanding how the human body responds to a drug introduced into its living tissues is an essential prerequisite for safe prescribing and when monitoring response to treatment. It ensures that the prescriber chooses the most appropriate medicine and drug formulation and, as far as possible, anticipates problems arising from inter-individual drug responses, interactions, and issues.

The 'focus boxes' used in several chapters are designed to encapsulate and present key content, emphasising important concepts and topic areas. 'Key points' boxes and 'key definitions' boxes have also been used to help navigation and to emphasise significant terms.

The pharmacology described here is anchored firmly in its scientific basis, but with a clear clinical slant. This textbook should be a useful resource for students and practitioners in health-related professions and would also be an appropriate resource for students in a range of life science programmes with an element of pharmacological content. Together with its companion book, *Ross and Wilson's Pathophysiology*, this text is designed to provide a fundamental but thorough grounding in the areas of disease and therapeutics. Both books have been written for you, the student; I hope this textbook meets your needs and is of direct and measurable benefit to your studies and your practice. I am happy to receive feedback, suggestions, and comments; academic resources are always improved by collaboration and discussion!

Allison Grant
March 2024

Acknowledgements

Without the (sometimes unseen but always appreciated) efforts of a range of people, this textbook would never have made it all the way from a few undefined ideas rattling around in my head to the finished product you now hold in your hands. I think of it as 'my book', because the time and effort required to prepare it has extended over 3 years, greedily consuming evenings and weekends and at times crowding out everything else going on in my life, though I am very conscious of and grateful for the support of family and friends and the huge role played by the team at Elsevier, because it would never have happened without them.

I thank Pauline Graham, formerly of Elsevier, who suggested and initiated the project in the first place. My gratitude is also due to Anne Waugh, who knows what I owe to her over the 20-plus years that we have been collaborators, co-authors, and friends. Thank you, Anne, for your time in reviewing some of this content and for everything else you've contributed to this project.

I thank all those at Elsevier who have had any part to play in the realisation of this project. I have no direct contact with the experts who deal with page layout, typesetting, or any of the other stages in converting my digital files, figure lists, and so on to the finished pages, but I thank you very much. In particular, I owe a huge debt of gratitude to Fariha Nadeem, who has been a constant, steady, and rock-solid support. I am also very pleased to thank Marie Dean, who managed to translate my coloured scrawls and scribbled instructions into the book's clear and colourful artwork.

I've been in higher education for a good few years now and taught thousands of students, and it is for you all that academics like me pick up our pens and write academic textbooks. Thank you for the inspiration. Stay curious, stay interested, keep reading, take nothing at face value, always look for the evidence base, always think 'but why…???', keep asking questions, don't expect me (or my academic colleagues) to have all the answers, and be prepared to go out and find the answers for yourselves. We are giving you the foundation, but you are the next generation and will be standing on our shoulders.

And finally, to my much-loved circle of family and friends, thank you for everything. None of you helped me write any of this, so you can't be blamed for any errors, but none of this would have happened without you.

Allison Grant
March 2024

For my sun, moon, and stars, Seona, Struan, and Will:
the adventures go on!!

The Story of Pharmacology

1

The history of human drug use from its earliest origins, for which we only have archaeological evidence, through the scientific revolution of the 18th and 19th centuries up to today's position as one of the key pillars of modern medicine, is one of the most interesting stories in science. One current definition of pharmacology from the British Pharmacological Society is 'the science of drugs and their effects on living systems'. A 'drug' can be defined as any chemical substance, natural or synthetic, that affects some aspect of the biology of a living system. This broad definition therefore encompasses not just the clinically useful drugs that are the subject of textbooks like this one aimed at students and practitioners in medical and healthcare professions, but also food additives, environmental pollutants, dyes and other chemicals, and a wide range of substances derived from the natural world, which includes some of the most toxic chemicals known. The conventional use of the word 'drug' implies a substance used to diagnose, treat, or prevent a medical condition as well as substances used recreationally, and the term 'clinical pharmacology' came into use in the 1950s to refer to all aspects of research, policy, safety, teaching, and use of drugs in humans.

THE ORIGINS OF PHARMACOLOGY

Mankind has had a long and fascinating relationship with chemical substances that affect some aspects of behaviour, feelings, or well-being. The earliest written record of the use of a drug is a scrap of Egyptian papyrus dating from 3500 BC describing alcohol production, but archaeological evidence from even earlier periods indicates that intoxicants were in use well before then.

The earliest recorded drugs were psychotropic agents used for recreational, ritual, and medicinal purposes, and include **alcohol**, **opium**, and **cannabis**. Alcohol was being fermented at least 10,000 years ago. Opium, the juice obtained from the seed head of the opium poppy (Fig. 1.1), was cultivated, distributed, and sold widely throughout large areas of the Middle East, Europe, and beyond. Its analgesic, euphoric, and sedative properties were well understood, as was its lethality: it was used to ease the passage into death and occasionally as a means to dispose of enemies. Archaeologists have found little opium flasks in graves and other archaeological sites, in the shape of the opium poppy seed head (Fig. 1.2), and analysis has shown that they contained opium and sometimes other psychoactive substances. Hemp has been in use for production of fibres for clothing and

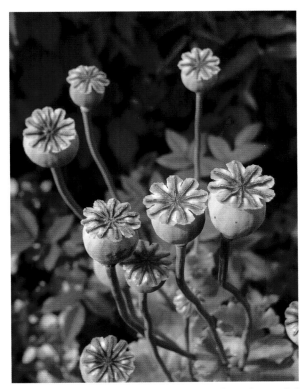

Fig 1.1 The seed head of the opium poppy. Once the petals have fallen off, exposing the seed head, opium is collected from vertical cuts made in the seed head. (From Garg A (2010) Implant dentistry, 2nd ed, Fig. 10.2. Philadelphia: Mosby.)

1

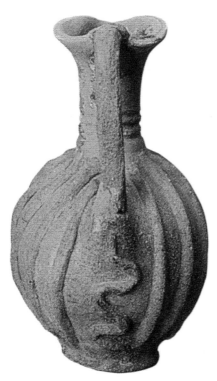

Fig 1.2   Clay vessel from Crete in the shape of the opium poppy seed head. (From Karageorghis V, Kanta A, Stampolides NC, et al. (2014). Kypriaka in Crete: from the bronze age to the end of the archaic period. Zurich: A.G. Leventis Foundation.)

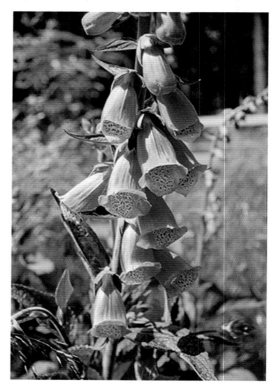

Fig 1.3   *Digitalis purpurea* (foxglove) (From Renneberg R (2023) Biotechnology for beginners, 3rd ed, Fig. 7.30. Philadelphia: Academic Press.)

rope for thousands of years. The use of cannabis, derived from hemp, also dates back to pre-history and was well-known in multiple cultures including ancient China, the Middle East, Greece, and Rome.

The plant kingdom was mankind's main source for medicinal and recreational drugs for thousands of years, and there is evidence that in some cultures, manufacturing took place on a large scale. In the late 2000s, a large kitchen dating from 2000 BC was found in Ebla in Syria, close to the city palace. There was no evidence of food remains, but there were traces of a range of plants used in medicine, including opium, chamomile (used as an anti-inflammatory), and heliotrope (used to treat infections), indicating a small-scale but well-established and well-organised drug preparation industry. In the era before written records, knowledge of useful plants and how to prepare extracts must have been part of a people's oral tradition. Development of traditional medicines over the centuries, with none of today's understanding of chemistry, physiology, genetics, or molecular biology, was largely a process governed by careful observation and trial and error. That is not to dismiss natural remedies as ineffective or without an evidence base: the use of opium as an analgesic and sedative in ancient cultures is proof of that. Many substances found in the natural world are highly potent: extracts of foxglove (*Digitalis purpurea*, Fig. 1.3) were used for centuries to treat dropsy. Dropsy is an obsolete term for oedema, which usually collects in the lower limb. Although it can be due to several conditions, one of the most common is heart failure, and the use of foxglove

extract, which contains **digitalis**, improved heart function and relieved the oedema. Digitalis is still used today to treat heart failure and some arrhythmias.

The scientific revolution of the 16th to 19th centuries brought rapid development across the biological, physical, and chemical sciences, driven by the change in thinking that is the scientific method—the process by which a researcher draws factual and substantiated conclusions after careful experimentation and rigorous testing of a hypothesis. Key to the emergence of pharmacology as a separate speciality were the advances made in chemistry, particularly organic chemistry, and physiology. As the early chemists learned how to extract, separate, synthesise, purify, and concentrate substances of interest, it became possible to test accurately measured drug quantities in biological systems. The first drug to be isolated from its crude extract was **morphine**, purified from opium by Friedrich Setürner in 1804 (Fig. 1.4). As physiological knowledge advanced, so did the understanding of what drugs were doing to the body and how they acted, and drug use in medicine began very slowly to move away from traditional, often arbitrary, frequently useless, and potentially lethal practices towards a more evidence-based approach to therapeutics grounded in observation, measurement, analysis, and pooled knowledge.

The development of analytical chemistry directly and indirectly produced whole new classes of drugs, many of which remain in widespread use. For example, the synthetic dye industry emerged in the mid-1850s and spawned a range of clinically important drug groups. The first dye to be used medicinally was **methylene blue**, the same dye used by Paul Ehrlich to demonstrate the presence of the blood–brain barrier (p. 12). In 1891, he was trying to stain the protozoa *Plasmodium*, which causes malaria, with methylene blue to study it under the microscope. He observed that the dye inhibited the activity of the protozoa and reasoned that it might be a useful agent to treat malaria in humans; as a result, methylene blue was used for this purpose until the early 20th century, when newer drugs superseded it. Phenothiazine antipsychotics such as **chlorpromazine**, antihistamines such as **promethazine**, tricyclic antidepressants such as **amitriptyline**, thiazide diuretics such as **bendrofluazide**, and sulphonamide antibacterials such as **sulphamethoxazole** are all derived from the synthetic dye industry.

In the first half of the 20th century, a plethora of new drugs appeared on the scene. Generally, they were found by accident; drugs developed as a side-line of the dye industry for example, or Alexander Fleming's chance observation that *Penicillium* moulds inhibited bacterial growth in his test plates, leading to the isolation of **penicillin** (Fig. 1.5). More targeted drug development became possible as research into the molecular basis of drug action rapidly advanced. Increasing knowledge of receptor science, enzyme structure, and molecular and cell biology expanded our understanding of how drugs interact with specific molecules to produce their biological effects.

Biologics

In the last 40 years or so, biotechnology has generated a wide range of new therapeutics called biologics. Biologics are drugs whose active substance is made by a living organism, including genetically engineered bacteria, and include antibodies, hormones, immunomodulators, vaccines, cytokines, blood products, and growth factors.

Pharmacogenomics

Advances in genetics have shone a bright light onto the relationship between our genes and disease, and on an individual's response to drugs. This new field, pharmacogenomics, is an important element in personalised medicine. It has been estimated that between 30% and 60% of drug treatments are ineffective because of genetically determined responses to the medication. Identifying important genetic variations between individuals allows optimal therapeutic choices to be made based on predicted drug responses and

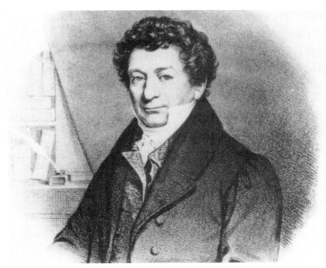

Fig 1.4   Friedrich Sertürner (From Göttmann F (1999) Paderborn - Geschichte der Stadt in ihrer Region. Band 2. Die frühe Neuzeit: gesellschaftliche Stabilität und politischer Wandel. Berlin: Schöningh.)

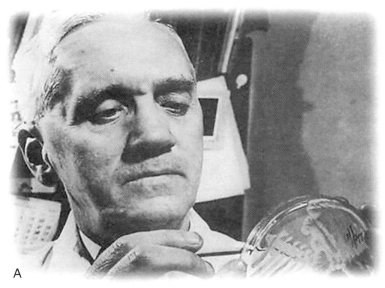
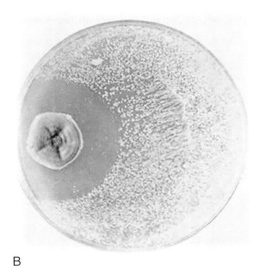

A   B

Fig 1.5   A. Alexander Fleming. B. A culture plate showing a large *Penicillium* mould on the left, surrounded by a clear area of agar into which the bacteria covering most of the plate cannot grow. Fleming concluded that the mould was producing a chemical toxic to the bacteria. (From Oria M and Raffin J (1971) Anatomie, physiologie, hygiène, 3rd ed, Hatier.)

likely side-effects. This principle is illustrated in Fig. 1.6. The group of patients shown in Fig. 1.6 all have the same disease, and all are being treated with the same dose of the same drug. Within this group, the patients depicted in green are predicted to respond well. The patients depicted in blue are predicted to respond poorly, if at all, and for these patients a different dose or a different drug would be a better choice. The patients depicted in red are predicted to experience significant toxicity, and this drug should not be used in these patients.

For instance, the gene that codes for the important drug-metabolising enzyme CYP2D6 commonly harbours mutations that can affect how effective the final enzyme product is. CYP2D6 metabolises a range of drugs including **anti-arrhythmics**, **antidepressants,** and **antipsychotics**, and for the 25% of the population in whom this enzyme is less active, their ability to metabolise these drugs is impaired and the risk of potentially dangerous side-effects at normal doses is increased. Clearly, genetic profiling information flagging up CYP2D6 deficiency in advance of prescribing would be very useful. Another example is serious hypersensitivity to **abacavir**, an antiviral used in HIV combination therapy. Around 5% of patients have a gene variant called *HLA-B*5701*, which increases the risk of a serious hypersensitivity reaction. Testing for this mutation allows the clinical team to make an informed choice regarding the risk-benefit ratio and has reduced the incidence of hypersensitivity reactions.

FROM BENCH TO BEDSIDE

The science underpinning the action of drugs is the foundation on which safe clinical pharmacology is based. It is useful to remember that the range of drugs used in medicine represents the tip of an iceberg; the bulk of the iceberg represents the vast amount of research time, money, and effort required to bring the drug into clinical use. Much of that research is done at the lab bench, so-called basic science. Fig. 1.7 shows the main stages of drug development.

THE DRUG DEVELOPMENT PROCESS

The average journey time of a drug from the lab bench to reaching the market is over 12 years, at a cost of over £1.1 billion. Typically, from an initial pool of 10,000 candidates, only one will be approved by the regulatory body, and only one in five drugs that reach the market will actually recoup the costs involved in its development.

In modern pharmaceutical science, the development of a new drug follows identification of a specific target. For example, if a lab-based research project in a university or a research institute studying the pathology of an inflammatory disease identifies a new enzyme that synthesises an inflammatory mediator, a drug that inhibits that enzyme might be a useful anti-inflammatory agent. The structure of the enzyme can be precisely determined, making it possible to design a range of compounds which could be expected to inhibit enzyme activity. This is called rational drug design. In addition, candidates from natural sources or compound libraries held by pharmaceutical companies may also be screened. Tens or possibly hundreds of thousands of potential candidates can be tested to see if they inhibit the enzyme. Of these initial screens, compounds with the most promising profiles are taken forward into more comprehensive studies. These are called lead compounds. Most screened compounds do not make it to this stage for one or more reasons; perhaps their molecular weight is too high, they demonstrate toxicity in cell lines or animal studies, they may not be potent enough, or they fail to show expected activity in animal studies.

PRE-CLINICAL DEVELOPMENT

The small number of candidate compounds, typically 10–20, that make it through the earlier stages are taken to preclinical development. This involves toxicity screening and pharmacokinetic assessment (absorption, distribution, metabolism, and excretion) in computer modelling, cell lines, and animal models. The test compounds will also undergo chemical assessment looking at formulation options and any limitations to large-scale synthesis. Drug candidates that perform satisfactorily in preclinical trials can go forward to clinical trials in humans.

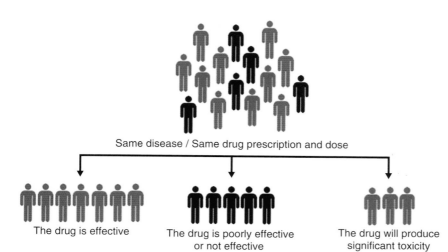

Same disease / Same drug prescription and dose

The drug is effective

The drug is poorly effective or not effective

The drug will produce significant toxicity

Fig 1.6 The advantages of predicting genetically determined drug responses. All patients have the same disease, and all are being treated with the same dose of the same drug. Green patients are good responders and should do well on the treatment. Blue patients will respond poorly or not at all, and this treatment is not the optimal choice. Red patients will experience significant toxicity and the treatment should be avoided. (Modified from Patrinos GP (2020) Applied genomics and public health, Fig. 6.1. Philadelphia: Academic Press.)

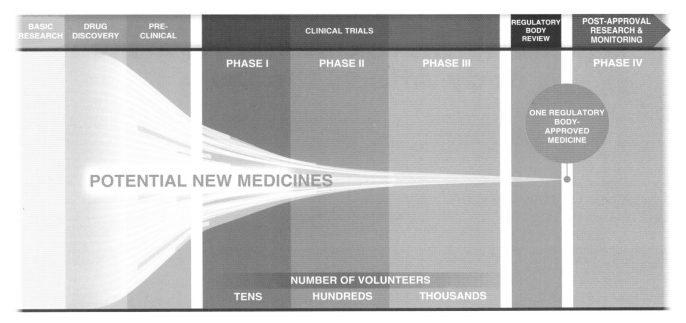

Fig 1.7 **The main stages in drug development.** (Reproduced from Profile, 2015 (2015) Pharmaceutical Industry, PhRMA, Washington DC.)

CLINICAL TRIALS

There are four main stages, and the candidate drug can be stopped at any stage if thought appropriate. In phase 1 studies, the candidate drug is given in small doses to a small group, usually 20 to 100, of healthy volunteers. The volunteers are monitored carefully for any adverse effects. In phase 2 studies, the drug is given to larger groups (100–500) of patients suffering from the condition(s) for which the candidate drug is thought to be potentially useful. Most drugs that fail at clinical trial do so during phase 2 studies, because evidence emerges of unacceptable adverse effects or toxicity, or the drug turns out to be inadequately potent. Phase 3 trials are much larger, double-blind, randomised clinical trials in which the candidate drug is tested at different doses in groups of thousands of patients against current treatments and/or placebo. Assuming the phase 3 trials show the drug to be effective, non-toxic, and not associated with unacceptable side-effects, the company can apply to the relevant national regulatory board for approval to bring it to market. Phase 4 trials are the processes by which the performance of drugs on the market are monitored and rare and/or chronic adverse effects picked up. They also include any special trials required to allow the drug to be licensed in specific groups of patients, e.g. children.

DRUG NAMES

A drug may have three names: its chemical name, its generic name, and its proprietary name.

The full chemical name is often long, unwieldy, and rarely appropriate for use in clinical settings. The recommendation to take two tablets of *N*-(4-hydroxyphenyl) acetamide for a headache would not mean much to most people; recommending two **paracetamol** tablets on the other hand is a much clearer and more familiar instruction.

The generic (non-proprietary) name of the active drug is the name approved by an expert regulatory body and used internationally. Paracetamol is the generic name for this drug assigned by the World Health Organisation and is the name used outside the US; it is called **acetaminophen** in the US because that is the generic name given to it by American regulatory bodies.

Proprietary names are assigned by a manufacturer to their own formulation of a drug. Paracetamol can be sold under the brand names Tylenol, Panadol, Metacin, Calpol, Crocin, Hedex, and others. It is important to realise that there is not always bioequivalence between two brands of the same dose of the same drug, meaning that depending on the formulation, preparations from different manufacturers may give different rates and extent of absorption. Plasma levels 1 hour after taking 500 mg of product A from one manufacturer may be very different to plasma levels 1 hour after taking 500 mg of exactly the same drug but as proprietary product B from another company. Changing from one brand to another can cause issues with drugs for which even slight changes in plasma levels can cause adverse effects, e.g. **anticoagulants** and **anticonvulsants**.

REFERENCES

Dollery, C.T., 2006. Clinical pharmacology-the first 75 years and a view of the future. Br J Clin Pharmacol 61 (6), 650–665.

Wainwright, M., 2008. Dyes in the development of drugs and pharmaceuticals. Dyes Pigm 76 (3), 582–589.

ONLINE RESOURCES

Adams, J.U., 2008. Pharmacogenomics and personalized medicine. Available at: https://www.nature.com/scitable/topicpage/pharmacogenomics-and-personalized-medicine-643/.

Genomics Education Programme, 2018. What is pharmacogenomics? Available at: https://www.genomicseducation.hee.nhs.uk/blog/what-is-pharmacogenomics/#tab-id-4.

Matyszak, P., 2019. Happy plants and laughing weeds: how people of the ancient world used – and abused – drugs. Available at: https://www.historyextra.com/period/ancient-history/ancient-drug-use-history-how-what-for-opium-hemp/.

Torjesen, I., 2015. Drug development: the journey of a medicine from lab to shelf. Available at: https://pharmaceutical-journal.com/article/feature/drug-development-the-journey-of-a-medicine-from-lab-to-shelf.

2 Pharmacokinetics: How the Body Affects the Drug

Pharmacokinetics is the umbrella term which describes how the tissues and organs of the body deal with biologically active drugs, sometimes simply put as 'what the body does to the drug'. The body is very good at dealing with foreign or unwanted substances, and an understanding of the physical and chemical principles governing these processes is an important part of clinical pharmacology. For example, pharmacokinetic data informs dosing regimens, predicts plasma levels (important to ensure that dose and dose frequency are appropriate), and guides a prescriber when inter-individual variability is likely to affect drug response. Discussion of the four key pharmacokinetic processes—absorption, distribution, metabolism, and excretion, often referred to by the mnemonic ADME—forms the core of this chapter, along with an explanation of relevant key concepts such as half-life and steady state.

DRUG MOVEMENT AROUND THE BODY

In general, drugs do not remain at their site of administration but travel to distant tissues; drug mobility is usually essential to achieving its therapeutic aim. The main biological barrier to drug movement between and through body compartments is the cell membrane.

THE CELL MEMBRANE

For drugs to move around the body, they must travel through sheets of body cells. For example, a swallowed drug is absorbed into the tissues of the wall of the small intestine and then across the walls of intestinal blood vessels into the bloodstream. To do this, the drug molecules must travel

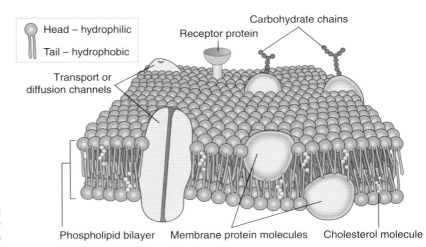

Fig. 2.1 The cell membrane. (From Waugh A and Grant A (2020) Ross & Wilson anatomy and physiology in health and illness, 14th ed, Fig. 3.2A. Oxford: Elsevier.)

through the layers of cells from the intestinal lumen to the bloodstream, and to do so must travel through the plasma membranes enclosing each cell. Fig. 2.1 shows the key features of the cell membrane. Cell membranes are semi-fluid sheets of phospholipid. A phospholipid molecule has two regions: two hydrophobic (water-repelling) lipid tails and a hydrophilic (water-attracting) head containing a phosphate group. Because body fluids, including both intracellular and extracellular fluids, are water-based, the phospholipid molecules align themselves into a bilayer, with the hydrophobic tails oriented inwards and the hydrophilic heads pointing outwards. Embedded in the membrane is a wide variety of proteins and carbohydrates, many of which are important drug targets and discussed in more detail in Chapter 3. Protein receptors allow the cell to respond to chemical signals such as hormones, growth factors, cytokines, and other substances in the extracellular environment, and these receptors are important targets for a very wide range of clinically important drugs. Additionally, the membrane is punctured with pores, channels, and pumps, which permits it to selectively transfer ions or molecules in or out of the cell.

DRUG TRANSFER ACROSS THE PLASMA MEMBRANE

Most drugs transfer passively across cell membranes by simple diffusion: that is, they travel down a concentration gradient from an area of high concentration to an area of low concentration (Fig. 2.2A). Advantages of simple diffusion are that energy is not required, and the transfer process is not saturable. This means that there is no rate-limiting step as there may be with carrier- or pump-driven transport mechanisms as described below. Taking absorption from the small intestine into the bloodstream as an example, drug levels in the intestine rise rapidly as a swallowed drug arrives from the stomach. Drug molecules therefore diffuse rapidly into the tract wall and across the walls of the blood vessels supplying it. Because the blood is constantly flowing, absorbed drug is rapidly carried away, keeping drug levels in the blood lower than drug levels in the tract lumen, and until most drug is absorbed from the intestine, there is a concentration gradient to ensure that drug diffusion and absorption continues. However, not all drugs travel equally well across plasma membranes. The main factors determining the efficiency of drug transfer through membranes are

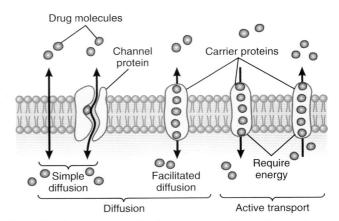

Fig. 2.2 Transport mechanisms across the cell membrane. A. Simple diffusion. B. Diffusion through ion channel. C. Facilitated diffusion. D. Active transport. (Modified from Hall JE and Hall ME (2021) Guyton and Hall textbook of medical physiology, 14th ed, Fig. 4.2. Philadelphia: Elsevier Inc.)

the lipid (fat) solubility, molecular weight (MW), and electrical charge (degree of ionisation) of the drug molecules.

Fat Solubility

The plasma membrane is essentially a lipid sheet, and to transfer rapidly from one side to the other, drug molecules must be fat-soluble. The more fat-soluble the drug, the faster and more efficiently it can transfer. Water-soluble drugs are repelled by the phospholipid bilayer and transfer slowly, and so travel less well through body tissues. Most drugs used in clinical practice are highly fat-soluble.

Molecular Weight

The plasma membrane is thin but densely packed, and larger molecules travel through it less easily than smaller molecules. Water molecules, despite being insoluble in fat, are so small (MW 18) that they travel freely through plasma membranes. To facilitate efficient movement around the body, drug molecules are generally small, with MWs less than 600, and drugs with a MW of 80,000 or more transfer very slowly, if at all.

Degree of Ionisation

The degree to which a drug molecule is ionised (electrically charged) affects its ability to transfer across cell membranes because it affects its water solubility and therefore its ability to pass through the lipid-rich cell membrane. The more highly ionised (charged) the drug is, the more water-soluble it tends to be, and it is repelled by membrane lipids, preventing its transfer. The degree of ionisation is affected by pH, as will be explored in more detail later; this is an important concept because there are significant differences in pH across different areas of the body.

Ion Channels

These channels allow ions to travel across the membrane to the other side (Fig. 2.2B). They are found in all cell membranes, but are particularly important in nerve and muscle cells, which rely on the movement of ions to generate and propagate electrical currents.

Facilitated Diffusion

As in simple diffusion, in facilitated diffusion drug molecules move passively down their concentration gradient, but at a faster rate because they are facilitated by a special carrier molecule in the membrane (Fig. 2.2C). Like simple diffusion, this is also a passive movement because no energy is required. The tissues richest in these carrier molecules are the intestines, kidney, and liver, the cells of which require to actively import a range of substances: the intestines for absorption, the kidneys for excretion, and the liver for metabolism. Carrier mechanisms allow relatively water-soluble drugs to transfer across plasma membranes, for example, the secretion of **penicillin** and **diuretics** into the filtrate in renal tubules. Other examples include **vitamin B_{12}** absorption in the intestine. These carrier mechanisms can represent a rate-limiting step in the transfer of drugs from one side of the membrane to the other. Once carrier mechanisms are fully saturated and operating at their maximal capacity, increasing drug concentrations does not increase transfer.

Active Transport

Active transport mechanisms use energy in the form of ATP to move a molecule from one side of the membrane to another and are useful when the drug is poorly lipid-soluble and diffusion rates are low (Fig. 2.2D). They also allow a drug to be moved against its concentration gradient, i.e. from low to high. Active transport mechanisms are frequently involved in the transfer of cytotoxic drugs including **5-fluorouracil**, as well as **iron** salts, **levodopa,** and **propylthiouracil**. A point worth noting regarding active transport mechanisms is that they have a maximum work rate, and so there is an upper limit on the speed of drug transfer: the mechanism can become saturated at higher drug concentrations.

pH, DRUG IONISATION, AND DRUG TRANSFER ACROSS MEMBRANES

pH is a measure of the acidity or alkalinity (basicity) of a solution. An acidic substance releases hydrogen ions (H^+, also called protons) when in solution; an acidic solution therefore is rich in H^+ ions. The higher the [H^+], the more acidic is the solution. A base binds H^+ ions and may release hydroxyl ions (OH^-) when in solution. The pH of a solution is measured using the pH scale (Fig. 2.3). The midpoint is assigned a value of 7 and represents pH neutrality, meaning the concentrations of OH^- and H^+ ions are equal. pH values below 7 represent increasing acidity as the value approaches 1; each whole value represents a tenfold increase in [H^+], so that a solution of pH 4 has 10 times as many H^+ ions as a solution of pH 5. pH values from 7 up to 14 represent increasing [OH^-] or increasing alkalinity.

Most drugs are weak bases, although some (e.g. **aspirin**, **warfarin**, **penicillin**) are weak acids. On arrival in the acidic environment of the stomach, because they are weak bases and H^+ ion acceptors, they pick up H^+ ions and become positively charged. This reduces their ability to travel across the stomach wall, and so they remain trapped in the stomach fluids. However, when they arrive in the small intestine, where the pH is much higher than in the stomach because the digestive juices are alkaline, they lose their H^+ and revert to their uncharged form. This increases their ability to cross plasma membranes, and as a result, they are absorbed across the intestinal wall into the bloodstream (Fig. 2.4A).

For drugs that are weak acids, the opposite applies. Arriving in the stomach, the drug molecules remain un-ionised (uncharged) because the gastric environment is already so rich in H^+ ions that they are unable to release their protons. As they remain un-ionised (uncharged), even though the stomach is not designed for absorption, some drug molecules diffuse into the tissues of the stomach wall and from there diffuse into the bloodstream. Once in the small intestine, where the pH is much higher, they give up their H^+ ions, acquiring a net negative charge, and their ability to cross the intestinal wall is greatly reduced (Fig. 2.4B). Having said that, most absorption of an acidic drug still takes place in the small intestine, because although ionisation of the drug slows its transfer across the tract wall, the total surface area of the small intestine is vast, which favours absorption and compensates for the slow transfer.

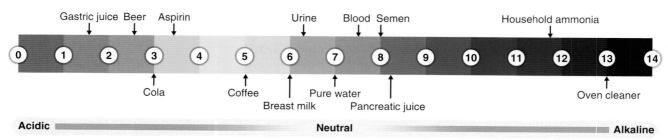

Fig. 2.3   The pH scale. (From Waugh A and Grant A (2020) Ross & Wilson anatomy and physiology in health and illness, 14th ed, Fig. 3.2A. Oxford: Elsevier.)

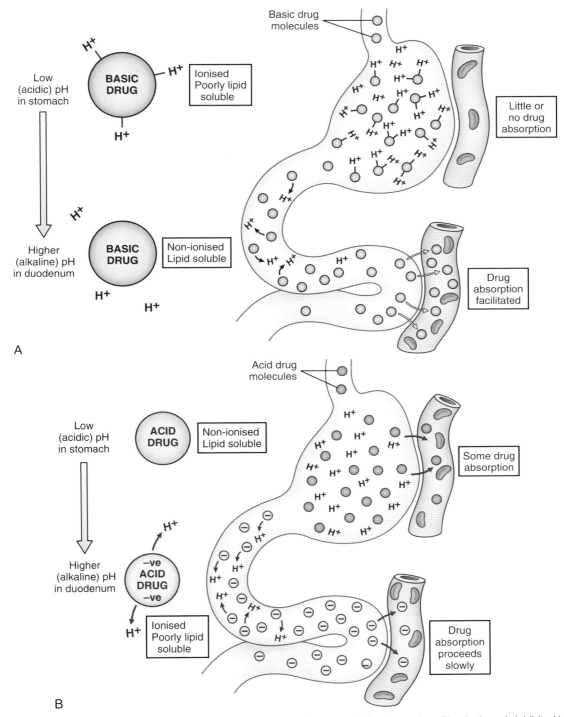

Fig. 2.4 The effect of pH on the ability of drugs to cross biological membranes. A. The absorption of basic drugs is inhibited in the stomach because the drug molecules attach H+ ions and become ionised, but it is facilitated in the small intestine, where they lose the H+ ions and revert to their uncharged form. B. The absorption of acid drugs is facilitated in the acidic environment of the stomach, where the molecules remain un-ionised, but it is slower in the alkaline environment of the small intestine, because they give up H+ ions and acquire a net negative charge.

pH PARTITIONING AND ION TRAPPING

The take-home message from the previous section is that acidic drugs tend to be attracted into and accumulate in basic environments, where they give up their H+ ions and acquire a net negative charge, reducing their ability to travel out of that environment. By the same reasoning, basic drugs tend to be attracted into and accumulate in acidic fluids: once in an acidic environment, they pick up H+ ions, acquiring a positive charge, which reduces their ability to cross membranes and escape. pH differences between body fluids therefore affect how acidic and basic drugs distribute between them. This is called pH partitioning and leads to ion trapping (Fig. 2.5). Altering the pH of body fluids can be useful in certain circumstances to facilitate the movement of a drug from one body fluid to another. For example, **aspirin** is weakly acidic and so will tend to remain in the blood plasma, which is weakly

alkaline (pH 7.4) in preference to the urine, which is weakly acidic (pH 6). In overdose, to accelerate urinary excretion of aspirin, a bicarbonate infusion may be given. The excess bicarbonate is excreted in the urine, causing a temporary rise (alkalinisation) in urinary pH and facilitating the movement of aspirin from the bloodstream into the renal filtrate.

DRUG DISPOSITION (ADME)

The four main pharmacokinetic processes (absorption, distribution, metabolism, and excretion) are described below individually for convenience and represented in Fig. 2.6, but it is important to remember that a drug present in the body will be undergoing all four processes simultaneously.

ABSORPTION

Absorption is the process by which drug molecules travel from their site of administration across biological membranes into the bloodstream. The term bioavailability refers to the percentage of administered drug that reaches the systemic circulation. Drugs given intravenously therefore have 100% bioavailability, but the figure is often much lower for drugs given orally, due to drug degradation in the intestine, first-pass metabolism (see below), and/or incomplete absorption. As described above, the properties of a drug molecule that promote absorption are small size, high fat solubility, and little overall electrical charge (an un-ionised state). Some drug molecules are too large, too water-soluble, and/or too highly charged to transfer across cell membranes, but this can be clinically useful. For example, **nystatin** is too toxic to be used systemically, but because it is not absorbed

Fig. 2.5 pH partitioning. Acid drugs are un-ionised in an acid environment and so can leave and enter a basic environment, where they ionise and are trapped. Basic drugs are un-ionised in a basic environment and so can leave and enter an acid environment, where they ionise and are trapped.

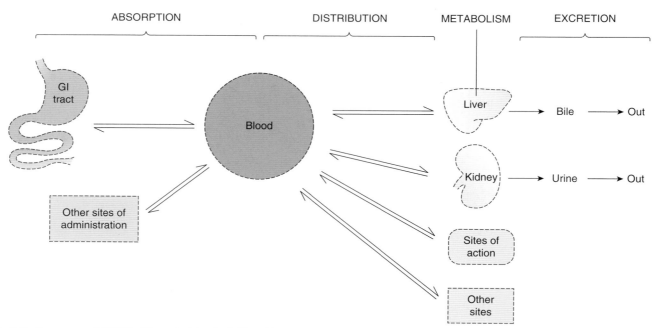

Fig. 2.6 Summary of ADME. GI, gastrointestinal. (From Burchum JR and Rosenthal LD (2016) Lenhe's pharmacology for nursing care, 9th ed, St. Louis: Elsevier.)

from the gut, it can be given orally to clear fungal infections of the gastrointestinal (GI) tract.

Most absorption of an orally administered drug takes place in the small intestine, and to get there it must pass through the stomach. The gastric environment is designed to be hostile to protect the body against potentially dangerous ingested substances: gastric fluids are strongly acidic, which denatures peptides and proteins, and contain the proteolytic enzyme pepsin. Some drugs are completely destroyed here, and others significantly are degraded. Enteric-coated formulations can protect the drug until it reaches the intestine.

The rate of gastric emptying is a major determinant of the speed at which a swallowed drug reaches the duodenum, and therefore factors that reduce gastric motility delay drug absorption. Gastric emptying is generally fastest when a drug is taken on an empty stomach with a glass of cold water. Gastric emptying is slowed in pain, in shock, in neuropathies (including diabetic neuropathy), and when there are foodstuffs in the stomach, especially fatty foods. Some drugs, including **opioids** and drugs with **antimuscarinic** activity, reduce gastric motility. Some foodstuffs can bind certain drugs, reducing their absorption; for example, **tetracyclines** should not be taken with dairy products because they bind the calcium present in these food items, forming an insoluble complex which cannot be absorbed.

Conditions that reduce blood flow through the GI tract, like heart failure, can also slow absorption.

DISTRIBUTION

Distribution is the transfer of a drug from the bloodstream into body tissues and fluids. Drugs do not distribute evenly throughout body tissues, and the main principles governing this are explained below. For example, water-soluble drugs tend to remain in the plasma, whereas very fat-soluble drugs are rapidly taken up and concentrated in body fat stores. Drug delivery is usually proportional to the blood flow: the higher the blood flow, the greater the drug delivery to the area. The kidneys, central nervous system (CNS), and liver receive a high proportion of cardiac output relative to their weight, and therefore can be exposed to particularly high levels of any circulating drug.

DISTRIBUTION INTO TISSUES AND FLUIDS

Drugs absorbed in the small intestine pass through the liver (see 'First-pass metabolism' below) into the systemic circulation. From here they distribute into other body tissues and fluids, and given enough time, the drug will equilibrate between these compartments (Fig. 2.7). For example, circulating plasma levels of a drug which enters the cerebrospinal fluid (CSF) will equilibrate between the blood and CSF, and, provided plasma levels remain constant, CSF levels will also remain constant. However, if plasma levels fall because dosing is stopped, drug levels in the CSF will also fall as drug redistributes from the CSF into the blood to maintain equilibrium. This two-way movement of drug is indicated in Fig. 2.7 by the two-way arrows.

Body fat (adipose) tissue is an important compartment when considering drug distribution because fat-soluble drugs are taken up and stored here. The percentage contribution to total bodyweight from fat varies considerably

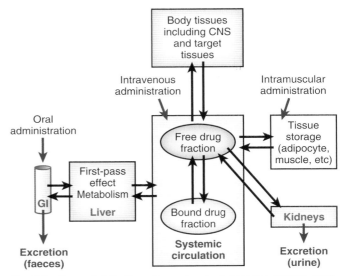

Fig. 2.7 Drug distribution. Drug absorbed from the plasma equilibrates between body tissues and fluids. CNS, central nervous system; GI, gastrointestinal. (Modified from Ha CE and Bhagavan NV (2023) Essentials of medical biochemistry, 3rd ed, Fig. 35.3. San Diego: Academic Press.)

and can make a significant difference to drug dosages and plasma half-lives.

Drug levels in the body are usually measured as plasma concentrations because it is easy and convenient to take blood samples; however, it must be remembered that probably only a small fraction of the drug is likely to be found in the blood because most of it will have distributed out of the plasma and into the tissues. Assuming the drug molecules are capable of efficient transfer across biological membranes, they are likely to access all body tissues and fluids, although this is influenced by how much of the drug is bound to plasma proteins and how much is free (see below). Because of this extensive distribution, very little of the administered dose reaches its target tissue.

Volume of Distribution

The volume of distribution (V_d) is an important concept in clinical pharmacokinetics because it gives an indication of how much of the total body drug has been retained in the plasma and how much has distributed into other body tissues and fluids. This is important when deciding what dose of drug to use to achieve a desired plasma level, and it determines the half-life (see below) of the drug.

> **Key concept**
>
> $$V_d = \frac{\text{amount of drug in the body}}{\text{plasma drug concentration}}$$

To calculate the V_d, plasma levels are measured following administration of a known quantity of drug. In a hypothetical example, 100 mg of drug A is given intravenously. After the drug has been allowed to distribute out of the blood and into the tissues, the drug plasma concentration is measured. In our hypothetical case, the plasma level of drug A is 1 mg/L. V_d is calculated by dividing the total amount of drug in the body (100 mg) by plasma levels of that drug (1 mg/L), giving a V_d of 100 L. This is the total volume of fluid that would be needed for our 100 mg of drug to achieve a homogenous plasma concentration of 1 mg/L. Clearly, the body does not possess 100 L of plasma, and so most of the drug must have left the plasma and entered other body compartments (Fig. 2.8A). Compare this to an intravenous (IV) 100 mg dose of hypothetical drug B. If the plasma concentration following administration of 100 mg of drug B is 20 mg/L, the V_d is 100 mg/20 mg/L, or 5 L. This shows that a much higher proportion of the drug has remained in the plasma and much less has distributed into peripheral tissues, and in this example, much lower doses of drug B are likely to be needed to reach a desired plasma level than drug A (Fig. 2.8B).

Therefore, the more of an administered dose of a drug that escapes from the plasma into other compartments, including body fat stores and general body tissues, the higher the V_d. Because the drug must be in the plasma to be cleared from the body, whether by metabolism or renal excretion, if most of the drug is elsewhere, then clearance is going to be slow and the plasma half-life (see below) long. High V_d values are therefore associated with long plasma half-lives, and drug A in the above example will likely have a much longer half-life than drug B.

SANCTUARY COMPARTMENTS

Drug distribution can be limited by membranes specially adapted to reduce their permeability. The placenta, for example, reduces the transfer of unwanted substances from the mother's bloodstream into the fetal circulation. The blood vessels supplying the testis are also less permeable than standard capillaries, to protect the sperm-producing stem cells from exposure to potentially toxic substances in the circulation. The largest sanctuary compartment comprises most of the brain and spinal cord and is protected by the blood–brain barrier.

The Blood–Brain Barrier

The first scientist to demonstrate that some substances circulating in the bloodstream cannot access large areas of the brain and spinal cord was Paul Ehrlich (1854–1915), who injected mice with methylene blue dye and noted that while other body organs stained heavily, the dye was excluded from most of the CNS. The specialised features of brain capillaries responsible for this protective mechanism are collectively called the blood–brain barrier (BBB). Fig. 2.9 shows the main features of the BBB compared with a typical blood capillary. Typical capillaries are porous, with loose and leaky junctions between the endothelial cells forming their walls, allowing rapid and free exchange of small molecules. Endothelial cells in brain capillaries are however joined at tight junctions, which are much less leaky, and capillaries are wrapped in an additional layer of extensions from astrocytes, providing an extra barrier to the movement of substances between the brain tissue and the blood. In addition, specific transporter mechanisms in the capillary wall can export any drug molecules that do escape into the brain and return them to the blood.

However, it must be emphasised that brain tissue is very lipid-rich, and the CNS has a very high blood supply. This means that most drugs reach the CNS, even if at lower concentrations than in the plasma, and transfer across the BBB increases as the dose rises. Many drugs, being small and fat-soluble, have no difficulty in crossing the BBB and equilibrate quickly between the CSF and the blood.

BODY FAT PARTITIONING

Because most drugs are fat-soluble, a proportion of a drug dose will be taken up into adipose tissue. Adipose tissue acts as a drug reservoir, and large quantities of drugs with particularly high fat solubility, like **benzodiazepines**, can accumulate here.

Drug Distribution in People with High Body Fat Content

People with high body fat content can store considerable quantities of fat-soluble drugs in their adipose tissue. At the start of a course of treatment, a large proportion of a fat-soluble drug can be rapidly taken up into fat stores, and plasma levels remain low until fat stores are saturated. It can therefore take longer to reach therapeutic blood levels, and if a rapid effect is needed, it may be necessary to give initial loading doses to bring plasma levels up rapidly. When the

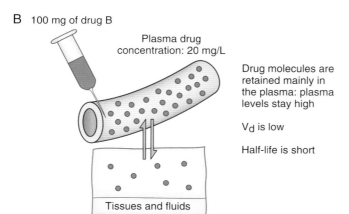

A 100 mg of drug A

Plasma drug concentration: 1 mg/L

Drug molecules distribute widely into body tissues and fluids: plasma levels stay low

V_d is large

Half-life is long

Tissues and fluids

B 100 mg of drug B

Plasma drug concentration: 20 mg/L

Drug molecules are retained mainly in the plasma: plasma levels stay high

V_d is low

Half-life is short

Tissues and fluids

Fig. 2.8 Relationship between volume of distribution, plasma levels, and half-life. A. When most drug leaves the circulation, plasma levels are low and the volume of distribution is high. B. When most drug stays in the circulation, plasma levels are high and the volume of distribution is small.

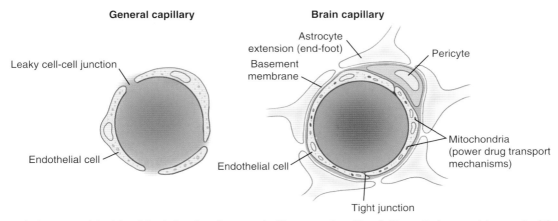

Fig. 2.9 The main features of the blood–brain barrier. Compared with a general capillary (left), capillaries supplying much of the brain feature tight junctions and an additional insulating layer of astrocyte foot processes. (Modified from Lundy-Ekman L (2023) Neuroscience, 6th ed, Fig. 26.12. St. Louis: Saunders.)

drug is withdrawn, as drug levels in the plasma fall, drug leaches out of adipose tissue and can keep blood levels high for an extended period even though drug administration has stopped. Older people, even those of a healthy weight, are also likely to store larger quantities of drug because ageing is usually accompanied by loss of lean tissue, and fat therefore contributes a larger proportion of body mass. This is one reason why drugs can accumulate more readily in older people.

Drug Distribution in People With Low Body Fat Content

Conversely, people with below average fat content may need below average drug doses because less is taken up into body fat and more remains in the plasma, resulting in higher blood drug concentrations.

PLASMA PROTEIN BINDING

Blood plasma contains a range of large-MW proteins, including albumins, globulins, and the clotting protein fibrinogen. Most plasma proteins are synthesised in the liver. Almost all drugs bind loosely and reversibly to plasma proteins, mainly albumin. This binding is not specific like drug-receptor binding; instead, it is a non-specific electrostatic attraction between negatively and positively charged groups on the drug and protein molecules. Bound drug (the 'bound fraction') cannot leave the bloodstream because the drug–protein complex is too large; this means that it does not get into the liver cells for metabolism and does not pass through the glomerular filter in the kidney. Bound drug is therefore protected from metabolism and renal excretion. Because it cannot leave the circulation, bound drug is also unable to reach its target tissue, and so, although it is chemically and biologically active, it is unable to produce its pharmacological effect. On the other hand, unbound drug, the so-called 'free fraction', is subject to metabolism and excretion and is free to leave the bloodstream and enter tissues (Fig. 2.10). The pharmacological effect of the drug is therefore exerted by the free fraction, and depending on the degree to which a drug is plasma protein-bound, the free fraction might be only a small proportion of the total drug present in the bloodstream.

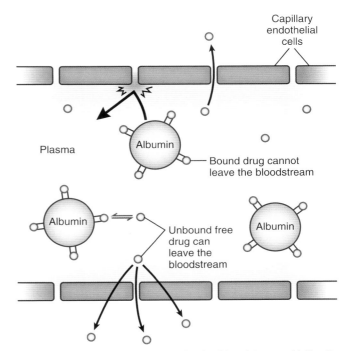

Fig. 2.10 Free and bound drug in the bloodstream. Unlike the free fraction, drug molecules bound to plasma proteins are unable to leave the circulation. (Modified from Lilley LL, Collins S, and Snyder J (2023) Pharmacology and the nursing process, 10th ed, Fig. 2.4. St. Louis: Mosby.)

For nearly all drugs at therapeutic concentrations, when administered regularly, the free and bound drug fractions reach an equilibrium, and the proportion of drug molecules bound to plasma proteins remains constant. This means that as plasma levels of the free fraction fall, drug molecules dissociate from their binding sites to maintain this equilibrium. For example, for a hypothetical drug that is 50% bound and 50% free, half the drug molecules are plasma protein-bound and half are free in the plasma. As the free drug is cleared from the plasma by metabolism or excretion, drug molecules dissociate from their plasma proteins to maintain

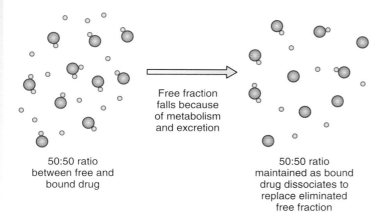

50:50 ratio
between free and
bound drug

Free fraction
falls because
of metabolism
and excretion

50:50 ratio
maintained as bound
drug dissociates to
replace eliminated
free fraction

Fig. 2.11 Equilibrium is maintained (50:50 ratio) between free and bound fraction as free drug is lost from the circulation by metabolism and excretion.

the 50:50 ratio (Fig. 2.11). For this reason, bound drug can be considered a 'reservoir', like drugs stored in body fat: present in the bloodstream, not pharmacologically active, but which can replenish and maintain plasma levels even after the drug is withdrawn.

Because there is normally an excess of plasma protein-binding sites available, even when multiple drugs are present in the plasma, they are generally not saturated. One important potential interaction however is between **warfarin** and **aspirin**, which compete for the same plasma protein-binding sites. The principle behind this potential interaction is shown in Fig. 2.12. Fig. 2.12A represents the situation in an individual stabilised on warfarin where the free and bound fractions have equilibrated. Warfarin in the plasma is usually more than 98% bound, meaning that fewer than 2% of the warfarin molecules in the blood are free. Introduction of aspirin (Fig. 2.12B) leads to competition between the drugs for the available binding sites, and the free fraction of each drug rises, increasing the risk of side-effects, e.g. warfarin-induced bleeding.

Factors that reduce plasma protein levels can reduce the bound fraction of a drug because fewer binding sites are available: for example, liver disease or protein malnutrition.

METABOLISM

Metabolism refers to any enzymatic alteration to the structure of the parent drug. Most body tissues can metabolise drugs to some degree, but the liver and kidneys are the main organs of metabolism, and liver and/or renal impairment can significantly reduce an individual's capacity to metabolise drugs. Conditions such as heart failure that reduce blood flow to the liver and kidneys can reduce delivery of the drug to these organs and reduce the rates of metabolism and clearance. Thyroid disease can also affect drug metabolism because thyroxine is an important regulator of metabolism. Hypothyroidism can reduce drug metabolism, whereas hyperthyroidism accelerates it, and drug doses may need to be adjusted accordingly in these conditions.

The ability of metabolising enzymes to keep up with rising plasma drug levels is not infinite; this is explored in more detail in the section headed 'First-order and second-order kinetics' below.

Liver cells (hepatocytes) are packed with metabolising enzymes responsible for the phase 1 and phase 2 reactions

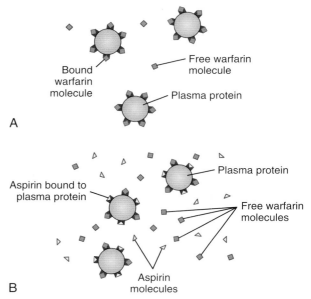

Bound warfarin molecule

Free warfarin molecule

Plasma protein

A

Aspirin bound to plasma protein

Plasma protein

Free warfarin molecules

Aspirin molecules

B

Fig. 2.12 **Warfarin and aspirin competing for plasma protein-binding sites.** A. Warfarin alone. B. Introduction of aspirin can displace bound warfarin and increase free warfarin levels, potentially causing adverse effects. (Modified from Howe T and Burton A (2021) Pharmacology for the surgical technologist, 5th ed, Fig. 1.14. St. Louis: Elsevier.)

described below. Hepatic metabolism therefore relies upon drugs being able to cross hepatocyte membranes and enter the cell. Because most drugs used in clinical practice have the chemical properties to do this (small, fat-soluble, and un-ionised), this is usually straightforward. Larger, highly charged, and more water-soluble drug molecules such as **penicillin**, **digoxin**, and the aminoglycoside antibiotics (e.g. **gentamicin**) cannot enter hepatocytes and so are poorly metabolised. The body relies on renal excretion (see below) to clear such drugs.

Because the biological activity of a drug is usually tied very closely to its precise chemical shape and structure, metabolism often reduces or abolishes a drug's pharmacological action. However, the primary function of metabolism is not actually to deactivate drugs, but to make them more water-soluble and enhance their excretion in the urine. Any product of a metabolic step is called a metabolite.

In terms of activity, there are three possible scenarios by which metabolism can affect drugs:
- An active drug is metabolised to one or more inactive metabolites. This is frequently the case because, as explained above, changes to the drug's chemical structure usually alter its biological activity.
- An active drug is metabolised to one or more active metabolites. Sometimes metabolites retain significant pharmacological activity. This prolongs the drug's duration of action. Examples include many benzodiazepines, e.g. **diazepam**, and opioids, e.g. **morphine**, **codeine**, and **diamorphine**.
- An inactive drug is metabolised to one or more active metabolites. A drug given in an inactive form is called a pro-drug and it relies on metabolism to produce the active form. Important pro-drugs include **zidovudine**, **acyclovir**, **enalapril**, and **cyclophosphamide**.

The two types of metabolism are phase 1 and phase 2 reactions (Fig. 2.13).

PHASE 1 METABOLISM

Phase 1 reactions increase the water solubility of the parent molecule by adding or exposing one or more charged groups: these are usually oxidation, reduction, or hydrolysis reactions. The metabolite is often more reactive than the parent molecule, which prepares it for a phase 2 reaction. This can mean that the metabolite is more toxic than the original drug: for example, **cyclophosphamide**, **paracetamol**, **ethanol**, and **halothane** all produce highly toxic metabolites which must undergo immediate further metabolism to render them harmless.

The Cytochrome P450 Enzyme Family

The cytochrome (CYP) P450 superfamily of enzymes contains 57 members classified into four main families (CYP1–CYP4), and each family is further subdivided. The main CYP enzymes involved in drug metabolism are shown in Fig. 2.14. They perform phase 1 reactions by oxidising their target molecule. CYP enzymes are found in the liver, the wall of the GI tract, and multiple other tissues, and it is likely that they metabolise around 90% of the most commonly used drugs. Genetic variation in the ability to produce CYP enzymes is an important factor in an individual's ability to metabolise drugs. Poor metabolisers clear drugs more slowly and are more likely to experience side-effects, whereas rapid metabolisers clear drugs very quickly and may not respond to normal doses.

Other Phase 1 Enzymes

A range of other enzymes perform phase 1 reactions. Examples include esterases in the plasma which hydrolyse **aspirin** (acetylsalicylic acid), removing the acetyl group and releasing salicylic acid. Alcohol dehydrogenase is one of the enzymes that metabolises **ethanol**; it oxidises alcohol, producing acetaldehyde, which is even more toxic than alcohol itself, and which is further broken down into harmless substances. Monoamine oxidase (MAO) is involved in the breakdown of the neurotransmitters **noradrenaline**, **dopamine**, and **serotonin**. MAO inhibitors such as **phenelzine** have been used for decades as antidepressants although

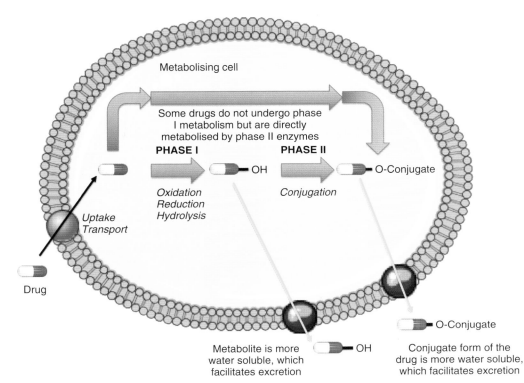

Fig. 2.13   Phase 1 and phase 2 metabolism. (Images used to generate this figure were modified from Servier Medical Art, licensed under Creative Commons Attribution 3.0 Generic License, http://smart.servier.com/)

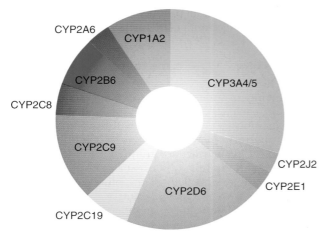

Fig. 2.14 The main CYP enzymes involved in drug metabolism. CYP, cytochrome (The data for the chart were taken from Zanger UM and Schwab M (2013) Cytochrome P450 enzymes in drug metabolism: regulation of gene expression, enzyme activities, and impact of genetic variation. *Pharmacology and Therapeutics*, 138 (1), 103–141.)

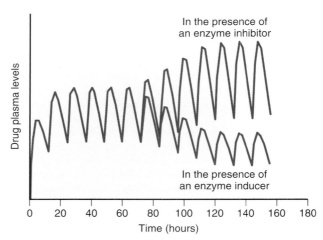

Fig. 2.15 Changes in plasma levels of a hypothetical drug following the introduction of an enzyme inhibitor or an enzyme inducer. Inhibition of metabolism increases drug concentrations, and induction of metabolism reduces them. (Modified from Atkinson A Jr, Abernethy D, Daniels C, et al. (2007) Principles of clinical pharmacology, 2nd ed, Fig. 15.2. San Diego: Academic Press.)

their use nowadays has largely been supplanted by newer drugs.

PHASE 2 METABOLISM

Phase 2 reactions may follow a phase 1 reaction, or the parent drug may undergo phase 2 metabolism directly. The water solubility of the drug or its metabolite is further increased by adding a water-soluble group such as an acetyl group or glucuronate. Adding another group to the drug is called conjugation. As with phase 1 reactions, there is significant genetic variation in people's ability to undergo phase 2 reactions: for example, acetylation is the main mechanism by which several drugs, e.g. **isoniazid**, **hydralazine**, **procainamide**, and **sulphonamides**, are metabolised. Poor acetylators metabolise these drugs significantly more slowly than fast acetylators.

INDUCERS AND INHIBITORS

An enzyme inducer increases the activity of a metabolising enzyme, and an enzyme inhibitor reduces it. Enzyme induction therefore increases the metabolism of an affected drug and reduces its plasma levels, and so is likely to reduce its expected activity, potentially to a level where there is no therapeutic effect. Enzyme inhibition suppresses metabolism and so slows the clearance of an affected drug, increasing plasma levels, enhancing its action, and increasing the risk of adverse effects. Fig. 2.15 shows the changes in plasma levels of a hypothetical drug when an inhibitor or an inducer is introduced. An important exception to this is when the affected drug is a pro-drug and relies on metabolism to activate it. In this circumstance, inhibition of metabolism actually reduces the therapeutic action of the drug by preventing its activation.

Induction and inhibition of metabolising enzymes, especially CYP enzymes, are important causes of interactions. Table 2.1 lists some important inducers and inhibitors. Polypharmacy increases the likelihood that one drug may affect the metabolism of another, but note that foodstuffs, alcohol, so-called 'natural' therapies, and cigarette smoking are

Table 2.1 Examples of Enzyme Inhibitors and Inducers

Inhibitors	Inducers
Cimetidine	Some anticonvulsants including phenytoin, carbamazepine, and primidone
Chloramphenicol	Alcohol
Erythromycin	Rifampicin
Allopurinol	Cigarette smoking
Ribonavir	
Ciprofloxacin	Spironolactone
Isoniazid	St. John's wort
Some foodstuffs including grapefruit and grapefruit juice	Some foodstuffs including Brussels sprouts, broccoli, barbecued meats

also implicated. For example, broccoli, smoking, and grilled foods induce CYP enzymes, whereas grapefruit juice contains flavonoids which inhibit CYP enzymes and reduce the metabolism of a range of drugs including **calcium-channel blockers**, **oestrogens,** and **statins**.

Autoinduction is the property of a drug to induce its own metabolising enzymes. When this happens, the drug's half-life reduces with time. For example, the half-life of an initial dose of **carbamazepine** can be up to 48 hours, but it falls to 10–20 hours on repeated administration because the liver rapidly increases the levels of CYP enzymes to metabolise it.

FIRST-PASS METABOLISM

This refers to any metabolism of an orally administered drug occurring between the intestine and systemic circulation (Fig. 2.16). Significant drug loss can occur in the hostile gastric environment because of the low pH and the action of the proteolytic enzyme pepsin. The main site of absorption is the small intestine, whose walls are packed with digestive enzymes, and the drug can be degraded here. Substances

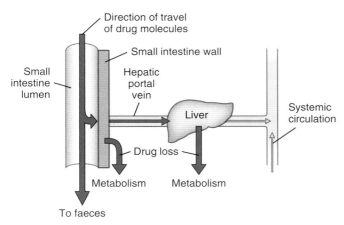

Fig. 2.16 First-pass metabolism. (Modified from Townshend A, Worsfold P, and Poole C (2005) Encyclopedia of analytical science, 2nd ed, Fig. 3. Oxford: Elsevier.)

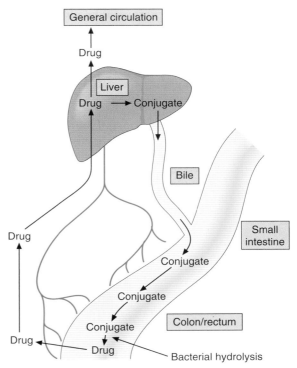

Fig. 2.17 Enterohepatic recycling. A drug may be conjugated in the liver and be passed into the bile. Once in the colon, bacteria may metabolise the drug–conjugate complex, releasing the lipid-soluble drug again, which can then be reabsorbed into the circulation. (From Waller DG, Sampson A, and Hitchings A (2022) Medical pharmacology and therapeutics, 6th ed, Fig. 2.13. Oxford: Elsevier.)

absorbed from the stomach and most of the intestine travel in the hepatic portal vein to the liver, the organ most strongly associated with first-pass metabolism. The liver has an important role in detoxification of unwanted substances and regulating the levels of key blood constituents, and so this arrangement ensures that potentially toxic substances including drugs, or materials absorbed in excess from the intestines, pass first through the liver before being delivered into the systemic circulation. After passing through the liver, the blood then travels in the hepatic vein to the inferior vena cava.

For some drugs, like **glyceryl trinitrate**, the liver removes 100% of an absorbed drug, so oral bioavailability is zero. Other drugs, such as **morphine**, are not completely eliminated, but most of the dose is destroyed and only a small proportion of the drug reaches the systemic circulation.

The veins draining the upper and lower parts of the GI tract do not empty into the hepatic portal vein but deliver their blood directly into the systemic circulation. Drugs absorbed across the membranes of the mouth and the rectum are therefore not exposed to first-pass metabolism. For this reason, **glyceryl trinitrate** is given sublingually. Drugs are often given rectally for reasons other than avoidance of first-pass metabolism, e.g. for a local anti-inflammatory action in haemorrhoids or anal fissures. However, avoiding first-pass metabolism can be a significant advantage when administering drugs rectally for systemic absorption; **analgesics, sedatives,** and **anticonvulsants** may all be given by this route to maximise the amount of drug reaching the circulation.

EXCRETION

Excretion is the removal of drugs or their metabolites from the body. The main route of excretion for most drugs is via the kidney, but drugs may be excreted in any body fluid or tissue, including bile, faeces, breast milk, hair, nails, sweat, and exhaled droplets.

FAECAL EXCRETION

Orally administered drugs that are poorly absorbed remain in the GI tract and are excreted in the faeces. In addition, some drugs conjugated in the liver are passed into the bile,

which is then secreted into the duodenum. Conjugated drugs can pass through the intestines and be excreted in the faeces, but some can be reabsorbed via enterohepatic recycling.

Enterohepatic Recycling

Conjugated drugs, which are now very water-soluble, can be passed into the bile and from there into the intestines. They travel in this form through the tract, too water-soluble to be reabsorbed. In the colon however, the environment changes: this region is richly populated with a range of bacteria, producing enzymes which can split the drug from its conjugated group, releasing the original fat-soluble drug molecule. The drug is therefore reabsorbed across the tract wall, keeping drug levels in the bloodstream high (Fig. 2.17). Enterohepatic recycling prolongs plasma levels of a range of drugs, including **morphine, digoxin,** and some **antibiotics**.

RENAL EXCRETION

The main functions of the kidney include regulation of the composition of body fluids and the excretion of unwanted substances, including drugs and their metabolites. Renal physiology is discussed in more detail in Chapter 9, and the anatomy of the kidney and its functional unit, the nephron, are shown in Figs. 9.1 and 9.2. Low-MW substances are filtered under pressure out of the bloodstream into the glomerular capsule, forming filtrate which travels through the nephron towards the collecting duct. The nephron has three segments: the proximal convoluted tubule, the loop of the nephron (loop of Henle), and the distal convoluted tubule. From here, urine, the final product, drains into the renal pelvis and ultimately into the ureter towards the bladder. As the filtrate passes through the nephron, important substances like glucose are reabsorbed from the filtrate back into the bloodstream, and unwanted substances like ammonium ions are actively secreted out of the bloodstream into the filtrate for excretion in the urine. The amount of drug present in the urine therefore depends on how much is filtered at the glomerulus, how much is reabsorbed from the filtrate, and how much is secreted into the filtrate. Fig. 2.18 summarises these processes, although except for the glomerulus, for clarity, it does not show the different regions of the nephron. A significant degree of metabolism may also take place as the drug passes through the renal tissues.

Filtration

Small-MW drugs and metabolites are filtered out of the bloodstream into the filtrate, although they do not necessarily stay there. Drugs bound to plasma proteins are not filtered because the drug–protein complex is too large. Drug molecules too large to cross the glomerular filter also stay in the bloodstream and do not enter the filtrate.

Reabsorption

As the blood flows from the glomerular capillaries into the peritubular capillaries supplying the remainder of the nephron, further exchange of drugs and their metabolites may take place. Filtered drugs that are very water-soluble remain in the filtrate, but if they retain some lipid solubility, they may be reabsorbed across the tubule wall and return to the bloodstream. Water-soluble drugs like **digoxin** and **gentamicin** are poorly metabolised because they cannot diffuse into hepatocytes and so escape metabolism and arrive in the kidney in their active forms. As the filtrate passes through the nephron and most of the water is reabsorbed, they become progressively more concentrated. **Gentamicin** causes significant renotoxicity because of this. An additional consideration here is that the body relies on renal clearance to get rid of drugs that are not metabolised, and so renal function must be carefully assessed when these drugs are used. Some drugs are actively reabsorbed, piggybacking on carrier and transport mechanisms used to reabsorb nutrients and other substances the body needs to retain, but this is not of much clinical importance as few drugs are not reabsorbed this way.

Urinary pH also influences drug reabsorption into the bloodstream. Normal urine has a pH of 5–6, and so acidic drugs will tend to stay un-ionised (uncharged) and be reabsorbed into the plasma (pH 7.4). Basic drugs will tend to ionise in the acid urine and so be less able to diffuse out of the tubule back into the bloodstream, promoting their excretion in the urine (see section on pH and pH partitioning above).

Secretion

Drugs too large to pass through the glomerular filter may be actively secreted out of the bloodstream into the tubule,

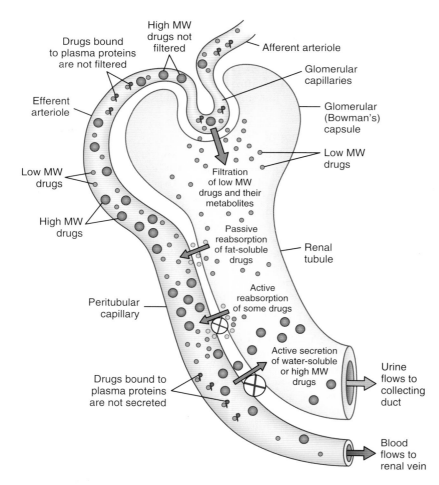

Fig. 2.18 Filtration, absorption, and secretion of drugs in the renal tubule. MW, molecular weight.

allowing the kidney to clear unwanted substances that escape filtration: examples include **furosemide**, **metformin**, **digoxin**, many **antivirals**, and **penicillin**. The transporters responsible for secretion are saturable, meaning that they have a maximum work rate. If two or more drugs are competing for the same transport mechanism and the transport maximum is reached, then the level of both drugs in the blood may rise. This is an important source of drug interactions: for example, secretion of **digoxin** is reduced when co-administered with **verapamil** or **amiodarone**, because these drugs compete for the digoxin transporter, increasing plasma digoxin levels. Plasma protein binding protects most drugs from secretion, although diuretics including **furosemide** are actively secreted in their bound form; this is the route by which they reach the lumen of the nephron, where they exert their pharmacological effect (p.174 and Fig. 9.6).

HALF-LIFE AND STEADY STATE

Plotting plasma levels following oral, intramuscular (IM), and IV administration of a single dose of a drug against time gives curves similar to those shown in Fig. 2.19. The curves demonstrate three phases. The absorption phase shows plasma levels rising. Here, absorption from the IM injection and the oral preparation in the GI tract is proceeding, and so although as soon as the drug hits the bloodstream it begins to distribute into the tissues, there is a net gain into the blood, and plasma levels rise. The absorption phase seen with the IV curve does not actually represent absorption and is very steep, because the drug is being delivered directly into the bloodstream. Peak plasma levels are reached when the amount of drug being delivered into the bloodstream is equal to the amount being removed by distribution, metabolism, and excretion. Most orally administered drugs reach peak plasma levels within 1–3 hours of dosing; absorption from an IM site is usually faster than from the gut, so this curve peaks more quickly. Following the peak, irrespective of the route of administration, plasma levels begin to fall.

This is the elimination phase, and drug is leaving the bloodstream because of distribution, metabolism, and excretion.

HALF-LIFE

The half-life ($t_{1/2}$) of a drug is the time required for its concentration to reduce by 50%. It can be measured in any body fluid or tissue, but in practice for convenience it is generally measured in the plasma. It is an important pharmacokinetic measurement, although it is not applicable in every situation (see saturation kinetics below).

The relationship between half-life and plasma levels is shown in Fig. 2.20. The *x*-axis shows time, and the *y*-axis shows drug levels, measured in percentage of the starting drug concentration. After one half-life, the drug level has fallen by half and is now 50% of the starting concentration. After another half-life, the drug level has fallen by another 50% and is now only 25% of starting levels. Another half-life later, the drug concentration is now 12.5% of the original.

Bear in mind that drug half-lives, in absolute time, vary hugely. For example, the plasma half-life of **penicillin** is less than half an hour, whereas the half-lives of some **antidepressants** and some **anticonvulsants** can be days. Plasma half-lives are affected by a range of factors. Rapid metabolism and/or excretion shorten the plasma half-life; penicillin's short half-life is due to exceptionally efficient renal clearance. Conversely, poor metabolism and/or sluggish renal excretion extend half-lives. Very fat-soluble drugs which are stored in large amounts in adipose tissue, or drugs which are highly plasma protein-bound, also tend to have long half-lives because of these significant drug reservoirs: when the drug is withdrawn, plasma levels can remain high for an extended time as drug lost to elimination processes is replaced by drug leaching from these stores.

First-Order (Linear) Kinetics and Zero-Order (Saturation) Kinetics

Drug metabolism is an important contributor to a drug's plasma half-life. For most drugs given at therapeutic doses, metabolising enzymes process the drug at a rate proportional to its concentration. This means that as drug levels rise,

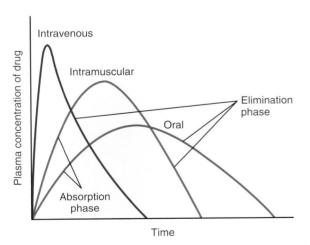

Fig. 2.19   A typical plasma concentration curve following a single dose of a drug, given orally, intramuscularly, and intravenously. (Modified from Page C, Anand R, and DeWilde S (2022) Trounce's clinical pharmacology for nurses and allied health professionals, 19th ed, Fig. 1.2. Oxford: Elsevier.)

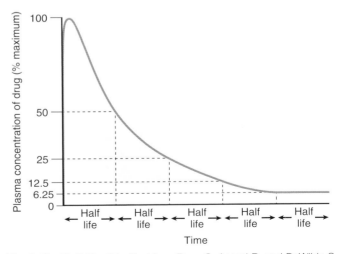

Fig. 2.20   Half-life. (Modified from Page C, Anand R, and DeWilde S (2022) Trounce's clinical pharmacology for nurses and allied health professionals, 19th ed, Fig. 1.2. Oxford: Elsevier.)

metabolism increases as well, and there is a direct and predictable relationship between drug concentration and the rate of metabolism. As long as drug levels remain within a certain range, metabolising enzymes can cope, and metabolism obeys the half-life rule as shown above. This is called first-order or linear kinetics because there is a direct, linear relationship; if the plasma level is 100 μg/mL, after one half-life, 50% will have been metabolised, reducing the original plasma levels to 50 μg/mL, and after another half-life the 50 μg/mL level is reduced by half to 25 μg/mL, and so on. When drug metabolism follows linear kinetics, predicting changes in plasma drug levels is more straightforward. This can be clinically useful. For example, when switching from one drug to another, it may be important to predict how long it will take for the first drug to disappear from the circulation and when the second drug may be safely started. In general, a drug's plasma levels become so low that its biological effects are lost after 5–6 half-lives (Fig. 2.20).

In some cases, this direct relationship between drug levels and metabolism is lost. This is usually because the metabolising enzymes become saturated: that is, they are working at their maximal capacity and cannot work any harder. This is called saturation or zero-order kinetics.

Metabolism switches from first- to zero-order kinetics with any drug if the concentration rises high enough, but fortunately this does not happen with most drugs within normal therapeutic drug ranges. However, for some drugs, including **phenytoin**, **salicylates**, and **sodium valproate**, enzyme saturation occurs within the therapeutic range. This presents a problem in drug management, because when the enzyme's maximum work rate is exceeded, additional drug accumulates in the plasma, and plasma levels rise rapidly and steeply. When adjusting doses of drugs in this scenario, special care is needed, because even a small dose increase can result in sudden onset of toxicity. In addition, there is significant variability between individuals, adding further unpredictability. Fig. 2.21 shows the effect of increasing dose on plasma levels of phenytoin in three patients. The black line shows the shape of curve expected if phenytoin

metabolism followed first-order kinetics: there is a proportionate, predictable, and steady rise in plasma levels as the daily dose increases. At lower doses, all three curves show this relationship, but at plasma concentrations below therapeutic levels, drug metabolism is maximal and additional drug accumulates, sending plasma levels sharply and steeply upwards. Patient 1 reaches the maximum therapeutic plasma level of 80 μM at around 200 mg daily; for patient 3, the corresponding dose is nearly 500 mg, showing significant inter-individual variation.

STEADY STATE AND THE THERAPEUTIC DOSE RANGE

In most clinical situations drugs are given not as a single dose but as a course of treatment, either in the short, medium, or long term, and the concept of steady state becomes important.

Steady state is the situation where drug levels remain consistently within a certain range. IV infusion gives constant plasma levels with little fluctuation, but oral administration gives a steady state curve featuring a series of peaks and troughs because of the time lapse between individual doses. Plasma levels peak shortly after an administered dose, and they begin to fall as distribution, metabolism, and excretion clear it from the circulation. The lowest point, the trough, is reached just before administration of the next dose. Dosing intervals are usually informed by the drug's half-life, and frequently doses are given at time intervals close to its half-life: drugs with long half-lives are given less frequently and drugs with shorter half-lives need to be given more frequently.

Fig. 2.22 shows changing plasma levels following repeated administration of three different doses of a hypothetical drug at half-life intervals. The sub-therapeutic dose (10 μmol/kg), therapeutic dose (30 μmol/kg), and

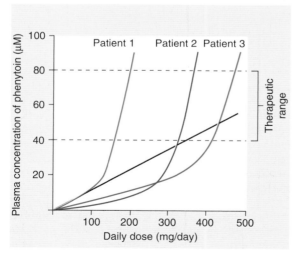

Fig. 2.21 Saturation kinetics. (From Waller DG, Sampson A, and Hitchings A (2022) Medical pharmacology and therapeutics, 6th ed, Fig. 2.13. Oxford: Elsevier.)

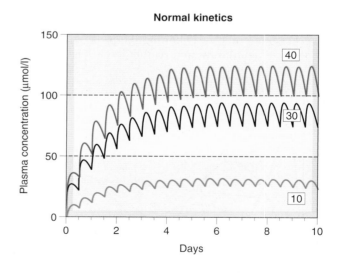

Fig. 2.22 Steady state with repeated oral dosing. Steady state is achieved with all three doses shown, although only 30 μmol/kg gives steady state in the therapeutic range. 40 μmol/kg exceeds the therapeutic range and is likely to cause toxicity. 10 μmol/kg is too low a dose to achieve therapeutic drug levels. (Curves were calculated with the Sympak pharmacokinetic modelling program written by Dr. J G Blackman, University of Otago.)

supra-therapeutic dose (40 μmol/kg) are shown. The desired therapeutic range, 50–100 μmol/L, is also shown. Steady state is achieved after five or six doses. This means that a drug with a half-life of 4 hours will reach steady state within 24 hours, but a drug with a half-life of 24 hours may take nearly a week. To reduce the time to achieve steady state for drugs with long half-lives, a loading dose can be given to initiate therapy; this accelerates the rise in drug plasma concentration and steady state is reached more quickly (Fig. 2.24).

The therapeutic dose range is the interval between the upper desired plasma level, above which toxic effects are likely, and the lowest desired plasma level, below which the drug is unlikely to exert a therapeutic action. Steady-state plasma levels should normally fall within this range. The dose and the dosing frequency should be such that peak levels do not reach toxic levels and (usually) that trough levels do not fall so low that the therapeutic action of the drug is lost, i.e. that the steady-state range remains within the therapeutic dose range for the drug.

THERAPEUTIC DRUG MONITORING

For the drugs for which even small increases in plasma concentrations can cause toxicity, it is sometimes useful to regularly measure plasma levels, especially at times when dose adjustments are being made. Typical examples include **digoxin**, **gentamicin**, **methotrexate**, and **phenytoin**.

ADMINISTRATION

Choosing the appropriate route of administration is crucial to ensure optimal drug delivery to the desired target site with minimal side-effects. Oral administration is often the best choice, with the added benefit of often being the cheapest option, but in some situations an alternative route may be better.

DRUG FORMULATIONS

The active drug is only one component of a medicine. The term given to the combination of the active drug with other ingredients is its formulation. The formulation determines the medicine's physical properties and the pharmacokinetics of the drug, including its stability, palatability, solubility, particle size, rates of absorption, and rate of release. It should not be assumed that one manufacturer's formulation of a drug, even across equivalent doses, will give identical plasma levels and effects to another's, and care should be taken when switching formulations of certain drugs, including **anticonvulsants** and **digoxin**.

Ingredients other than the active drug are called excipients and generally contribute about 90% to the bulk of the final product. Typical excipients include stabilisers, colourants, diluents, binding agents, and coatings and films used to seal tablets and capsules. An ideal excipient is biologically inert, non-toxic, and non-allergenic, but this ideal is rarely achieved, and excipients can cause adverse reactions to medicines. A number have been associated with allergic responses: for example, **lanolin** (wool fat) used as an emulsifier in some topical preparations, the colouring agent **tartrazine**, and the antioxidants **sodium metabisulphite** and **propyl gallate**.

Different formulations of the same drug allow it to be given by different routes, to modify its rate of release from the site of delivery or to target specific cells or tissues. **Hydrocortisone**, for example, is formulated differently in preparations intended for oral, IV, or topical use. Acid-sensitive drugs, e.g. **omeprazole,** may be formulated as enteric-coated tablets or capsules to protect them against gastric juices and to release the drug in the alkaline environment of the small intestine. Conversely, drugs irritant to the stomach, including **non-steroidal anti-inflammatory drugs**, can be enteric-coated to help protect the gastric lining. Drugs given by IM injection may be formulated in an oil base to give a depot in the muscle, from which the drug is released over an extended period, removing the need for frequent injections. Examples include **contraceptive** preparations and **antipsychotic** medications. Other modified formulations include sustained or slow-release preparations, which release their drug slowly in the intestines and keep plasma levels high over an extended period.

Formulation technology is becoming progressively more sophisticated, producing a number of novel drug delivery vehicles. For example, liposomes are tiny, artificially engineered spheres made of lipid, used to deliver drugs that may be poorly absorbed or poorly delivered into cells because of low lipid solubility or large MW (Fig. 2.23). Fat-soluble (hydrophobic) drugs can be inserted into the lipid bilayer, and water-soluble (hydrophilic) drugs can be enclosed within the liposome. For example, many **anticancer drugs** are much more water-soluble than lipid-soluble, so their ability to cross biological membranes is limited. Packaging the drug in liposomes, which readily cross membranes, greatly enhances drug delivery to its target. In addition, the outer surface of liposomes can be coated with molecules that bind specifically to target cells, allowing the drug to be selectively delivered to the desired location. The advantage of this, for example in cancer chemotherapy, is obvious: cytotoxic drugs cause significant damage to healthy cells as well as malignant cells, so targeted therapy reduces general toxicity. Liposomes modified with polyethylene glycol (PEGylated) are more stable than standard liposomes and reduce the uptake of liposomes by macrophages in the liver and spleen, prolonging the drug's presence in the bloodstream.

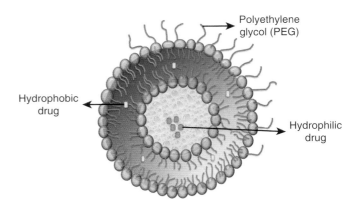

Fig. 2.23 The basic structure of a liposome. (From Dua K, Hansbro PM, Wadhwa R, et al. (2020) Targeting chronic inflammatory lung diseases using advanced drug delivery systems, Fig. 6. San Diego: Academic Press.)

ORAL ADMINISTRATION

Advantages of oral administration include convenience and ease. For people with difficulty swallowing tablets or capsules, liquid formulations are often available, although some may taste unpleasant. Oral administration is not an option for patients who are unable or unwilling to swallow, who are actively vomiting, or whose consciousness is lost or impaired. Additionally, acid-sensitive drugs are destroyed in the stomach and protein-based drugs are digested or degraded here. If blood flow to the GI tract is reduced, i.e. in acute pain, developing shock, or heart failure, oral absorption of medication is slowed. Malabsorption and inflammatory conditions of the GI tract can also reduce absorption.

Because it usually takes some time for plasma levels to rise, oral administration is not ideal if a rapid response is needed. To accelerate the rise in plasma levels following oral administration, an initial loading dose may be used: this increases the concentration gradient between the intestinal lumen and the bloodstream and speeds up drug transfer into the blood (Fig 2.24).

TOPICAL ADMINISTRATION

Topical absorption means the drug is applied directly to a body surface or membrane. Often this is the preferred route when localised drug action is needed, e.g. **hydrocortisone** cream for a skin allergy. A range of drugs, including **anti-inflammatories** and **antimicrobials,** can be formulated for direct application to the eye or ear canal. One important advantage of topical application for local effect is that lower drug concentrations are required, and although some drug is likely to be absorbed into the circulation, exposure of other body tissues to the drug is greatly reduced. Application of drugs to the skin and internal mucosal surfaces, e.g. buccal (tucked into the pouch between the cheek and teeth), nasal, vaginal (per vagina, PV), or rectal membranes, may also be useful for a local effect, but sometimes the drug is intended to be absorbed across the membrane and reach the systemic circulation. Drug absorption across the healthy skin barrier (transdermal absorption) is generally slow, but this can be advantageous in some circumstances, giving slow

and sustained drug release; examples of drugs that can be given in skin patches include **fentanyl**, **nicotine**, and **contraceptive hormones**.

The mucous membranes of the mouth and rectum have a good blood supply, and drugs are generally absorbed reasonably well here. Rectal (per rectum, PR), sublingual (SL, under the tongue), and buccal administration have the advantage that absorbed drug is not subject to first-pass metabolism (see above). Rectal administration may be an alternative route for drugs that are destroyed in or irritant to the stomach, like **non-steroidal anti-inflammatory agents**. It may also be used when the oral or IV routes are not available or potentially hazardous, for example the use of **benzodiazepines** to terminate a seizure, or in severe vomiting or gastric stasis.

INTRAVENOUS ADMINISTRATION

Drugs given directly into the bloodstream are usually injected into a vein (IV) rather than an artery (intra-arterial, IA) because veins are thinner and easier to penetrate, tend to run more superficially under the skin so are more accessible, and carry blood under lower pressure so bleeding from the site is usually less likely. First-pass metabolism is bypassed, and bioavailability is 100%. There is no risk to the drug from gastric acid degradation, the onset of drug action is rapid, and providing venous access is available, this route permits medication delivery when the patient is asleep or unconscious. Drugs may be given as a one-off (bolus) dose and/or a continual infusion and stopped immediately at any time. Potential risks include infection, bleeding, and local tissue damage, especially if an in-situ cannula dislodges and infusion continues into local tissues rather than the vein.

IA injection is used to target delivery of a drug to a particular organ, e.g. **cytotoxic drugs** can be injected directly into a tumour's arterial blood supply.

INTRAMUSCULAR ADMINISTRATION

The main skeletal muscles used for IM injection (Fig. 2.25) are the gluteal muscles of the buttock, the deltoid muscle which forms the fleshy part of the shoulder, and the vastus

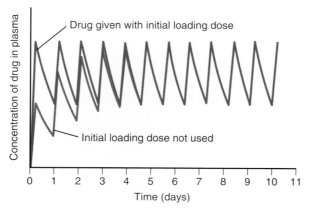

Fig. 2.24   Blood drug levels following a loading dose compared to standard dose. Therapeutic drug levels are reached more quickly when a loading dose is used. (Modified from Taylor K and Aulton M (2022) Aulton's pharmaceutics, 6th ed, Fig. 22.8. Oxford: Elsevier.)

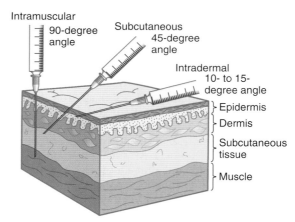

Fig. 2.25   Intradermal, subcutaneous, and intramuscular injection. (From Bonewit-West K (2012) Clinical procedures for medical assistants, 8th ed. St Louis: Saunders.)

lateralis of the thigh. Skeletal muscle has a good blood supply and drug absorption is usually reliable; IM administration may be suitable if the patient cannot take medication orally or other routes are not suitable. Depot formulations given as deep IM injection release active drug slowly over an extended period, but it must be borne in mind that the drug cannot then be withdrawn, and adverse effects may therefore be prolonged. Risks include infection, bleeding, and damage to adjacent structures if the injection is too deep or not accurately placed, and of course it is likely to be painful. Absorption from the muscle is reduced if blood flow to skeletal muscle falls, for example in developing shock.

SUBCUTANEOUS/INTRADERMAL ADMINISTRATION

Immediately below the epidermis of the skin lies the dermis and below that lies the subcutaneous tissue, which is rich in poorly perfused adipose tissue (Fig. 2.25). Subcutaneous injection therefore delivers the drug into a very fat-rich environment with little blood flow, so drugs given this way are absorbed slowly into the bloodstream; this is ideal when sustained blood levels are required: **insulin** and **heparin** are routinely given by this route. Only small volumes (up to 2 mL) can be delivered by a single subcutaneous injection, but some drugs, e.g. **opioid analgesics** in terminal care, can be administered by subcutaneous infusion. In situations where skin blood flow is reduced, such as in developing shock,

absorption from subcutaneous tissue can be significantly impaired. Potential complications include infection and abscess formation, and in the case of repeated injections in the same site, degenerative tissue changes (lipodystrophy).

Intradermal administration (Fig. 2.25) is infrequently used to give drugs. One example of its use is in allergy testing, in which potential allergens are instilled into the dermis.

INHALATION

Inhalation of drugs is usually used to deliver drugs locally into the airways, but occasionally for systemic drug administration, e.g. inhaled **general anaesthetics**. Inhalation, for example, of **anti-inflammatory drugs** and **bronchodilators** in obstructive airway disease such as asthma gives targeted delivery and allows drug doses to be kept small. It must be borne in mind that airway tissues have a good blood supply, and drug absorption into the systemic circulation is a real possibility, especially at higher doses and with frequent administration. Delivery of drugs by inhalation is discussed in more detail on p. 158.

INTRATHECAL AND EPIDURAL ADMINISTRATION

Fig. 2.26 shows the placement of the needle for intrathecal and epidural administration of drugs.

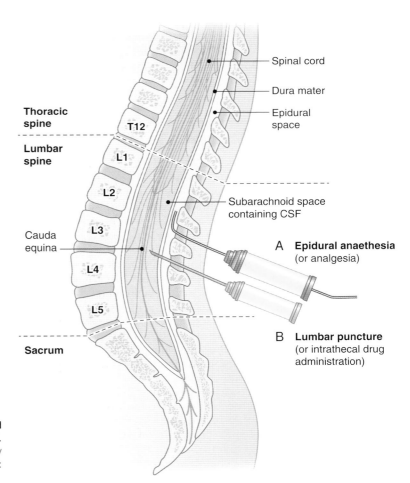

Fig. 2.26 Sites of needle placement for intrathecal and epidural drug administration. CSF, cerebrospinal fluid. (From Waugh A and Grant A (2020) Ross & Wilson anatomy and physiology in health and illness, 14th ed, Fig 7.14. Oxford: Elsevier.)

Intrathecal administration is delivery of drug directly into the subarachnoid space, which is filled with CSF. This bypasses the blood-brain barrier and allows therapeutic agents, e.g. **contrast media**, **anaesthetics**, **analgesics**, **antibiotics**, or **cytotoxic drugs**, to be introduced directly into the CNS. The needle is inserted between adjacent vertebrae and punctures the dura and arachnoid mater to deliver the drug directly into the CSF, which circulates around and through the brain carrying the drug with it. Potential complications include bleeding, introduction of infection into the CSF, and CSF leakage.

Epidural administration is delivery of a drug into the epidural space, which lies between the vertebrae and the dura mater. The arachnoid mater is therefore not punctured. Drugs instilled into the epidural space do not circulate, because there is no CSF in the epidural space, and epidural administration is most frequently used to introduce **anaesthetics** or **analgesics** around spinal nerve roots, giving loss of sensation, including pain, from the legs and lower body regions served by the affected nerves. It is commonly used to eliminate the pain of labour and childbirth. Complications include the introduction of infection or accidental puncturing of the arachnoid mater, which would allow the drug to access the CSF.

ADMINISTRATION INTO BODY CAVITIES

Occasionally, drug delivery into body cavities or specific structures is used: for example, intra-articular injection of **anti-inflammatory steroids** into the joint cavity can relieve pain and stiffness in arthritis. Drugs that inhibit the growth of abnormal blood vessels in macular degeneration can be given directly by intraocular injection into the vitreous humour of the eye. Intraosseous (into the medullary cavity of the bone) delivery is used particularly in paediatrics when IV access is not available.

DRUG INTERACTIONS

Drug interactions refer to the situation where a drug interferes with some aspect of the pharmacokinetic or pharmacodynamic properties or behaviour of another. They are a common cause of problems and adverse effects with drug therapy, and consideration should always be given to interactions caused by foodstuffs, non-prescription medicines, and herbal and natural remedies.

It must also be borne in mind that not all interactions are harmful or unwanted. For example, beta agonists like **salbutamol** and anti-inflammatory steroids such as **budesonide** are regularly used together in maintenance treatment of asthma. In combination, the therapeutic effects of these two drugs synergise and enhance each other (see also p.166 and Fig. 8.11).

Pharmacokinetic interactions occur when a drug interferes with the disposition of another in the body, and several examples are discussed in earlier sections of this chapter. Pharmacodynamic interactions occur when a drug interferes with the biological activity of another, often by antagonising or acting additively to it. Pharmacodynamic principles are the subject of Chapter 3, but pharmacodynamic interactions are discussed here for consistency. This section does not attempt to provide a comprehensive list of all important drug interactions because the list of potential and confirmed interactions is vast, but rather offers a selection of examples to illustrate the main principles. A suitable drug formulary should always be consulted for detailed information on potentially hazardous drug combinations.

PHARMACOKINETIC INTERACTIONS

Drugs can interfere with another's absorption, distribution, metabolism, or excretion. Most pharmacokinetic interactions are due to one drug interfering with another's metabolism, and this is discussed above.

ABSORPTION

Dairy products, which are rich in calcium, interfere with **tetracycline** absorption because the calcium complexes with the drug to form an insoluble complex. Drugs that reduce gastric motility, e.g. **opioids**, and drugs with antimuscarinic properties, e.g., some **antihistamines** and **antidepressants**, slow the rate of absorption of other drugs because they impair drug delivery into the small intestine. **Adrenaline** co-injected with a **local anaesthetic** acts as a vasoconstrictor, reducing the loss of the anaesthetic from the area in the bloodstream and prolonging its effect, and is thus useful in longer procedures.

DISTRIBUTION

Drugs may potentially compete for plasma protein-binding sites: the standard example, **aspirin** and **warfarin**, is discussed above.

EXCRETION

Drugs that impair renal function or reduce renal blood flow can reduce excretion of other drugs and increase their circulating blood levels. Carrier mechanisms in the renal tubule that secrete particular drugs may be inhibited by competing drugs. For example, **non-steroidal anti-inflammatory drugs** inhibit the secretion of **methotrexate** and can increase methotrexate levels in the blood.

PHARMACODYNAMIC INTERACTIONS

Drugs can interfere with each other's physiological activity in a range of ways because pharmacodynamic processes are so complex. Some interactions are beneficial and exploited clinically, and some are not. The most serious drug interactions can be lethal.

BENEFICIAL INTERACTIONS

The combined use of analgesics with different mechanisms of action, e.g. **codeine** and **paracetamol**, is common. The analgesic action of the drugs is additive and allows the doses of the individual drugs to be kept lower than if each was being used alone, reducing the likelihood of adverse effects. Another example of a therapeutically exploited interaction is the use of reversal agents when two drugs compete for the same binding site, for example, when **naloxone** or another opioid antagonist is used to reverse **morphine** overdose.

UNWANTED/DANGEROUS INTERACTIONS

Sometimes both drugs have the same biological effect, and when used together, produce an excessive response: for example, the risk of haemorrhage is increased when drugs that increase bleeding times, including **warfarin**, **heparin**, and **aspirin**, are used together. Another example is the use of dopamine receptor agonists such as **ropinirole** to treat Parkinson's disease and dopamine receptor antagonists such as **olanzapine** in the treatment of psychiatric disorders: this drug combination is avoided as they directly interfere with each other's pharmacological action. Many diuretics, including **furosemide**, predispose to hypokalaemia, which increases the risks of **digoxin** toxicity.

PHARMACOKINETIC SPECIAL SITUATIONS

Even in health, drug disposition can vary significantly between individuals.

OLDER AGE

Physiological processes tend to decline in older adults. Gastric emptying may be slower, delaying drug delivery into the small intestine. Age-related reduction in liver and kidney function may affect metabolic and excretory mechanisms in healthy older people, although there is significant variability in the degree to which this affects drug disposition, and patients should be carefully assessed on an individual basis. First-pass metabolism may be reduced, increasing the amount of an orally administered drug reaching the general circulation and necessitating a reduction in drug dose. From the age of 50 years, the glomerular filtration rate (GFR) may be reduced by 25% and by 50% by 75 years, reducing renal drug excretion.

Plasma protein levels are lower in older people, potentially increasing the drug-free fraction and necessitating lower doses, especially at the start of a course of drugs or when drugs are being administered in an acute setting. In general, the adipose–lean body mass balance tips towards the deposition of adipose tissue, increasing the potential for drug accumulation in body fat stores. Older people may be more sensitive to the central effects of drugs, including sedation, confusion, amnesia, and impaired cognition.

BABIES AND CHILDREN

There are significant differences between children and adults in the pharmacokinetic disposition of drugs. In addition, ADME processes change with the developing child, and distinction must be made between a premature baby (born before 37 weeks of gestation), a neonate (up to 4 weeks old), an infant (between 4 weeks and 1 year of age), and a child (up to 11 years of age). Great care must therefore be taken in neonatal and paediatric drug therapy: this is definitely a situation where children are not just small adults!

Physiological processes in the very young may be immature, particularly in prematurity. Topically applied drugs are absorbed more readily because children's skin is thinner and there is less subcutaneous fat. Oral administration may not be the best way to give drugs because GI motility is sometimes erratic, especially if the baby is ill. Gastric emptying times may not reach young adult values until about 6 months of age. Gastric pH is higher in babies, so drugs which are normally subject to significant acid degradation, e.g. **penicillin**, are better absorbed. Drug elimination is slow because liver and kidney function is immature at birth.

It can take up to 2 years for full liver function to be achieved, and metabolic patterns for a particular drug in children may be different in adults. Importantly, drug metabolism and half-life changes according to the age of the child and the developmental stage of the liver. For example, some members of the CYP450 family are relatively more important in metabolising some drugs in children than in adults, which perhaps counterintuitively means that the half-life of the drug may be shorter in the child than the adult and can change according to the developmental stage of the liver. For example, the half-life of **phenytoin** in the adult is typically 20–30 hours. In the neonate, its typical value is 30–60 hours. This falls to 2–7 hours in neonates, as one particular CYP enzyme matures, and extends to 2–20 hours in children. With other drugs, metabolism in babies and children is lower at all stages than in adults.

The GFR in the newborn is only 20% of adult values, which generally increases to young adult level within 6 months. Fully mature renal excretion of drugs may not be achieved until 18 months of age. Plasma protein levels do not reach young adult levels until about 3 months of age, and the free fraction of drug can be elevated in very young babies. Central effects of drugs in the very young are likely to be exaggerated, partly because the blood-brain barrier does not fully mature until around 4 months of age, but also because the brain is proportionately larger in children than in adults and so receives a greater blood supply.

PREGNANCY

Drug use in pregnancy presents possible dangers to two people: the mother and the baby. Fetal liver and kidney function are immature throughout pregnancy, and so the baby is largely reliant on the mother to eliminate circulating drugs. Even in a healthy pregnancy, physiological changes affect the pharmacokinetic profiles of drugs. Pregnancy-associated nausea and vomiting can limit the usefulness of orally administered drugs. Blood volume rises in pregnancy, diluting plasma proteins and potentially increasing the free fraction. Cardiac output rises, increasing blood flow through the kidney and liver, and potentially accelerating drug elimination. In addition, hepatic metabolism increases because enzyme levels rise, which also speeds up drug clearance. When therapeutic drugs must be used in pregnancy, particular care must be taken in monitoring the health of both the mother and the baby.

GENETIC VARIABILITY

A significant source of inter-individual variation in metabolism is genetically determined, discussed in more detail above. However, genetic differences can also affect receptor populations, absorption mechanisms, and hypersensitivity responses and affect both how the body deals with the drug as well as how the drug affects the body. Identifying important genetic differences in pharmacokinetic and pharmacodynamic profiles and using this information in planning and prescribing drug therapy is becoming slowly but increasingly a part of personalised medicine. One drug may be chosen over another because it is known that the patient will metabolise it better, is likely to have a better clinical response to it, or is likely to have less severe adverse effects with it. This is truly a situation of the story being written in the genes!

REFERENCES

Fernandez, E., Perez, R., Hernandez, A., et al., 2011. Factors and mechanisms for pharmacokinetic differences between pediatric population and adults. Pharmaceutics 3 (1), 53–72.

ONLINE RESOURCES

Haywood, A., Glass, B.D., 2011. Pharmaceutical excipients – where do we begin? Aust Prescr 34, 112–114. Available at: https://www.nps.org.au/australian-prescriber/articles/pharmaceutical-excipients-where-do-we-begin.

Le, J., 2022. Overview of pharmacokinetics. MSD Manual. Available at: https://www.msdmanuals.com/en-gb/professional/clinical-pharmacology/pharmacokinetics/overview-of-pharmacokinetics.

Pharmacology Education Project, 2023. Clinical pharmacokinetics. Available at: https://www.pharmacologyeducation.org/clinical-pharmacology/clinical-pharmacokinetics.

Yartsev, A., 2024. Required reading: pharmacokinetics. Deranged Physiology. Available at: https://derangedphysiology.com/main/cicm-primary-exam/required-reading/pharmacokinetics.

Pharmacodynamics: What the Drug Does to the Body

3

INTRODUCTION TO PHARMACODYNAMICS

Pharmacodynamics is the umbrella term describing the mechanisms by which drugs exert their effects on body tissues, sometimes simply put as 'what the drug does to the body'. The response of the body to a typical drug is likely to be complex. A drug given to treat a specific condition or to relieve a specific symptom will frequently produce additional, usually unwanted adverse effects, often affecting the function of organs or systems that are not the desired target of the drug and often at drug doses in the desired therapeutic range. A sound grasp of basic pharmacodynamic principles is essential to understanding why this occurs.

THE LEVELS OF DRUG ACTION

Drug action can be considered at different levels. Although the effects of a drug are often assessed or measured by its success in achieving an intended aim, like relief of a headache with **paracetamol** or reduced blood pressure when taking an antihypertensive such as **ramipril**, its action is almost always via specific molecular targets: for example, a cell-surface receptor, an enzyme, or an ion channel controlling the movement of specific ions in or out of the cell. Understanding drug action at the molecular level not only facilitates understanding of the therapeutic action of the drug, but also sheds light on the potential for adverse effects. Fig. 3.1 shows an example of the different levels of action of **salbutamol**, a bronchodilator drug used in asthma (see also p. 164).

At the whole-person level, salbutamol relieves the physiological and emotional distress of an impending asthma attack; it improves alveolar ventilation, ensuring adequate oxygenation of the blood and elimination of carbon dioxide. This clearly has beneficial consequences for all body organs. At the (respiratory) system level, salbutamol increases airway diameter to maximise air flow. At the tissue level, it relaxes bronchial smooth muscle tissue, dilating the airway. At the cellular and molecular level, salbutamol is a beta (β) receptor agonist. It binds directly to β receptors on bronchial smooth muscle cells and activates them, triggering a series of biochemical events within the cell which ultimately reduce intracellular calcium (Ca^{2+}) levels. Because Ca^{2+} is essential for muscle contraction, bronchial smooth muscle relaxes and the airway dilates.

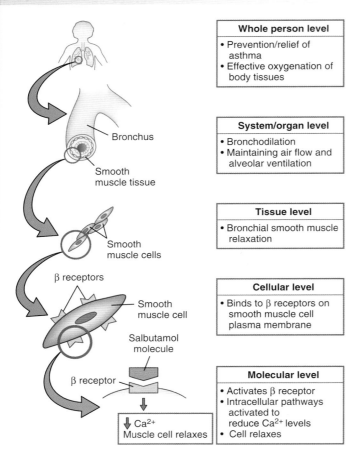

Whole person level
• Prevention/relief of asthma • Effective oxygenation of body tissues

System/organ level
• Bronchodilation • Maintaining air flow and alveolar ventilation

Tissue level
• Bronchial smooth muscle relaxation

Cellular level
• Binds to β receptors on smooth muscle cell plasma membrane

Molecular level
• Activates β receptor • Intracellular pathways activated to reduce Ca²⁺ levels • Cell relaxes

Fig. 3.1 The levels of drug action. Drug action can be examined on the whole person, on the physiological system, in a specific organ, at the tissue/cellular level, and at the molecular level. The figure uses salbutamol as the example.

cell-surface proteins (receptors), or they may enter the cell, cross the nuclear membrane, and bind to one or more genes, either inhibiting or activating gene expression and production of the gene-specific protein. In doing so, they alter the cell's activity, which in turn alters the activity of the tissue and the organ to which the affected cells belong. Sometimes a drug target is a body enzyme. A drug may bind to and affect (usually inhibit) the enzyme's activity, blocking a step in a metabolic pathway. Other drugs may affect the transport of substances across the cell membrane, inhibiting the ability of the cell to regulate its internal environment. The precise chemical structure of the drug molecule is usually critical to its ability to interact with its molecular target, and alterations to this can abolish the drug's pharmacological activity.

DRUG RECEPTORS

KEY DEFINITIONS

- Ligand:
  the general term for any chemical binding to a receptor.
- Agonist:
  a drug which binds to a receptor and activates it. Using a 'lock and key' analogy, the drug is the equivalent of a key which fully engages a lock (the receptor) and can either lock or open it.
- Antagonist:
  a drug which binds to a receptor and blocks it. Using a 'lock and key' analogy, an antagonist acts like a key that is a close enough match to enter a lock but not a close enough fit to operate it. However, while this 'false' key occupies the lock, it prevents a 'true' key from being inserted, and so the lock is useless.

This explains why salbutamol is useful in asthma, but put in a wider context, it also explains why adverse effects of the drug may include tachycardia and hypertension. β receptors are found in a number of body tissues; they belong to the adrenoceptor family (Table 3.1), receptors which respond to the sympathetic mediators, **adrenaline** and **noradrenaline**. The sympathetic nervous system prepares the body for fight or flight, and bronchodilation is part of that response: dilating the airways improves airflow to the lungs and supplies the additional oxygen required in a physiologically stressful situation. However, salbutamol may also activate β receptors in the heart, increasing the rate and force of cardiac contraction and raising blood pressure, also important components of the sympathetic response. Understanding the underlying mechanism of action of a drug at the cellular/molecular level therefore explains why β agonists should be used with care, if at all, in people with cardiovascular disease.

PRINCIPAL TARGETS OF DRUG ACTION

Most drugs act through one or more general mechanisms: for example, they may bind to and activate or block

The human body is a community co-operative composed of around 30 trillion cells, each occupied with its specialised function, but not living in isolation: all work together to maintain homeostasis and health. This requires that every cell must interact with and respond to chemical signals such as hormones, neurotransmitters, growth factors, and inflammatory mediators in its local environment. One of the most important mechanisms allowing this complex communication system to work are the populations of receptor molecules present on the cell surface (see Fig. 2.1) and within the cell, including nuclear DNA receptors. It is important to remember that these receptors are present to mediate endogenous physiological activities, and so drugs are usually either mimicking or blocking an endogenous function, i.e. acting as agonists or antagonists at the receptor (Fig. 3.2). The example of **salbutamol** in Fig. 3.1 illustrates this point: β-receptor agonists bind to receptors whose physiological function is to mediate sympathetic responses. Another example is the use of opioid analgesics like **morphine** in pain control. Two groups of naturally occurring substances with analgesic activity, the **endorphins** and **enkephalins**, are found in the central nervous system and in some peripheral tissues, particularly in nerve pathways concerned with the transmission and processing of

Table 3.1   Important Receptor Families and Some of Their Subtypes

Main Endogenous Ligand		Main Subtypes	Main Locations/Functions
Adrenoceptors: adrenaline (Adr)/noradrenaline (NA)	α receptors	α_1 (three further subtypes) α_2 (three further subtypes)	Central and peripheral nervous system (CNS and PNS, respectively); blood vessels
	β receptors	β_1 β_2 β_3 β_4	CNS and widespread in body tissues. β_1: main type in heart (NA/Adr increase heart rate), β_2: main type in airway smooth muscle (NA/Adr cause bronchodilation.)
Cholinergic receptors: acetylcholine (ACh)	Muscarinic (M)	M_1, M_2, M_3, M_4, M_5	See Table 4.1
	Nicotinic (N)	three subtypes	CNS and PNS; N_M found at neuromuscular junction (synapse between a voluntary (motor) nerve and skeletal muscle)
Histamine		H_1, H_2, H_3, H_4	See Table 4.2
Serotonin (5-HT)		5-HT$_{1-7}$ Multiple subtypes, especially of the 5-HT$_1$ and 5-HT$_2$ receptor	All widespread in CNS. Some types found in blood vessels and gastrointestinal smooth muscle. 5-HT$_2$: main type in platelets (5-HT aggregates platelets.)
Gamma-amino butyric acid (GABA)		$GABA_A$ $GABA_B$	Widespread in brain; GABA is always inhibitory.
Dopamine		D_{1-5}	CNS, heart, and kidneys. D_2: main type in vomiting pathways and in nigrostriatal pathway involved in voluntary muscle control. D_1: main type in mesolimbic (reward) pathways
Opioid: endogenous opioids		MOP: μ-opioid receptor DOP: δ-opioid receptor KOP: κ-opioid receptor	MOP: main type in pain pathways and also the main opioid side-effects: sedation, miosis, respiratory depression

5-HT, 5-hydroxytryptamine

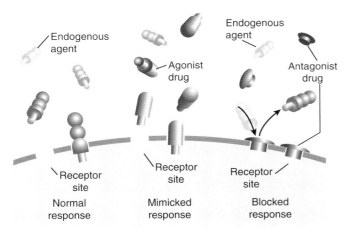

Fig. 3.2   The action of an endogenous agent, an agonist, and an antagonist at a receptor. (Modified from Lilley LL, Collins S, and Snyder J (2023) Pharmacology and the nursing process, 10th ed, Fig. 2.7. St. Louis: Mosby.)

Excitatory and Inhibitory Receptor Responses

It feels intuitive that the binding of an agonist to a receptor should activate a process or in some way excite or stimulate some aspect of the cell's behaviour. However, it is important to realise that drug–receptor binding may either stimulate or inhibit a response in the target cell, depending on the nature of the receptor and the biochemical mechanisms to which the receptor is linked. For example, in the central nervous system, it is important that neuronal activity can be suppressed as well as activated; like a dimmer switch controlling light levels in a room, it permits finely tuned control of nerve activity. The **endorphins**, **enkephalins**, and **morphine** discussed earlier are agonists (they activate the MOR) but the effect produced in their target cells is inhibitory, and they reduce the transmission of pain signals. Another example is gamma-amino butyric acid (**GABA**), an important inhibitory neurotransmitter widespread in the central nervous system. It reduces nerve activity by acting as an agonist at its GABA receptor on chloride (Cl$^-$) ion channels on nerve endings (see ion channels below) and opens the channel; the entry of negatively charged Cl$^-$ ions inhibits the nerve and reduces its firing rate. Benzodiazepines like **diazepam** and **midazolam** are in widespread clinical use as sedatives, anxiolytics, and anticonvulsants: they work by enhancing GABA's action (see also p. 61). On the other hand, **acetylcholine** (ACh), a neurotransmitter found widely in both the central and peripheral nervous systems, is usually excitatory, and it stimulates its target cell.

pain signals. They are agonists at mu (μ) opioid receptors (MORs) present on nerves in pain pathways, and shut down transmission there, diminishing pain signals. Morphine and other opioid drugs are agonists at MORs and activate the same pain-relieving mechanisms as the internal analgesics.

Specificity, Selectivity, and Receptor 'Families'

Receptor Specificity

Receptors are usually protein molecules folded into complex and specific three-dimensional shapes. This means they can only bind chemicals that have a complementary shape and 'fit' the receptor binding site, like a lock and a key. The ability of a ligand such as a neurotransmitter, hormone, or drug to discriminate between different receptor types and to bind to one and not another, even if the two are structurally very similar, is called specificity and is essential in normal healthy body function. For example, there are currently more than 100 known neurotransmitters in the human nervous system, each with its own particular and precise range of roles to play in the sophisticated and finely tuned neurological control of body physiology. It is essential that each is only active at its own receptors and does not affect receptors for other transmitters because this would significantly disrupt this intricate and complex control network. In clinical pharmacology, drug specificity is very important, because the more specific the drug is for its intended receptor, the less likely it is to cause unwanted adverse effects through binding to other receptor types. The lower the drug–receptor specificity, the greater the risk and incidence of adverse effects unrelated to the drug's intended therapeutic aim. Many drugs are not absolutely specific for their target receptor and affect other receptor types. Fig. 3.3A shows that older (first-generation) antihistamines, such as **chlorphenamine**, block H_1 histamine receptors, the mechanism by which they exert their anti-inflammatory effect. However, although the fit is not perfect, they also bind to and block muscarinic cholinergic receptors in the autonomic nervous system. Unwanted antimuscarinic effects (p. 51), including dry mouth, sedation, and blurred vision, are therefore common with these drugs. There is no interaction with, for example, dopamine receptors, because there is no molecular fit.

Receptor 'Families' and Receptor Selectivity

A further important consideration regarding receptor populations for any particular ligand is that they are not homogeneous throughout the body, giving rise to the concept of 'receptor families'. Receptor families contain two or more receptor subtypes, all responding to their principal ligand, but which differ slightly in structure and may be differentially distributed in different tissues and associated with different functions. A knowledge and understanding of receptor subtypes is important in clinical pharmacology because the use of drugs selective for particular subtypes narrows their therapeutic target, usually improving their clinical performance and reducing the risk of adverse reactions. The ability of a

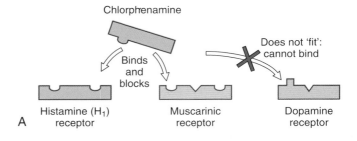

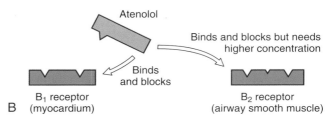

Fig. 3.3   Specificity and selectivity. A. Specificity. Older antihistamines, e.g. chlorphenamine, typically bind to and block other receptor types as well as histamine H_1 receptors. Blocking muscarinic cholinergic receptors gives the antimuscarinic side-effects characteristic of these drugs. Other receptor types, e.g. dopamine receptors, are not affected. B. Selectivity. Atenolol binds to and blocks both β_1 and β_2 adrenoceptors but achieves best fit with β_1 receptors. At higher doses, however, it blocks both.

drug to discriminate between subtypes of the same receptor is called selectivity. Important receptor families and some of their clinically important subtypes are summarised in Table 3.1. Although the expanding array of receptor subtypes in some families, e.g. serotonin (5-hydroxytryptamine/ 5-HT), may seem overwhelming, this research area has paved the way for the design of increasingly targeted drugs.

For example, consider the histamine receptor family. Currently four histamine receptor subtypes have been identified, named H_1, H_2, H_3, and H_4. Although they are all in some way involved in immunity and body defence and they all respond to histamine, they are not distributed evenly throughout histamine-responsive tissues, and they mediate different functions of histamine. The pharmacology of histamine and its receptors is discussed in more detail in Chapters 6 and 10, but let us use the example here to briefly illustrate the point that different receptor subtypes mediate different functions of the same chemical and can be blocked by different drugs. H_1 receptors are found in blood vessels and secretory epithelia (e.g. the linings of the nose), and histamine acting here produces the standard signs and symptoms of allergic inflammation: an insect bite gives red, swollen, itchy skin, and hay fever gives a runny nose and red, itchy eyes. Antihistamines like **chlorphenamine** and **cetirizine** block H_1 receptors and relieve these symptoms. H_2 receptors are found in the stomach, and histamine acting here increases gastric acid secretion, another important defence mechanism. However, antihistamines have no effect on H_2 receptors; a different class of drugs, the H_2 receptor blockers including **cimetidine** and **famotidine**, are used to reduce gastric juice secretion in conditions associated with excess acid production.

Increasing dose can affect the specificity and selectivity of a drug. For example, the β-receptor family all respond to **adrenaline** and **noradrenaline**, but different subtypes are found in different tissues. The myocardium in the heart has mainly β_1 receptors, and airway smooth muscle has mainly β_2 receptors. Some β-blockers, for example **atenolol**, have relative selectivity for β_1 cardiac receptors and bind preferentially to this subtype over other subtypes (Fig. 3.3B). However, as atenolol doses increase, its effects on other subtypes become more significant, including β_2-mediated bronchoconstriction, which may be a problem in people with obstructive airways disorders such as asthma.

Reversible and Irreversible Drug–Receptor Binding

The term 'binding' used to refer to drug–receptor interactions might suggest that a drug molecule arrives at the target receptor and locks onto it, like someone sitting down in a chair and staying there. However, in physiology, this arrangement would not work because it would limit the degree of control possible over the interaction and the subsequent biological action. Physiological systems need to be able to exert moment-to-moment control over their activity, and ligand–receptor interactions in living systems are reversible. Drug molecules actually bind to and release from their receptor repeatedly, like someone bouncing up and down in their chair. However, the time frame for each binding is very short—a tiny fraction of a second—and so a drug molecule binds, releases, binds, releases, many times each second. The more drug molecules present, the greater the proportion of receptor sites occupied at any one time and the greater the drug response.

Competitive Antagonism

This model of drug–receptor interactions explains why a reversal agent can be used to block the action of a drug already in the system. For example, **naloxone** is a MOR (Table 3.1) antagonist that can be used to reverse an opioid overdose. Because the opioid molecules bind and dissociate from their MORs multiple times a second, naloxone molecules can also bind while the receptor is momentarily free. This is called competitive antagonism (Fig. 3.4), because the reversal agent competes with the opioid for receptor occupancy, and while naloxone molecules are present in appropriate concentrations at the receptors, they limit opioid binding and reduce opioid effects.

Irreversible Drug–Receptor Binding

Examples of this are fairly rare in clinical pharmacology; most drug–receptor interactions are reversible as described above. **Aspirin** (acetylsalicylic acid) binds irreversibly to its target enzyme, cyclo-oxygenase, as described in Chapter 6, which means that a once-daily low dose (75 mg) produces a sustained and effective anti-platelet action. **Omeprazole** (p. 186), used to reduce gastric acid secretion, irreversibly inhibits the proton pump in gastric parietal cells. A single dose of omeprazole reduces gastric acid secretion for up to 2 days, increasing to 5 days when the drug is used regularly.

Regulation of Receptor Numbers

Receptor proteins are synthesised on the cell's ribosomes and transferred to the plasma membrane. Receptor numbers are controlled by the cell and can be increased (upregulated) or decreased (downregulated) as required. In the absence of any drug with activity at a receptor type

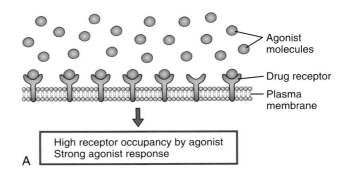

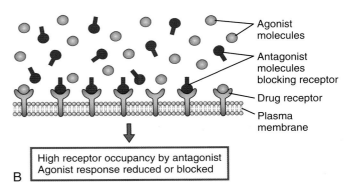

Fig. 3.4 Competitive antagonism, showing reversal of morphine with naloxone. A. Morphine alone. B. Morphine is displaced from its receptors because naloxone is competing for binding.

(which may upregulate or downregulate receptor numbers as described below), the main factor determining receptor numbers is the presence (or absence) of its physiological ligand. In general, if the ligand concentration falls, the cell will usually upregulate receptor numbers to compensate for reduced receptor stimulation and to bring the signal back up to its normal range. On the other hand, if the concentration of the ligand goes up, increasing receptor stimulation, the cell responds by downregulating receptor numbers to dampen the excessive signal.

Regular or sustained exposure of tissues to a drug acting on a particular receptor can induce the cells to adjust their receptor numbers to control their sensitivity to a signal. For example, prolonged use of an antagonist and the consequent receptor blockade can induce a tissue to upregulate its receptor numbers (Fig. 3.5A). This may cause problems when the antagonist is withdrawn. For example, medium- to long-term use of a β-blocker like **propranolol** may upregulate β_1 receptors in the myocardium. If propranolol is suddenly withdrawn, tachycardia and hypertension can follow because with its increased β-receptor population, the myocardium is more sensitive to the effects of sympathetic stimulation.

On the other hand, overuse of β-agonist bronchodilators such as **salbutamol** in asthma can reduce its effectiveness, because in the constant presence of the drug, the smooth muscle cells of the airway downregulate their receptor population to reduce the excessive signal (Fig. 3.5B). The individual with asthma finds that they must use their inhaler more frequently to relieve or prevent their symptoms, downregulating receptor numbers even further and establishing a vicious cycle.

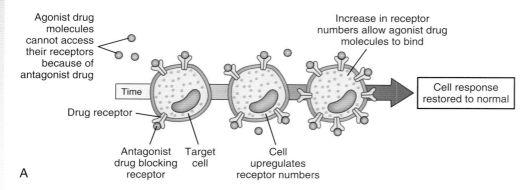

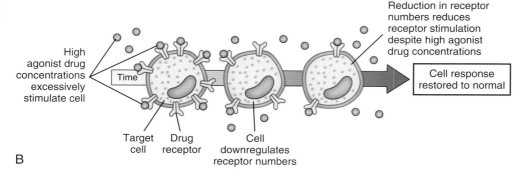

Fig. 3.5 Upregulation and downregulation of receptor numbers. A. Upregulation when receptors are blocked by an antagonist. The reduced signal causes the cell to synthesise more receptors. B. Downregulation when a cell is exposed to high concentrations of an agonist. The cell reduces its receptor numbers to dampen the excessive signal. (Modified from Power-Kean K, Zettel S, El-Hussein MT, et al. (2023) Huether and McCance's understanding pathophysiology, Canadian edition, 2nd ed, Fig. 18.3. Toronto: Elsevier Canada.)

RECEPTORS AND THEIR ACTIONS

Most clinically relevant drug receptors are found on the cell membrane and allow the cell to respond to chemical signals in the extracellular environment. Some drugs, e.g. **steroid hormones**, cross the cell membrane and bind to cytosolic receptors, from where they travel into the nucleus and bind to receptor sites on DNA, either stimulating or inhibiting the production of proteins coded for in the cell's genes. Some receptors are an integral part of the structure of ion channels (see below), and when their ligand binds to them, they open or close the channel, regulating ion movements across the cell membrane. This is especially important in excitable tissues such as nerve and muscle which rely on ion movements to generate and transmit electrical signals. Fig. 3.6 shows the main locations of cellular receptors.

Cell-Surface Receptors

Drug–receptor binding on the cell membrane is only the first stage in a chain of steps which convert the interaction of the drug with its receptor to its final biological effect. It could be likened to speaking to a receptionist at the front door of an office block, which is only the first step in making it to your appointment with someone on the fifth floor. The receptionist must trigger a chain of communication within the building, perhaps by telephoning or emailing someone to let them know you have arrived, or by asking an assistant to take you in the lift to the correct floor. A similar chain of messages is triggered by drug–receptor binding. Drug–receptor binding usually initiates a conformational change in the receptor which triggers a series of biochemical communication steps within the cell, transferring the message from the receptor to intracellular mechanisms that will produce the final cellular response. These are called transduction

mechanisms, and there are several different types. Only G protein-coupled receptor mechanisms are discussed here in more detail because they are particularly important.

G Protein-Coupled Receptors

Around a third of therapeutically important cell-surface drug receptors are linked to a special protein called a G protein, which is bound to the internal surface of the cell membrane. They are therefore called G protein-coupled receptors (GPCRs). They are a large and diverse receptor family, including receptors for many neurotransmitters, inflammatory mediators, and peptide hormones. A GPCR is formed from a long protein chain, folded seven times, and embedded in the cell membrane. One end is exposed on the outer surface of the cell membrane and acts as the drug receptor. The internal end of the receptor protein is directly linked to the G protein (Fig. 3.7). G proteins are sometimes called **g**o-between proteins because they act as intermediaries between the cell-surface receptor and the final stage in the sequence of events transmitting the drug's message into the cell's interior. The final stages in the communication chain, responsible for generating the final effect of the drug on the cell, are called second-messenger pathways.

Second-Messenger Pathways. The two most important second-messenger pathways are the cyclic AMP (cAMP)/adenylate cyclase system and the phosphatidyl inositol/phospholipase C systems. Although the biochemical cascades are different for each, they both involve the activation of intracellular enzymes called kinases. Kinases are key enzymes in the regulation of protein activity in the cell. They convert ATP to ADP, releasing energy-rich phosphate groups which phosphorylate and activate or inactivate a wide range of cellular enzymes and other proteins, including ion channels

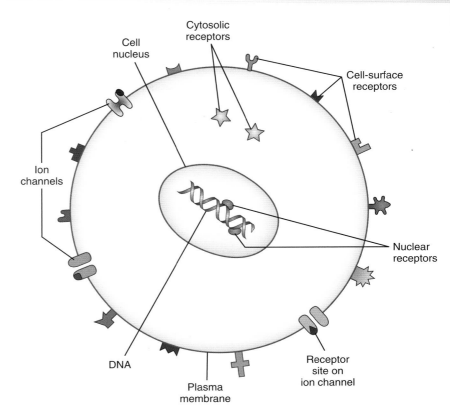

Fig. 3.6   The main locations of drug receptors.

and transport proteins. There are hundreds of different kinase subtypes in the human cell, reflecting their central role in cellular biochemistry and metabolism.

Adenylyl Cyclase/cAMP Pathway. ATP is converted to cAMP by the action of the enzyme adenylyl cyclase (Fig. 3.7). cAMP is a very important second messenger with multiple functions in the cell: for example, it controls a wide range of cellular functions, including growth, differentiation, energy metabolism, and muscle contraction. Adenylyl cyclase is constantly active, and so cAMP levels are controlled by the family of phosphodiesterase enzymes (PDEs), which destroy cAMP (and the related second-messenger nucleotide, cyclic guanosine monophosphate, cGMP). A range of drugs including **sildenafil** (p. 179, used mainly for erectile dysfunction) and **theophylline** (p. 165) are PDE inhibitors used clinically; by blocking PDE, cAMP/cGMP levels in the cell rise.

Inhibitory and Stimulatory G Proteins. Two important subtypes of G protein are an inhibitory (G_i) and a stimulatory (G_s) form. If the receptor is coupled to a G_i protein, it exerts an inhibitory effect on the cell. For example, MORs (Table 3.1), to which endogenous opioids like endorphins and opioid analgesics like **morphine** attach, are linked to G_i proteins. MORs are found, among other locations, on nerve endings at synapses within pain pathways, and they modulate pain signals in the brain and spinal cord. Binding of either the endogenous opioid or an exogenous opioid drug to a MOR activates the G_i protein, which in turn inhibits synaptic transmission here and blocks the pain signal. On the other hand, if the receptor is coupled to a G_s protein, its effect is excitatory. An example is the β adrenoceptor, which responds to **adrenaline** and **noradrenaline** and β agonists such as **salbutamol**. Activation of the β receptor

activates adenylyl cyclase, increases cAMP levels, and among other effects, phosphorylates a range of enzymes important in metabolic pathways (Fig. 3.8).

Nuclear Receptors

Some drugs, e.g. **steroid** hormones, do not bind to a cell-surface receptor. They are highly fat-soluble, so they cross the plasma membrane and bind to their receptor, called a steroid-binding protein, in the cytosol. The drug–receptor complex then crosses the nuclear membrane and binds directly to a specific binding site on one or more genes contained within the cell's DNA. This may activate the gene, resulting in the production (transcription) of a molecule of messenger RNA (mRNA). The mRNA molecule leaves the nucleus and attaches to ribosomes in the cytoplasm, which produce the protein that the gene encodes (Fig. 3.9). Alternatively, steroid binding to a gene may switch the gene off and halt protein production. For example, anti-inflammatory glucocorticoids such as **hydrocortisone** switch off genes that code for pro-inflammatory proteins and activate genes that code for proteins that suppress inflammation. The onset of action of drugs which affect gene expression is often slow because it takes time for the target protein levels to either rise or fall sufficiently to make a difference to cell function.

ION CHANNELS

Ion channels embedded in the cell membrane open and close to control the flow of ions such as Ca^{2+}, sodium (Na^+), and Cl^- across the cell membrane. Opening the channel allows ions to travel down their concentration gradient and

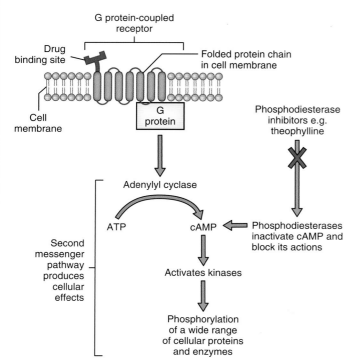

Fig. 3.7   G protein-coupled receptors and the cyclic AMP (cAMP) second-messenger system. Phosphodiesterases (PDEs) block adenylyl cyclase and reduce cAMP levels. PDE inhibitors therefore increase cAMP levels and increase its cellular effects.

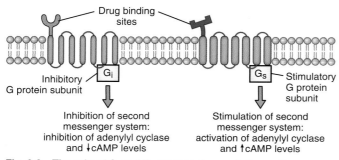

Fig. 3.8   The role of G_i and G_s proteins in regulating cell responses to G protein-coupled receptors. G_i, inhibitory G protein; G_s, stimulatory G protein.

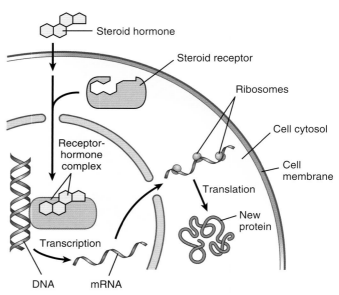

Fig. 3.9   The mechanism of action of steroid drugs. (Modified from Jones R and Lopez KH (2006) Human reproductive biology, 3rd ed, Fig. 1.5. San Diego: Academic Press.)

either enter or leave the cell. Because ions are electrically charged, their movement in or out of the cell regulates the electrical excitability of the cell and allows nerve and muscle cells to generate and propagate electrical signals. Sodium and calcium channels permit Na^+ and Ca^{2+} respectively to flow into the cell, which depolarise (activate) nerve and muscle cells. Potassium (K^+) channels allow K^+ to leave the cell, which hyperpolarises (desensitises) an excitable cell, making a nerve, for example, less able to fire. Chloride channels allow Cl^- to enter the cell, which hyperpolarises it, making nerve cells less likely to fire. Generally, drugs which affect ion channel function have a rapid onset of action because they cause an immediate change in ion concentrations in the cell.

Drugs affecting ion channel function usually work in one of two ways: they may bind to a receptor site attached to

the channel and regulate the channel opening, or they may bind directly to the channel protein and physically block the channel opening.

Drugs Which Bind to a Receptor Site on the Channel

Ion channels are formed from several protein subunits assembled around the central channel pore. Receptor sites on one or more of the subunits control the opening and closing of the channel. Some neurotransmitters including **ACh** acting on nicotinic receptors and **GABA** operate this way, permitting very fast control (in milliseconds) of synaptic transmission. GABA (p. 16) is an important inhibitory transmitter in the brain, and it hyperpolarises neurons, reducing synaptic transmission. It binds to a subunit on Cl^- ion channels on nerve endings, opening them and increasing the entry of inhibitory Cl^- ions into the nerve. Benzodiazepines like **midazolam** bind to a different receptor site on the Cl^- channel and enhance the inhibitory effect of GABA, prolonging channel opening, increasing Cl^- flow into the nerve, and further reducing its excitability. This underpins the sedative, anxiolytic, and anticonvulsant action of this group of drugs.

Drugs That Block Ion Channels

Local anaesthetics like **lignocaine** block Na^+ channels in nerve axons. The influx of positively charged Na^+ ions into the axon generates the electrical current that sweeps along the nerve as the action potential, and when a local anaesthetic molecule plugs the channel and prevents sodium entry, the nerve is silenced. Ca^{2+}-channel blockers like **verapamil** and **nifedipine** have been used for decades to treat cardiovascular disease and hypertension. They prevent Ca^{2+} entry into cardiac and smooth muscle cells; deprived of Ca^{2+}, the cells become less excitable. Cardiac contractility is reduced, producing an anti-arrhythmic action, and vascular smooth muscle relaxes, reducing blood pressure.

RECEPTOR DESENSITISATION AND DRUG TOLERANCE

Drug tolerance is the reduction in the response to a drug seen with continued administration. It is a very common phenomenon and can cause significant problems in therapeutics. It usually occurs over a period of time and generally develops more quickly at higher drug doses. As tolerance develops, higher and higher drug doses are needed to achieve the same effect, and at its extreme it may mean that the drug response is completely lost; the tissue is now said to be refractory.

Tolerance may be due to, for example, increased metabolism because sustained drug levels induce hepatic enzymes (p. 16). However, as explained above, cells exposed to persistently high drug levels reduce (downregulate) receptor numbers to reduce the excessive receptor signalling. This too can cause tolerance. Another mechanism by which tolerance can develop is if the receptors themselves become less sensitive to the drug. This is called receptor desensitisation and can occur after even a single dose of a drug: for example, tolerance to the analgesic effects of **morphine** can be seen after only a single dose. Loss of receptor sensitivity can be due to an uncoupling of the receptor from its second-messenger systems; the drug can still bind but cannot activate internal pathways, like cutting the wire from a doorbell, and its effect is lost.

MEMBRANE TRANSPORT MECHANISMS

To control the composition of its cytosol, a cell must be able to regulate what enters and leaves. For this purpose, the plasma membrane is populated with a range of pumps and carriers, which import essential substances like glucose. One example of a tissue where such transport mechanisms are important is the kidney: in the renal tubule, ion-specific pumps and co-transport mechanisms control reabsorption or secretion of key electrolytes. Some diuretics, including the **thiazides** and the **loop diuretics**, work by interfering with Na^+ transport mechanisms in the tubule wall and increase Na^+ excretion; increasing Na^+ levels in the urine pulls water with it and increases urine volume.

Other important membrane pumps include the Na^+/K^+ ATPase pump (sometimes just called the $Na^+–K^+$ pump). This pump is found in the membrane of all body cells. It operates continuously, exchanging Na^+ for K^+ across the membrane. By pumping Na^+ out of the cell and pumping K^+ into the cell, it maintains high Na^+ concentrations in the extracellular fluids and high K^+ concentrations inside cells. Extracellular Na^+ concentrations regulate water distribution and cell volume, and the Na^+/K^+ gradients across the cell membrane maintain the electrical excitability of nerve and muscle tissue. **Digoxin** inhibits this pump in cardiac muscle cells, reducing the contractility of the myocardium; it is used to treat some cardiac arrhythmias and to reduce cardiac workload in heart failure.

Another example is the proton pump, which exchanges hydrogen (H^+) ions for K^+ in parietal cells in the gastric lining. It concentrates H^+ in gastric fluids, maintaining the low (1–2) pH of normal stomach fluids. Proton-pump inhibitors like **omeprazole** are used to reduce gastric acidity in conditions such as acid reflux.

ENZYMES

Enzymes are biological catalysts and speed up chemical reactions inside and outside cells without themselves being changed: the ultimate recyclers! The body contains tens of thousands of enzymes, each driving one or more steps in the millions of chemical reactions taking place every second. Drugs can themselves be enzymes: for example, **streptokinase** is a thrombolytic drug used to break down a blood clot blocking a coronary or cerebral artery and restore blood flow. More commonly, drugs affecting enzyme action are inhibitors and block the enzyme; for example, **ibuprofen** blocks the enzyme cyclo-oxygenase, which produces pro-inflammatory prostaglandins. This is the basis of ibuprofen's anti-inflammatory action, but because prostaglandins have additional physiological functions, inhibiting their production causes a range of other side-effects (see Chapter 6).

NON-MAMMALIAN CELL TARGETS

Not all drugs target some aspect of human cell function. For example, osmotic diuretics, e.g. **mannitol**, work by increasing the osmotic pressure of filtrate in the kidney tubules, which passively pulls water from the bloodstream into the tubule to be excreted in the urine. Antimicrobial drugs target infecting or invading organisms. A key tenet of antimicrobial therapy is that the drug should have as little impact on host cells as possible, while being sufficiently toxic to the infecting organism to treat the infection.

ASSESSMENT OF DRUG ACTION

Assessing the effectiveness, safety, and nature of drug action is an important aspect of drug development and testing, as well as evaluating its performance when approved for use.

Affinity, Efficacy, and Potency

The affinity of the drug to its receptor is a measure of how strong the drug–receptor attraction is. Drugs with high affinity spend more time bound to the receptor than drugs with lower affinity. This usually means that the drug is more potent and that a lower concentration of drug is needed to produce a given response. Efficacy, on the other hand, is the power of the drug, once bound, to activate the receptor. Agonists, by definition, have affinity and efficacy because they bind and activate their receptor. Antagonists, on the other hand, must have affinity but no efficacy; i.e. even though they bind to their receptor, they cannot activate it.

Potency describes the relationship between drug concentrations and a given response. The lower the drug concentration needed to produce a given response, the more potent the drug is said to be. To illustrate, imagine you have two hypothetical antihypertensive drugs, A and B. Both drugs in clinical trials reduce average systolic blood pressure by 10 mmHg, but the dose of drug A needed to do this is 100 mg compared to 10 mg for drug B. Drug B is therefore the more potent of the two.

DOSE–RESPONSE RELATIONSHIPS

In general, there is a direct relationship between drug dose and the biological response it produces: the higher the dose, the greater the effects, both therapeutic and unwanted. This can be quantified using dose–response (DR) curves, which demonstrate key features of drug action including the therapeutic range and the maximally effective dose. The y-axis plots the drug response under consideration. The x-axis of the DR curve shows drug concentrations, usually plotted as their logarithms (logs) to allow a wide range of values to be plotted along a shorter axis, and gives a characteristic sigmoid (S)-shaped curve with a central linear portion (Fig. 3.10).

DR curves can be constructed to show the activity of a drug in a lab-based experiment; for example, to show how increasing drug concentrations inhibit the activity of a specific enzyme (in which case it is more properly known as a concentration–response curve) or to show the effect of a drug in a living system. Fig. 3.10 shows a DR curve presenting the relationship between increasing dose of a hypothetical diuretic drug and the increase in daily urine output. It clearly shows that as drug concentration rises, there is a steady rise in urine output. It also shows that below the point marked with one star, the drug shows little or no effect: this is the sub-therapeutic drug range. Above the point marked with two stars, the diuretic effect plateaus, and increasing the dose to supra-therapeutic levels gives no further clinical benefit. In this example, the therapeutic range (sometimes called the therapeutic window), which is the dose range across which maximal therapeutic benefit is likely to be obtained, is also shown. It is important that drug concentrations in body tissues, usually measured in the plasma, fall within the therapeutic range. If they fall below the

therapeutic minimum, the drug is unlikely to produce its desired benefits. If they exceed the therapeutic maximum, the risk of adverse effects increases. It is important to realise that for most drugs, some adverse effects may occur even when plasma levels fall within the therapeutic range. Whether or not this is acceptable to the patient and the clinical team is likely to depend upon the situation. Significant unwanted effects occurring within the therapeutic range may be tolerated if the disease is serious or if other treatment options are limited; for example, cytotoxic agents used in cancer can produce horrible adverse effects which may be accepted because the treatment may be life-saving.

The ED_{50} (the dose producing an effective therapeutic response in half of a test population) is also shown on this graph. The ED_{50} is important when calculating the therapeutic index (TI; see below).

THERAPEUTIC INDEX

DR curves can be used to show the relationship between dose and likely toxicity. The TI, in its simplest form, is a measure of the difference between the therapeutic dose of a drug and the dose likely to cause a particular adverse effect. It is calculated as a ratio of the toxic dose to the effective dose. The closer the toxic dose is to the therapeutic dose, the closer the ratio is to 1. A low TI therefore indicates that adverse effects are likely to be seen at drug doses close to the therapeutic dose. Higher TI values indicate a wider difference between therapeutic and toxic doses, which is clearly more desirable.

Fig. 3.11 demonstrates this relationship for the same hypothetical diuretic drug shown in Fig. 3.10 and used to treat high blood pressure. Its standard DR curve is shown in green. It has two known unwanted effects: renal toxicity and hair loss. We can plot the DR curve showing the relationship between drug dose and hair loss; this is shown in orange. We can see that the two curves are very close together, so that for most doses across the therapeutic range, there is also likely to be hair loss. The DR curve showing the relationship between drug levels and kidney toxicity is shown in grey. This curve is significantly shifted to the right, showing that renal toxicity is likely only at supra-therapeutic drug doses.

It seems obvious from simply eyeballing the graph that hair loss is a much more common adverse effect than renal toxicity, but the TI is a quantitative value usually calculated as a ratio. The TI is expressed as the ratio between the TD_{50}, which is the dose of the drug producing the adverse effect in half of a test population, and the ED_{50}, and it is calculated as TD_{50}/ED_{50}. The closer the TD_{50} is to the ED_{50}, the higher the risk of the given side-effect. If TD_{50} and ED_{50} are the same or very close, the ratio is 1 or close to 1, and the toxic effect is pretty much guaranteed to occur at therapeutic doses. For example, if the TD_{50} is 20 mg and the ED_{50} is 10 mg, the TI is $20/10=2$, which is low and suggests a high likelihood of the adverse effect occurring. However, if the TD_{50} is much higher than the ED_{50}, the ratio is much higher and reflects a greater safety margin with respect to toxicity. For example, if the TD_{50} is 1000 mg and the ED_{50} is 1 mg, the TI is $1000/1=1000$.

It is important to realise, however, that not all adverse effects are seen more frequently or more severely with increasing dose. Allergic and anaphylactic drug reactions can occur even after minimal exposure, and cough, a common and

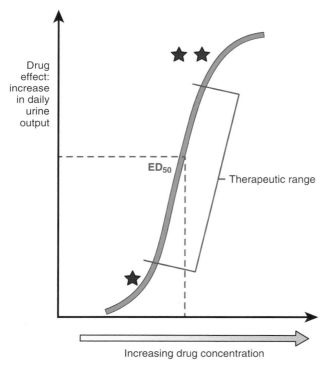

Fig. 3.10   Dose–response curve for a hypothetical diuretic drug, showing the therapeutic range and the ED_{50}.

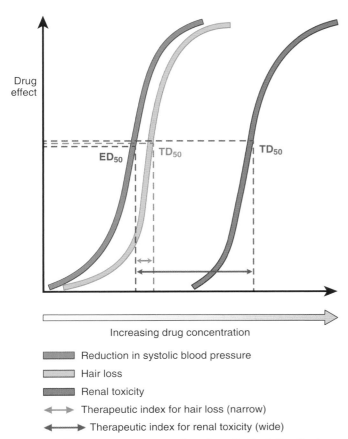

Fig. 3.11   Dose–response curves for a hypothetical diuretic drug, illustrating a narrow therapeutic index for hair loss and a wide therapeutic index for renal toxicity.

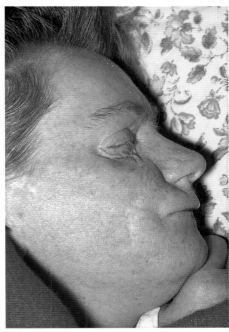

Fig. 3.12   Facial rash from penicillin hypersensitivity. (From Cawson R and Odell EW (2008) Cawson's essentials of oral pathology and oral medicine, 8th ed, Fig. 35.2. Edinburgh: Churchill Livingstone.)

troublesome side-effect of angiotensin-converting enzyme (ACE) inhibitors like **captopril**, is not dose-dependent. In these circumstances, DR curves and TI are not relevant.

ADVERSE DRUG REACTIONS

Adverse drug reactions (ADRs) are common, often troublesome, and occasionally catastrophic. Management of unwanted effects caused by one drug by prescribing additional drugs is an important cause of polypharmacy, which in turn greatly increases the risks of further side-effects and interactions. For example, Ca^{2+}-channel blockers like **verapamil** can cause acid reflux, which can be troublesome enough to require the addition of a proton-pump inhibitor like **omeprazole** to the prescription. ADRs are a common reason for people to consult their healthcare provider and are the cause of a significant proportion of hospital admissions. Risk factors for ADRs include renal and liver insufficiency, female sex, serious illness and/or immunocompromise, extremes of age, and polypharmacy.

MECHANISMS OF ADVERSE DRUG REACTIONS

ADRs can usually be classified into one of four main groups. Any given drug may have unwanted effects in one or more of these groups.

IMMUNOLOGICALLY MEDIATED ADVERSE DRUG REACTIONS

Sometimes the drug itself or one of the constituents of a medicine (for example, lanolin in topical preparations) triggers an allergic response. There are four types of allergies (the Coombs and Gell classification), and all are implicated in immunological drug reactions. Drugs may cause reactions in more than one category: for example, **penicillin** and other β-lactam antibiotics can cause type I, II, and III reactions. Some unwanted effects may seem to be immune-mediated but are not; for example, **opioids** can cause itch in some people. This is not an allergic reaction as might intuitively be supposed but is due to a direct effect of the opioid on mast cells, which synthesise histamine: **morphine** binds to the mast cell and stimulates histamine release. Immune-mediated ADRs are more common in women and in people with a history of allergy.

Type I: Immediate Hypersensitivity

This form of allergy is associated with excessive IgE levels and histamine release from mast cells, and it causes conditions like hay fever and anaphylaxis, the most dangerous form of allergy. The organ most commonly affected in type I allergic reactions is the skin (Fig. 3.12). A range of drugs including **aspirin**, **penicillin** and other antibiotics, and **monoclonal antibodies** cause immediate hypersensitivity reactions.

Type II: Cytotoxic

In type II drug-mediated allergic reactions, the drug binds to a component of the plasma membrane of a particular cell type, e.g. platelets, erythrocytes, or connective tissues, which makes the cell a target for immune attack. **Penicillin**, **cephalosporins**, **thiazide diuretics**, oral **hypoglycaemics**, and phenothiazines like **chlorpromazine** can cause haemolytic anaemia by this mechanism: the drug binds to erythrocyte membranes and stimulates an immune response which destroys the red cells. **Penicillamine** can cause myasthenia gravis and systemic lupus erythematosus by type II-mediated reactions.

Type III: Immune-Complex Mediated

In type III drug-mediated immune reactions, the body makes antibodies to the drug, which bind to the drug molecules in the bloodstream, forming large immune complexes. Immune complexes may deposit in a range of tissues and organs and trigger an immune response against that tissue, damaging and possibly destroying it. For example, **hydralazine** and **sulphonamides** can cause a systemic lupus erythematosus-like syndrome.

Type IV: Delayed

Delayed-type drug-mediated immune reactions involve the activation of T-cells directed against the target; this can take hours or days, and so the immune response is not immediate. Topical **antihistamines** can cause contact dermatitis by a type IV mechanism, and pulmonary toxicity caused by **bleomycin**, **sulphonamides**, and **amiodarone** is thought to be type IV-mediated. Stevens–Johnson syndrome (Fig. 3.13A) and toxic epidermal necrolysis (TEN; Fig. 3.13B; see below) are also examples of type IV reactions.

PHARMACOLOGICALLY MEDIATED ADVERSE DRUG REACTIONS

These ADRs are caused by known pharmacological actions of the drug, including both therapeutic and non-therapeutic effects. They are very common. For example, **antihypertensive drugs** can cause hypotension, and **diuretics** can cause dehydration; these are both instances where the adverse effect is due to an overextension of the desired therapeutic effect. Another example is **aspirin**-induced bronchoconstriction, likely to be particularly problematic in people with asthma. Although bronchoconstriction is not the intended therapeutic aim of aspirin administration, which is usually used for either its antiplatelet or anti-inflammatory activity, its effect on the airways is well understood and predictable (p. 120).

BIOCHEMICALLY MEDIATED ADVERSE DRUG REACTIONS

A drug may interact with cell molecules other than their target molecule and interfere with some aspect of cell structure or biochemistry. For example, one of the hepatic metabolites of **paracetamol** is a reactive and highly hepatotoxic substance called N-acetyl-p-benzoquinone imine (NAPQI), which irreversibly binds to key proteins in the liver cell and induces necrosis. Drugs, for example **cytotoxic agents** used to treat cancer, which affect the structure of DNA (i.e. are mutagenic) interfere with cell division and are associated with significant ADRs, including birth defects and the development of further cancers.

COMMON ADVERSE DRUG REACTIONS

Tissues with high metabolic activity and/or high cell turnover rates are often most likely to be adversely affected by drugs. ADRs are easiest to spot when they occur quickly following drug treatment, and when they are common, significant, and/or

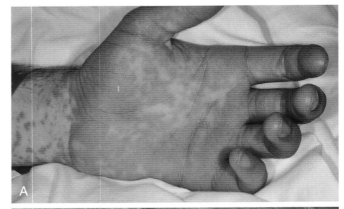
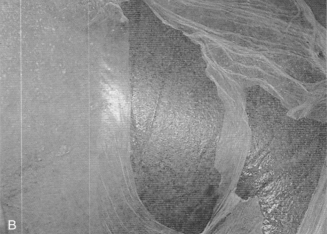

Fig. 3.13 A. Stevens–Johnson syndrome caused by carbamazepine. B. Toxic epidermal necrolysis. (From (A) Paller A and Mancini A (2011) Hurwitz clinical pediatric dermatology, 4th ed, Fig. 20.21. St. Louis: Elsevier, and (B) Micheletti R, James W, Elston D, et al. (2023) Andrews' diseases of the skin clinical atlas, 2nd ed, Fig. 2.41. Oxford: Elsevier.)

unusual. For example, a drug that causes a mild, non-itchy rash on the back which does not appear until a few days after the initiation of treatment might not even be noticed, but if it turns the urine bright purple on the day after treatment starts, the link between the drug and the adverse effect is likely to be made immediately!

HEPATIC ADVERSE DRUG REACTIONS

The liver is metabolically very active, and because its key functions include metabolism and excretion of unwanted substances, hepatocytes concentrate drugs and so are exposed not only to high levels of the parent drugs but also to potentially toxic metabolites. Many agents, including **halothane**, **paracetamol**, **statins**, **chlorpromazine**, **ketoconazole**, and **sodium valproate**, are strongly associated with drug-induced liver injury. With all drugs, care should always be taken when there is known or suspected liver impairment, including age-related decline in liver function in healthy older people.

RENAL ADVERSE DRUG REACTIONS

The kidney concentrates unwanted substances within the renal tubules, which exposes its tissues to high levels of drugs and drug metabolites, some of which are actively renotoxic. Many drugs, including **non-steroidal anti-inflammatory drugs, proton-pump inhibitors,** and **ACE inhibitors**, can impair kidney function. Drugs that are poorly metabolised in body tissues, for example **furosemide, streptomycin,** and **digoxin**, are concentrated in the kidney in their active form, and can cause considerable toxicity. Care should always be taken when there is known or suspected renal impairment, including age-related decline in kidney function in healthy older people.

CUTANEOUS ADVERSE DRUG REACTIONS

A wide range of drugs, including **anticonvulsants, antibiotics**, and **non-steroidal anti-inflammatory agents**, cause skin reactions. Sometimes these are delayed following starting the offending medication, so the link is not always obvious. Cutaneous ADRs range from a mild, possibly itchy rash to potentially lethal conditions such as Stevens–Johnson syndrome and its more widespread form, TEN. In Stevens–Johnson syndrome (Fig. 3.13A) and TEN (Fig. 3.13B), the epidermis sloughs away from the dermis and there are painful erosions of mucous membranes, e.g., in the mouth and the urogenital tract. It carries a 25% mortality rate and is particularly associated with **anticonvulsants, allopurinol**, and **sulphonamides**.

RED BONE MARROW TOXICITY

The red bone marrow produces around 2 million new red blood cells every second, the highest rate of new cell production of any of the body's tissues. It also produces platelets and white blood cells. With such high turnover, the red bone marrow is a particular target for drugs which inhibit cell division, in particular **cytotoxic drugs** used in cancer treatment, which cause neutropenia, anaemia, and thrombocytopaenia. Red cells and platelets may be involved in immune reactions to drugs, leading to anaemia and thrombocytopaenia. Haemolytic anaemia is a recognised side-effect of a range of drugs including **diclofenac, piperacillin**, and the **cephalosporin** antibiotics. Immune-mediated platelet destruction causing thrombocytopaenia include **quinine, sulphonamide antibiotics, heparin**, and **vancomycin**. **Chloramphenicol** carries a small but significant risk of irreversible complete bone marrow failure (aplastic anaemia); the mechanism is not known.

REPRODUCTIVE FUNCTION

The use of both prescription and non-prescription drugs in pregnancy presents potential risks to the developing baby. Most drugs, being fat-soluble, cross the placenta and many do so in significant concentrations. The decision to prescribe new drugs or to continue with pre-existing prescriptions in pregnancy or in women wishing to become pregnant must be carefully weighed up in terms of the risk-benefit ratio to both mother and child. In the first 3 months, while the baby's cells and tissues are differentiating and the organ systems are being laid down, drugs may cause fetal abnormalities; drugs that do this are called teratogens. Significant teratogens include **ethanol**, many anticonvulsants including **phenytoin** and **valproate**, **cytotoxic drugs**, **warfarin**, **ACE inhibitors**, **methotrexate**, and **retinoids**. In the second two trimesters, when organogenesis is completed, ADRs on the fetus are often similar to those seen post-natally: for example, **anticoagulants** increase the risk of bleeding, **oestrogens** can feminise male fetuses, and **ACE inhibitors** can interfere with fetal kidney function. **Ethanol** can cause significant developmental retardation at all stages of pregnancy, including low birthweight and facial and cardiac malformations.

Quantitative and evidence-based data on the effect of drugs on mother and baby during pregnancy and in breastfeeding women is often limited, because for obvious reasons it is not ethical to include pregnant women in clinical trials. In general, the use of drugs in pregnancy should be avoided if possible, especially in the first trimester. If drug treatment is unavoidable, the lowest possible doses of long-standing drugs that are believed to be safe should be used.

Some drugs can interfere with sperm production and ideally should be avoided in men trying to father a child. These include **ethanol**, **opioids**, **anabolic steroids**, and **cytotoxic agents**.

NERVOUS SYSTEM ADVERSE DRUG REACTIONS

The brain represents only 2% of total bodyweight, but it receives 12% of the cardiac output. Despite the blood–brain barrier (see Fig. 2.9), which is at best an imperfect protection for the brain, this means that brain tissues are exposed to significant drug levels. Central ADRs include sedation, visual impairment, seizures, confusion, sleep disorders, and cognitive impairment.

CLASSIFICATION OF ADVERSE DRUG REACTIONS

The ABCDE (Rawlins–Thomson) classification system is convenient and easily remembered.

TYPE A (AUGMENTED) REACTIONS

These are unwanted effects that are extensions of the drug's known pharmacological activity: for example, hypoglycaemia with **insulin**, bradycardia with **beta-blockers**, hypokalaemia with **loop diuretics**, peptic ulceration with **non-steroidal anti-inflammatory drugs**, and bleeding with **anticoagulants**. They are generally predictable, dose-dependent, and reversible on withdrawal of the drug or reduction of dose. Type A are the most common type of ADRs.

TYPE B (BIZARRE) REACTIONS

These unwanted effects are not dose-related. They are not linked to the drug's known pharmacological activity and often involve an immunological reaction to it: for example, **penicillin** allergy is a type B reaction. Although in many cases they are unpredictable, there may be indications that an individual may be at increased risk: for example, a history of allergy may indicate an increased risk of drug allergy. In general, type B reactions are more severe than type A reactions, and because they are rare, they are often not picked up until after a drug has been licensed for clinical use.

TYPE C (CHRONIC) REACTIONS

Type C reactions are associated with chronic drug use and may themselves be persistent: for example, gum hyperplasia seen with **phenytoin** and growth retardation in children treated with **corticosteroids** are type C reactions.

TYPE D (DELAYED) REACTIONS

These ADRs do not appear until after the drug is withdrawn and may not appear until years later: for example, the development of blood malignancies later in life following cytotoxic treatment for an unrelated cancer when younger, and post-antibiotic rashes.

TYPE E (END-OF-DOSE) REACTIONS

These are the ADRs seen after a drug is withdrawn, for example, withdrawal syndromes when **opioids** or **benzodiazepines** are stopped and adrenal insufficiency when a medium- to long-term course of **corticosteroids** ends. These reactions can often be avoided or ameliorated if the drug is withdrawn slowly (stepped down) over a period of time.

DRUG DEPENDENCE

Substance dependence occurs when an individual is unable to function without regular intake of a substance, experiences distress when deprived of it, and continues to use the substance despite associated problems. It is frequently associated with recreational drugs, including **ethanol**, but can also arise with drugs used therapeutically, including **opioid analgesics**, **antidepressants**, and **benzodiazepines**.

It is characteristic of human behaviour that we like to repeat pleasurable and rewarding experiences. The evolution of powerful reward pathways, seen across the animal kingdom and not just in humans, ensures the continuation of the species because it reinforces essential survival behaviours such as eating, sexual and reproductive activity, and parent–child bonding. The key nerve pathways in the brain responsible for regulating reward-related behaviour are found in the mesolimbic system, and the main neurotransmitter involved in promoting rewarding behaviours is **dopamine**. Although other brain centres are also involved, the key areas associated with reward are the ventral tegmental area (VTA) in the midbrain and the nucleus accumbens (NA), located anteriorly to the VTA (Fig. 3.14A). The VTA projects dopamine-releasing neurones to the NA, which is the main centre for reward-orientated learning and behaviour. Dopamine, acting on D_1 receptors in the NA, reinforces activities found to be positive, beneficial, or enjoyable and increases the likelihood that the behaviour will be repeated.

A range of drugs via a direct or indirect action on the VTA increase dopamine levels in the NA and so increases the likelihood that the drug will be taken again (Fig. 3.14B). Repeated use of the drug produces sustained elevated dopamine levels in reward pathways and brain structures, which over time leads to neuroadaptive changes, which may be

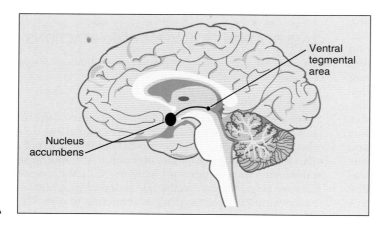

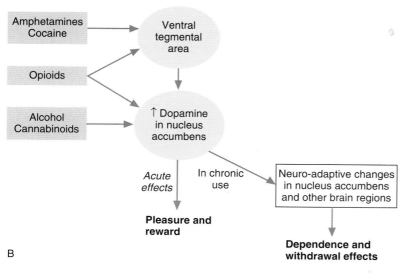

Fig. 3.14 The reward pathway. A. The ventral tegmental area and the nucleus accumbens. B. The action of drugs that cause dependence on dopamine levels in the nucleus accumbens. ((A) Modified from National Institute on Drug Abuse. The Neurobiology of Drug Addiction. Available at http://www.nida.nih.gov/pubs/teaching/Teaching2/Teaching.html, and (B) from Waller DG, Sampson A, and Hitchings A (2022) Medical pharmacology and therapeutics, 6th ed, Fig. 54.1. Oxford: Elsevier.)

irreversible. The reward pathways become tolerant of consistently elevated dopamine levels and cannot function without them. When drug levels fall, and dopamine levels fall as a consequence, unpleasant withdrawal effects motivate the individual to repeat their drug-taking.

WITHDRAWAL SYNDROMES

Withdrawal syndromes are collections of signs and symptoms seen when a drug is discontinued, and they can be severe: for example, delirium tremens following **alcohol** withdrawal can necessitate intensive care support, and seizures following **benzodiazepine** withdrawal can be life-threatening.

REFERENCES

Pasternak, A.L., Ward, K.M., Luzum, J.A., et al., 2017. Germline genetic variants with implications for disease risk and therapeutic outcomes. Physiol. Genomics 49 (10), 567–581.

ONLINE RESOURCES

Farinde, A., 2023. Overview of Pharmacodynamics. Available at: https://www.msdmanuals.com/en-gb/professional/clinical-pharmacology/pharmacodynamics/overview-of-pharmacodynamics.
Pharmacology Education Project, 2024. Clinical Pharmacodynamics. Available at: https://www.pharmacologyeducation.org/clinical-pharmacology/clinical-pharmacodynamics.
Yartsev, A., 2024. Required Reading: Pharmacodynamics. Available at: https://derangedphysiology.com/main/cicm-primary-exam/required-reading/pharmacodynamics.

4 Drugs and Neurological Function

INTRODUCTION

The nervous system controls multiple aspects of body function, and because of this, drugs that affect neurological processes often have significant and widespread effects.

NERVE CONDUCTION AND SYNAPTIC TRANSMISSION

Neurones are specialised cells that generate and conduct electrical impulses (action potentials), allowing them to communicate with each other and to control activity in muscles, glands, and other organs. A typical nerve cell has a cell body, which has multiple fine extensions called dendrites and contains the nucleus, as well as an extended filament called an axon, which conducts the action potential (Fig. 4.1A). The axon terminates in a sheaf of tiny extensions called axon terminals, each of which comes into very close association (but not direct contact) with the dendrites of another neurone, or with a target cell of peripheral tissue, e.g. smooth muscle or a gland. Some nerve axons have a myelin sheath, which increases the speed of nerve conduction.

The Synapse

A nerve cell does not physically make contact with other nerve or target cells: the tiny gap between an axon terminal and the dendrite of another neurone, or the axon terminal and a target cell, is called the synaptic cleft and the site of connection is called the synapse. The nerve conducting an action potential towards the synapse is called the pre-synaptic neurone, and the cell receiving the action potential is called the post-synaptic cell (Fig. 4.1B).

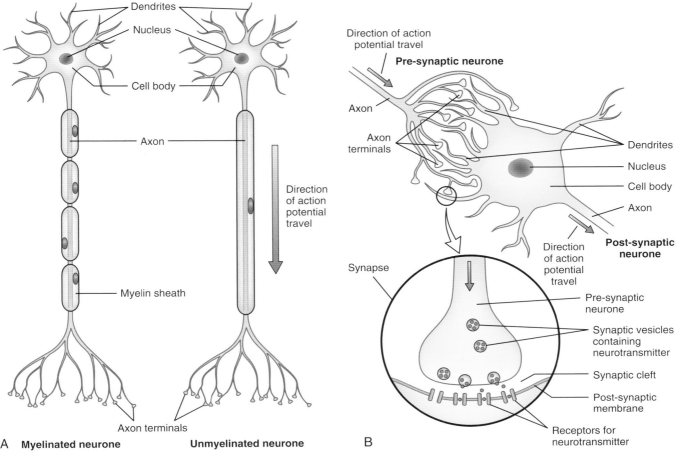

Fig 4.1 A. Nerve cell structure. B. General structure of a synapse. (Modified from Waugh A and Grant A (2018) Ross & Wilson anatomy and physiology in health and illness, 13th ed, Figs 7.2 and 7.7. Oxford: Elsevier.)

Without physical contact between pre- and post-synaptic membranes, the electrical action potential cannot be directly transmitted from cell to cell. Instead, the pre-synaptic axon terminal synthesises a chemical called a neurotransmitter, which is released in response to the arrival of an action potential. Neurotransmitter molecules diffuse across the narrow synaptic cleft and bind to receptors on the post-synaptic membrane. This produces a response in the post-synaptic cell, which may be activated or inhibited depending on the neurotransmitter and the nature of the post-synaptic receptors. Inhibitory neurotransmission is an essential component of neurological control and an important target for clinically important drugs. Neurotransmitter synthesis, release, and action on its receptors are very important drug targets.

Termination of Neurotransmitter Action
Nervous control is fast and flexible, allowing body functions to be rapidly activated or inhibited and finely tuned and controlled. Neurotransmitter levels in the synapse must therefore be tightly regulated. Once released, a neurotransmitter requires only a fraction of a second to diffuse across the synaptic cleft and activate its receptors and must be immediately removed so that its action can be rapidly terminated if required. There are two main ways in which this happens at the synapse, both of which are important targets for drug action.

Re-uptake Pumps. Specialised pumps and carriers in the pre-synaptic nerve cell membrane are in continuous opera-

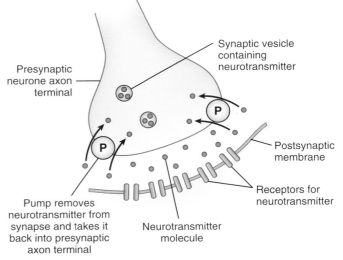

Fig 4.2 Removal of a neurotransmitter from the synapse by re-uptake pumps. (Modified from Burchum J and Rosenthal L (2022) Lehne's pharmacology for nursing care, 11th ed, Fig. 35.1. St. Louis: Saunders.)

tion, constantly removing the transmitter from the synapse and taking it back up into the pre-synaptic nerve (Fig. 4.2). Sometimes the transmitter is then simply repackaged into vesicles, allowing it to be reused—an efficient recycling mechanism! Sometimes the pumps are found on the post-synaptic membranes, in which case the transmitter is then broken down by enzymes in the post-synaptic cell. Drugs that block these pumps increase neurotransmitter levels in the synapse and prolong its action. Key examples include **tricyclic antidepressants** and **serotonin-specific re-uptake inhibitors** (SSRIs).

Degradative enzymes. Enzymes in the synapse or in either the pre- or post-synaptic cells destroy the transmitter. Important examples of drugs that inhibit these enzymes, therefore increasing transmitter levels in the synapse and prolonging its activity, include anti-cholinesterase drugs like **neostigmine**, which prolong the action of acetylcholine (ACh), and monoamine oxidase (MAO) inhibitors like **phenelzine** and **selegiline**, which prolong the actions of noradrenaline (NA) and related monoamine neurotransmitters.

Generation and Conduction of Action Potentials

Action potentials, the electrical signals that sweep along nerve and muscle membranes at speeds of up to 100 m/s, are generated and propagated by the transfer of electrically charged particles (ions) across the cell membrane through specific ion channels. When the concentration of an ion is higher on one side of the membrane than the other, a potential is said to exist, because there is the potential that the ions will move across the membrane until their concentrations are equal on both sides. This ion movement generates an electrical signal measured in volts (or in the case of cells, millivolts, because the electrical potentials are small). Nerve cells control their electrical activity by opening and closing specific ion channels, regulating ion transfer from one side of the membrane to the other. In nerves, the main ions involved are sodium (Na^+) and potassium (K^+), both positively charged ions (cations). Although these are the principal players in nerve action potential generation, other electrically charged ions, both cations and negatively charged ions (anions), are present, and changes in their movement across the membrane also affects its electrical state. Examples include chloride (Cl^-) and calcium (Ca^{2+}) ions.

The Resting Membrane Potential and the Sodium–Potassium Pump

When the nerve is resting, i.e. not firing, there is a potential difference across the membrane called the resting membrane potential, because Na^+ and K^+ ion concentrations on either side of the membrane are unequal. Na^+ is concentrated outside the cell, and K^+ is concentrated inside the cell, and this is maintained by the sodium–potassium (Na^+/K^+) pump. This pump, found in cell membranes of all body cells, is a critically important mechanism in maintaining Na^+, K^+, and water balance between intracellular and extracellular fluids. It constantly pumps Na^+ leaking through the membrane into the cell back out, and K^+ that leaks out of the cell back in. The resting membrane potential in neurones is -90 mV: that is, the interior of the cell is negatively charged compared to the outside of the cell, because although K^+ is concentrated in the cell, so are Cl^- ions and intracellular proteins, most of which carry a negative charge.

The Nerve Action Potential *(Fig. 4.3)*

In the resting neurone, K^+ and Na^+ channels are closed. Activation of the nerve is initiated at the post-synaptic membrane when an excitatory neurotransmitter binds to its receptors. This opens Na^+ channels in the nerve cell membrane, and Na^+ floods into the cell down its concentration gradient. This

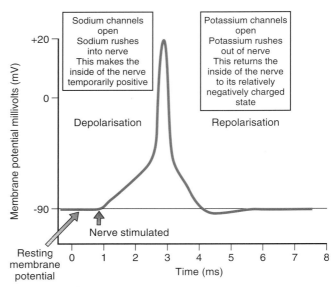

Fig 4.3   The nerve action potential. The nerve is depolarised when sodium channels open in the membrane, allowing sodium to flood into the nerve. Repolarisation occurs when potassium channels open, allowing sodium to flood out of the nerve. (Modified from Herlihy B (2022) The human body in health and illness, 7th ed, Fig. 10.6. St. Louis: Elsevier.)

influx of positively charged ions reverses the charge inside the cell, which goes from negative to positive. This is called depolarisation, and as each area of the neuronal membrane depolarises, it triggers opening of adjacent Na^+ channels, so that the action potential travels along the nerve axon towards the axon terminal. The Na^+ channels are open for only a tiny fraction of a second, and close almost immediately. At this point, the K^+ channels open and K^+ floods out of the cell down its concentration gradient. The rapid efflux of these positively charged ions returns the charge inside the cell to negative compared to the outside. This is called repolarisation.

The membrane potential is now back to where it was before activation, at about -90mV, but the distribution of Na^+ and K^+ ions is reversed, because they are now on opposite sides of the membrane from where they started. Na^+ is rapidly driven out of the cell and K^+ pulled back in by the continuous action of the Na^+/K^+ pump, restoring the original excitability of the nerve. Interfering with ion movements across the nerve cell membrane eliminates the action potential and prevents nerve conduction. **Local anaesthetics** block the Na^+ channels in nerve cell membranes, preventing Na^+ flow and silencing the nerve.

THE NEUROTRANSMITTERS OF THE NERVOUS SYSTEM

Conventionally, the nervous system is considered in two parts: the central nervous system (CNS) comprising the brain and spinal cord, and the peripheral nervous system (PNS), comprising nerves and associated tissue carrying nerve impulses between the CNS and body tissues.

THE PERIPHERAL NERVOUS SYSTEM: THE AUTONOMIC AND SOMATIC DIVISIONS

The PNS is considered in two functional divisions: the somatic and autonomic divisions. The somatic nervous system is under voluntary control and supplies skeletal muscle. The synapse between a motor nerve and a skeletal muscle fibre is called the neuromuscular junction. The autonomic nervous system (ANS), on the other hand, is not under voluntary control and regulates the huge range of physiological and biochemical activity constantly operating below the level of consciousness. This includes control of the smooth muscle found in the walls of passageways and hollow organs, e.g. regulating blood vessel and airway diameter and the motility of the gastrointestinal tract. The ANS also influences the rate and strength of the heartbeat, the secretion and activity of many glands, and essential metabolic functions relating to energy production and storage (e.g. blood glucose levels). Drugs that affect ANS function therefore often have a wide range of often predictable actions and side-effects.

The Autonomic Nervous System

The ANS is further divided into two branches: the sympathetic and the parasympathetic. Most body structures receive both sympathetic and parasympathetic innervation, whose effects usually oppose each other. Sympathetic nervous system (SNS) activity tends to prepare the body for physical activity and emotional, psychological, and pathological stressors, and supports the body during these episodes. This may be something as trivial as preventing a fall in blood pressure when going from sitting to standing, or a major event like surgery or a systemic infection. Parasympathetic nervous system (PSNS) activity, on the other hand, is usually associated with states of physical rest and low stress. Autonomic nerve supply to the main body organs and its actions are shown in Fig. 4.4. Sympathetic pathways leave the spinal cord from

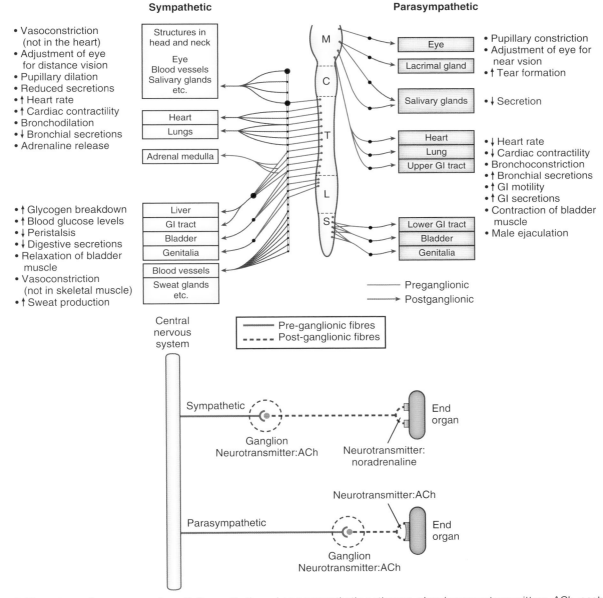

Fig 4.4 A. The autonomic nervous system. B. Sympathetic and parasympathetic pathways, showing neurotransmitters. ACh, acetylcholine; GI, gastrointestinal. (Modified from Ritter JM, Flower RJ, Henderson G et al. (2020) Rang & Dale's pharmacology, 9th ed, Fig. 13.1. Oxford: Elsevier; and Hemmings H and Egan T (2019) Pharmacology and physiology for anesthesia, 2nd ed, Fig. 13.2. Philadelphia: Elsevier.)

the thoracic and lumbar regions, and parasympathetic out-flow is from the cervical and sacral regions.

Autonomic pathways from the CNS to body tissues always contain two nerves (Fig. 4.4B). There are therefore two syn-apses per pathway, both potential targets for drug action. The first nerve, called the pre-ganglionic nerve, leaves the CNS and terminates in a ganglion (a collection of cell bod-ies), where it synapses with the cell body of the second nerve in the pathway, the post-ganglionic nerve. The ganglia of sympathetic pathways lie very close to the vertebral column, so the pre-ganglionic nerve is very short, and a long post-ganglionic nerve is needed to reach the target organ. How-ever, in the PSNS, the pre-ganglionic nerve is very long, re-quiring only a short post-ganglionic nerve to reach the target tissues. The neurotransmitter at sympathetic post-ganglionic nerve endings is noradrenaline (NA), and acetylcholine (ACh) is the transmitter at both sympathetic and parasympa-thetic ganglia and at parasympathetic nerve endings.

The receptors on which acetylcholine and noradrenaline act are not all identical but are subdivided into subtypes, found in different tissues (see also Table 3.1). Understanding the difference between the subtypes of autonomic receptors is important because some drugs act at one subtype and not others, which has a direct impact on their clinical action.

PHARMACOLOGY OF IMPORTANT NEUROTRANSMITTERS

A wide range of clinically important drugs work by inter-fering in some way with neurotransmitter activity, either by blocking, mimicking, or enhancing its effects. The number of known neurotransmitters currently stands at over 100, but some are more widespread than others. The most abun-dant neurotransmitters include **acetylcholine**, **dopamine**, gamma-aminobutyric acid **(GABA)**, **glutamate**, **noradrenaline,** and **serotonin**. Others have more restricted distributions but are still important drug targets, including **histamine** and the endogenous **opioids**.

Serotonin

Serotonin (5-hydroxytryptamine, 5-HT), has multiple phys-iological functions, including in the gastrointestinal tract and as an important platelet activator in clotting. The role of serotonin in these tissues is discussed in more detail in the relevant chapters. It is widespread in the CNS; it regu-lates mood and arousal, eating behaviours, vomiting, cogni-tive function, sleep, sensory pathways including pain, and body temperature; and it is hallucinogenic.

Serotonin Receptors

There are seven types of serotonin receptor, named 5-HT_{1-7}, and each type has multiple subtypes (see Table 3.1). All seven types are found in the brain, and the development of drugs that act selectively at particular subtypes has yielded drugs with specific clinical usefulness. For example, 5-HT_3 recep-tors are found in the area postrema in the medulla, which controls vomiting. 5-HT release by these nerves stimulates vomiting. **Ondansetron** is a selective 5-HT_3 antagonist and a potent anti-emetic. **Methysergide** is a 5-HT_2 antagonist used to treat migraine. 5-HT_{2C} receptors are found extensively in brain regions associated with mood and emotional responses, and stimulation of these receptors reduces dopamine levels and is associated with depressive states. Certain atypical anti-depressants, e.g. **trazodone**, block these receptors.

5-Hydroxytryptamine Synthesis and Breakdown

5-HT is synthesised from the amino acid tryptophan and, like noradrenaline and dopamine, is classified as a monoamine transmitter. It is removed from the synapse by re-uptake pumps (targeted by the **serotonin-specific reuptake inhibitors**) and is destroyed by monoamine oxidase, the same enzyme that destroys NA and dopamine. **MAO inhibitors** (MAOIs) are used as antidepressants.

Gamma-Aminobutyric Acid

GABA is the brain's main inhibitory neurotransmitter. It is widespread in the brain and controls a wide range of pathways and neurotransmitter activity. Drugs that increase GABA levels, e.g. **benzodiazepines** (BDZs), sedate, cause sleep, and reduce anxiety, aggression, and activity. They are also used to reduce the excessive, abnormal electrical dis-charge that causes seizures.

Gamma-Aminobutyric Acid Receptors

There are two types of GABA receptors: $GABA_A$ and $GABA_B$. When GABA binds to either of its receptors, it opens ion channels in the nerve cell membrane, allowing a flow of ions into the nerve cell that reduce its resting potential (Fig. 4.2), reducing its excitability and increasing the size of stimulus required to activate the nerve. $GABA_A$ receptors are linked to Cl^- channels (**BDZs** are $GABA_A$ agonists), and $GABA_B$ receptors are indirectly linked to K^+ channels (the antispasmodic **baclofen** acts here).

Gamma-Aminobutyric Acid Synthesis and Breakdown

GABA is synthesised in the pre-synaptic nerve from the amino acid glutamate. After release into the synapse, it is removed by specific re-uptake pumps in the pre-synaptic nerve membrane, allowing it to be recycled. Some clinically important anticonvul-sant drugs block GABA re-uptake (e.g. **tiagabine**) or breakdown (e.g. **vigabatrine**) and are discussed in the relevant section.

Dopamine

Dopamine is a neurotransmitter in both the PNS and CNS. It is an intermediate in the biosynthetic pathway for NA and adrenaline, so it too is a catecholamine (Fig. 4.12). Tyrosine is converted to dihydroxyphenylalanine (DOPA, specifically, L-DOPA or levodopa) by the enzyme tyrosine hydroxylase. Levodopa is converted to dopamine by DOPA decarboxylase. Dopamine in turn is converted to NA by dopamine β-hydroxylase, and noradrenaline to adrenaline by phenylethanolamine N-methyltransferase. Seventy-five percent of the brain's dopamine content is found in the nigrostriatal pathway, concerned with voluntary muscle control. Dopamine is also found in pathways concerned with behaviour, reward, motivation, and addiction; with vomiting; and with endocrine control. Key drugs in the treatment of Parkinson's disease and schizophrenia work by changing dopamine levels in the brain. Several dopa-mine antagonists, e.g. **domperidone** and **metoclopramide**, are used as anti-emetics.

Dopamine Receptors

There are two groups of dopamine receptors: D_1 and D_2. Dopamine, like many other neurotransmitters, has both inhibitory and excitatory actions depending on the nerve pathway involved. For example, it activates reward pathways

Focus on: Adrenergic Pharmacology

Noradrenaline is an abundant neurotransmitter, found in both the peripheral and central nervous systems. In the peripheral nervous system, it is released at sympathetic post-ganglionic nerve endings (Fig. 4.4B), and in the brain it is found in cardiovascular control pathways and in pathways regulating mood, alertness, reward, learning, and memory. NA is very similar chemically to the hormone **adrenaline**, acts on the same receptors, and produces the same effects. Chemically, both are catecholamines, derived from the amino acid tyrosine and consisting of an amine group bound to a catechol ring (Fig. 4.12). The term 'monoamine' is also used for transmitters derived from a single amino acid; the monoamine transmitters include **NA**, **dopamine,** and **serotonin**. Receptors that bind NA and adrenaline are called adrenergic receptors, and drugs that stimulate adrenergic receptors are called sympathomimetics, because they produce the same effects as NA and adrenaline.

Fig. 4.5 shows the effects of sympathetic stimulation on some key tissues, and the subtype of adrenergic receptor responsible. Most blood vessels constrict in response to sympathetic stimulation; this increases blood pressure and maintains blood flow, and this action is mediated by α_1 receptors. However, some blood vessels, for example, coronary arterioles and arterioles supplying skeletal muscle, contain β_2 receptors, which cause them to dilate. This ensures that during stress of whatever origin, the heart and skeletal muscle receive an increased blood supply to maintain performance. The radial muscle of the iris contracts to open the pupil and ensure adequate light for good vision. This is mediated by α_1 receptors. α_1 receptors in the GI tract reduce motility and secretions, because in a time of stress, digestion and absorption are not a priority. The liver contains α_1 and β_2 receptors, which both promote the breakdown of glycogen to increase blood glucose levels and ensure that key body tissues have an adequate energy supply. The airways dilate because of β_2 receptor activation in the smooth muscle in their walls, and the heart rate and cardiac contractility rise because of β_1 receptor activation in the myocardium. Both actions improve cardiorespiratory function and increase oxygen supply to the tissues. Some drugs acting on adrenergic receptor subtypes are shown in Fig. 4.6.

α_2 Receptors

α_2 receptors need a special mention. These receptors are found on pre-synaptic membranes and, perhaps counterintuitively, they oppose the action of sympathomimetics because they decrease NA release from the nerve terminal. They are part of the nervous system's

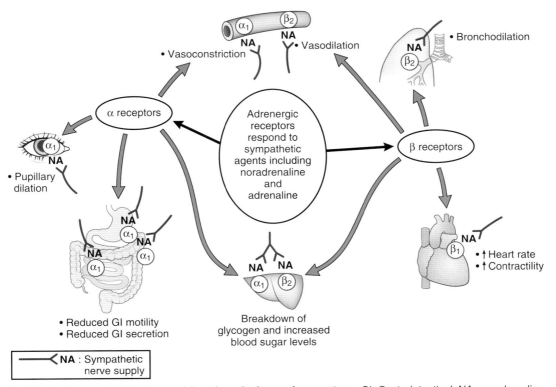

Fig 4.5 Subtypes, distribution, and function of adrenergic receptors. GI, Gastrointestinal; NA, noradrenaline.

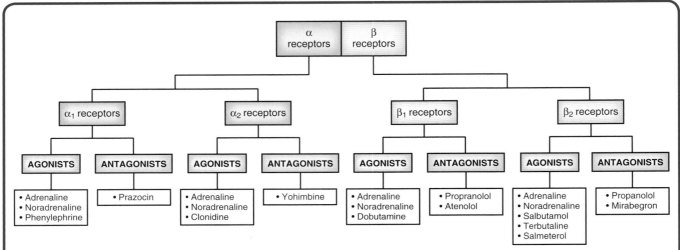

Fig 4.6   Examples of drugs acting on adrenergic receptor subtypes. (Modified from Partin AW, Dmochowski RR, Kavoussi LR, et al. (2020) Campbell Walsh Wein urology, 3rd ed, Fig. 145.4. Philadelphia: Elsevier.)

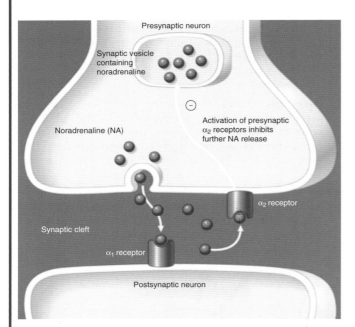

Fig 4.7   The role of α_2 receptors in reducing noradrenaline release from sympathetic nerves. (Modified from Rosenthal LE and Burchum JR (2021) Lehne's pharmacotherapeutics for advance practice nurses and physician assistants, 2nd ed. St. Louis: Elsevier.)

Removal of Noradrenaline From the Synapse

NA's action is terminated by two main mechanisms. Most is pumped back into the pre-synaptic nerve ending by re-uptake transporters (Fig. 4.2), and some is recycled and reused. Blockade of these pumps increases NA concentration in the synapse and prolongs its action, enhancing sympathetic effects. Re-uptake inhibitors, e.g. **SSRIs**, are used in depressive illness. In addition, NA is destroyed by two key enzymes: monoamine oxidase (MAO) and catechol-O-methyl transferase (COMT). Inhibitors of these drugs are clinically useful in depression and other disorders and are discussed in the relevant sections.

intrinsic control mechanisms; if sympathetic activity is high and NA levels in the synapse are elevated, this activates α_2 receptors which inhibit further NA release (Fig. 4.7). This is called autoinhibition. An example of an α_2 agonist in clinical use is **clonidine**, used sometimes in hypertension. **Yohimbine** is an α_2 antagonist not used clinically in the UK except in veterinary medicine but is available as a supplement in some herbal and complementary preparations to treat a variety of conditions including erectile dysfunction.

Focus on: Cholinergic Pharmacology

Acetylcholine, identified in 1913, was the first neurotransmitter to be discovered. It is widespread in both the peripheral and central nervous systems. In the PNS, it is released at sympathetic and parasympathetic ganglia and by the post-ganglionic neurone in parasympathetic pathways (Fig. 4.4B). It is also the neurotransmitter released by a somatic nerve supplying a skeletal muscle; this synapse is specifically called the neuromuscular junction. In the brain, ACh is found in pathways controlling voluntary muscle movement, memory and learning, and alertness. Receptors that bind ACh are called cholinergic receptors.

KEY POINT: CHOLINERGIC RECEPTORS

There are two main classes of cholinergic receptor: nicotinic receptors and muscarinic receptors. There are subdivisions of each. Nicotinic receptor subtypes are not discussed here. Muscarinic receptor subtypes are classified as M_1 to M_5.

Fig. 4.8 shows the distribution and activity of cholinergic receptors in key body tissues. All respond to ACh. Nicotinic receptors are found on skeletal muscle fibres at the neuromuscular junction. ACh released here acting on these nicotinic receptors causes skeletal muscle contraction. They are also found at the ganglia in both sympathetic and parasympathetic nerve chains in the PNS. They are widespread in the brain, where they are often responsible for regulating the release of other neurotransmitters. The main locations and functions of

the subtype of muscarinic receptors are also summarised in Table 4.1. Some drugs acting on cholinergic receptor subtypes are shown in Fig. 4.9. Most muscarinic agonists and antagonists cannot differentiate between the different subtypes and act on them all. This leads to unwanted and widespread side-effects, which often limits their use (see Focus on: Antimuscarinic Side-Effects box). Design and production of selective drugs that work only on one subtype could be of great clinical value.

Removal of Acetylcholine From the Synapse

The enzyme acetylcholinesterase (AChE) is the main mechanism by which ACh is removed from the synapse. It breaks ACh down into acetyl groups, which are destroyed, and choline, which is pumped back into the pre-synaptic nerve to produce more transmitter (Fig. 4.10). Drugs that inhibit the action of AChE, called anticholinesterases, therefore increase ACh levels in the synapse and prolong its action. Anticholinesterases are used therapeutically to reverse neuromuscular blockade and to improve cholinergic transmission in myasthenia gravis. Some anticholinesterase agents are among the most toxic on the planet. Organophosphates, e.g. **malathion**, are highly potent anticholinesterases used in low concentrations as insecticides. Other organophosphates have been used for much more sinister purposes: as agents of chemical warfare (now banned by the Geneva Convention) and for terrorist attacks, for example, the Tokyo subway atrocity of 1995, in which the anticholinesterase **sarin** killed 12 and injured thousands more. Excessive ACh levels stim-

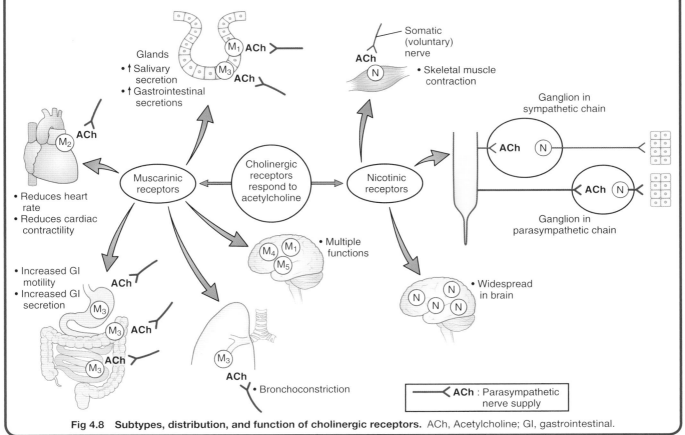

Fig 4.8   Subtypes, distribution, and function of cholinergic receptors. ACh, Acetylcholine; GI, gastrointestinal.

Table 4.1   Subtypes of the Muscarinic Receptor

Subtype	Location	Function
M_1	Central nervous system (CNS); glands	Widespread functions in CNS; stimulates glandular secretion
M_2	Heart	Slows heart rate and reduces cardiac contractility
M_3	Smooth muscle; glands	Increases gastrointestinal motility; stimulates glandular secretion; stimulates bladder contraction; bronchoconstriction
M_4	Mainly CNS	Widespread functions in CNS
M_5	Mainly substantia nigra of brain	Motor control (see Parkinson's disease)

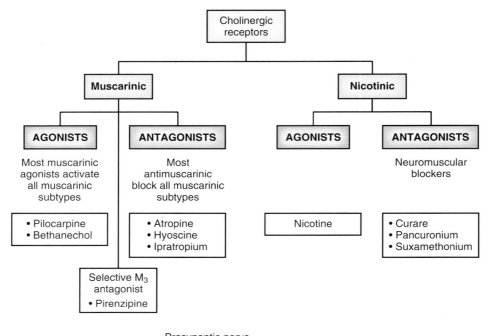

Fig 4.9   Examples of drugs acting on cholinergic receptor subtypes.

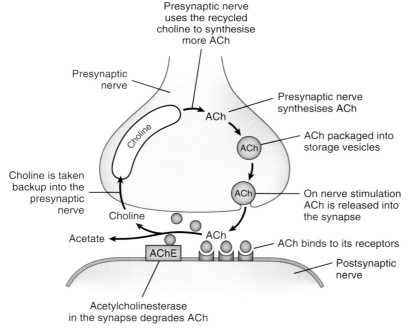

Fig 4.10   The action of acetylcholinesterase. ACh, Acetylcholine; AChE, acetylcholinesterase. (Modified from Rosenthal LE and Burchum JR (2021) Lehne's pharmacotherapeutics for advance practice nurses and physician assistants, 2nd ed, Fig. 12.6. St. Louis: Elsevier.)

ulate muscarinic and nicotinic receptors throughout the body, causing widespread disruption of organ function. This is reflected in a wide range of signs and symptoms including diarrhoea, nausea and vomiting, excessive salivation and tear formation, bradycardia, bronchoconstriction, and increased respiratory secretions.

Focus on: Antimuscarinic Side-Effects

The terms 'anticholinergic' and 'antimuscarinic' are often used interchangeably when talking about drugs used in medicine and their side-effects, but the explanation in the Focus on: Cholinergic Pharmacology box shows the difference between them. Muscarinic and nicotinic receptors are subtypes of the cholinergic receptor. Both respond to ACh, although their distribution and function are different, so that nicotinic receptor blockade gives a very different picture from muscarinic receptor blockade. Antimuscarinic drugs are themselves used for a range of conditions, to block the effects of parasympathetic nervous system 'rest and digest' activity in peripheral tissues, or to block muscarinic receptors in the brain. For example, the antispasmodic **oxybutynin** reduces bladder motility in some forms of urinary incontinence, **ipratropium** is a bronchodilator sometimes used in asthma, and **hyoscine** reduces secretions prior to surgery. Many commonly used drugs have antimuscarinic side-effects because, in addition to their therapeutic target, they block muscarinic receptors: these include **antihistamines**, **antidepressants**, **antipsychotics,** and **opioids**. Antimuscarinic side-effects can impose a significant and potentially dangerous burden, especially in elderly people, and they may be easily missed because they are so widespread and non-specific. The characteristic collection of antimuscarinic side-effects include:

- Cardiovascular system: The PSNS slows the heart rate, so antimuscarinic drugs cause tachycardia. Blood vessels in the skin dilate, causing flushing.
- Gastrointestinal system: The PSNS promotes digestive activity, so antimuscarinic activity reduces gastrointestinal motility, with delayed gastric emptying, vomiting, gastro-oesophageal reflux, and constipation. The production of digestive secretions, including saliva, is reduced, and dry mouth is a very common complaint. Reduced salivary production increases the risk of dental caries.
- Respiratory system: The PSNS contracts bronchial smooth muscle and causes bronchoconstriction. It also promotes the production of respiratory secretions, so antimuscarinic activity gives rise to bronchodilation and reduces respiratory secretions.
- Secretory activity: Sweat and tear production are reduced, resulting in dry skin and dry eyes.
- Smooth muscle: The PSNS promotes bladder contractility, and drugs with anti-muscarinic properties cause urinary retention and overflow incontinence.
- Central effects: ACh is widespread in the brain, and its activity is reduced by drugs with anti-muscarinic activity that cross the blood–brain barrier. This leads to sedation, confusion and cognitive impairment, hallucinations, and memory problems.

- Visual problems: The PSNS controls the ciliary muscle of the eye, which controls focussing of the lens, and constricts the circular muscle of the iris, constricting the pupil. Antimuscarinic side-effects therefore include blurred vision and widely dilated pupils. A consequence of these actions may be raised intraocular pressure and the development of glaucoma. When the circular muscle of the iris and the ciliary body are constricted by parasympathetic activity, the iris is stretched and thinned. This opens the canal of Schlemm in the iris–corneal angle, allowing aqueous humour to drain from the interior of the eye and keeping intraocular pressure within normal limits (Fig. 4.11A). Antimuscarinic agents dilate the pupil by allowing the iris to relax and bulge; this can obstruct the canal of Schlemm, block aqueous humour drainage, and predispose to closed-angle glaucoma (Fig. 4.11B). In some people, there is little space already between the cornea and the iris, and any drug with antimuscarinic effects is absolutely contraindicated because it can cause a rapid rise in intraocular pressure with permanent damage to the optic nerve.

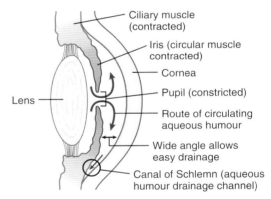

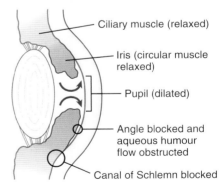

Fig 4.11   The effect of antimuscarinic drugs on aqueous humour drainage and intraocular pressure.

in the mesolimbic system, contributing to the development of addiction to euphoric substances such as **cocaine**. However, dopamine released by the hypothalamus inhibits the release of prolactin by the anterior pituitary and is the physiological 'brake' preventing breast development and lactation in males and in non-pregnant and non-lactating females (in this context it is called **prolactin inhibitory factor**; see Fig. 5.2).

Dopamine Synthesis and Breakdown

Because it is synthesised from an amino acid, dopamine, like NA and serotonin, is classed as a monoamine transmitter. The monoamine produced by a particular tissue depends on the enzymes available. Neurones that release dopamine as their transmitter do not contain dopamine β-hydroxylase, and so dopamine production is the terminal event in the pathway. However, in sympathetic nerves, dopamine is further converted to NA, and in the adrenal medulla, NA is converted to adrenaline (Fig. 4.12). Dopamine is removed from

the synapse of dopaminergic nerves by specific dopamine re-uptake pumps and broken down by MAO and COMT, the same enzymes responsible for NA and serotonin destruction.

Histamine

Histamine's best-known activity is as an inflammatory mediator in allergy, but it is also an important neurotransmitter in the CNS, with a role in sleep–wake rhythms, appetite, thermoregulation, and vomiting pathways. This is the reason why many antihistamines are sedative and explains why antihistamines are useful anti-emetics.

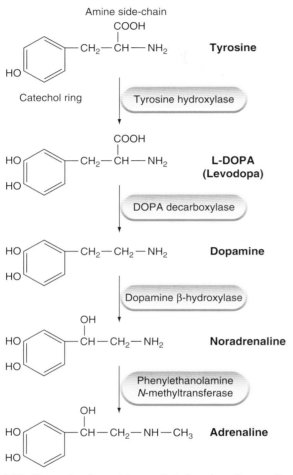

Fig 4.12 Dopamine is an intermediate in adrenaline synthesis. (Modified from Ritter JM, Flower RJ, Henderson G, et al. (2020) Rang & Dale's pharmacology, 9th ed, Fig. 14.1. Oxford: Elsevier.)

Histamine is synthesised from the amino acid histidine and broken down by enzymatic action following its release into the synapse.

Histamine Receptors

There are four main types of histamine receptors: H_1–H_4. Each type has a characteristic distribution in body tissues, relating directly to the different physiological roles of histamine. This is summarised in Table 4.2, and each is further discussed in relevant chapters. H_1, H_2, and H_3 receptors are all found in the brain and mediate the effects triggered by histamine released by histaminergic nerves. Some clinically important antagonists at the different subtypes of histamine receptors are also listed in Table 4.2. Note that the term 'antihistamine' is reserved for drugs that block H_1 receptors. Antihistamines (p. 122) are in widespread use as anti-allergy medications, sedatives, and anti-emetics. H_2 receptor blockers (p. 187) are used to reduce gastric acid levels.

Histamine and the Sleep–Wake Cycle. Histamine has an important role in the body's circadian rhythm. Histamine-releasing neurones originating in the posterior hypothalamus radiate widely throughout the brain, stimulating activity and promoting wakefulness. These nerves fire during the day and are silent at night. Blocking the action of histamine in the brain with antihistamines, e.g. **chlorphenamine** and **cyclizine**, produces sedation and sleep. Current research in the field of narcolepsy is investigating the use of drugs that target H_3 receptors to increase histamine levels in the brain and reduce daytime sleepiness. The first drug to be used successfully in this area is **pitolisant**, approved by the European Medicines Agency in 2016.

Table 4.2 Subtypes of the Histamine Receptor

Subtype	Location	Function	Clinically useful antagonists
H_1	Smooth muscle, secretory membranes, glands	Inflammation, often of allergic origin	Chlorphenamine
	Brain	Neurotransmitter	Cyclizine
			Cetirizine
H_2	Parietal cells in the stomach	Triggers gastric acid secretion	Ranitidine
	Heart	Increases heart rate	Famotidine
	Brain	Neurotransmitter	
H_3	Brain	Neurotransmitter	Pitolisant
H_4	Immune cells	Supporting the role of T- and B-cells in the immune response	-

Focus on: Dopamine and Parkinson's Disease

This disorder of voluntary muscle control was first described by Dr. James Parkinson in 1817. Voluntary muscle movement is normally very finely controlled, allowing for continuous, subconscious, smooth, co-ordinated, and sometimes split-second adjustments in skeletal muscle activity. Movement of the body or individual body parts requires stimulation of appropriate skeletal muscle groups and simultaneous relaxation of opposing muscle groups. For example, when flexing the arm at the elbow to pick up a book from a table, the biceps brachii must contract, but the triceps must relax. Voluntary muscle movement is initiated by the motor cortex in the brain, which is stimulated by the thalamus. The stimulatory input to the motor cortex from the thalamus is in turn regulated by the basal ganglia, collections of highly interconnected cell bodies deep in the brain that include the globus pallidus and the corpus striatum. The globus pallidus applies constant inhibition to the thalamus, preventing inappropriate skeletal muscle contraction. The corpus striatum in turn controls the globus pallidus. The corpus striatum receives input from the substantia nigra via a collection of nerves, collectively called the nigrostriatal pathway, which release dopamine at their nerve terminals in the striatum (Fig. 4.13 and 4.19). The function of dopamine in regulating the corpus striatum is complex, but its overarching effect is to stimulate the globus pallidus, increasing inhibition of the thalamus and ensuring that skeletal muscles are not inappropriately or excessively contracted, and appropriate skeletal muscle relaxation can take place. In PD, the neurones of the nigrostriatal pathway progressively degenerate and the dopamine content of the corpus striatum falls, giving the increased muscle tone and rigidity associated with the disorder. Pharmacological management focusses primarily on replacing the lost dopamine to restore the key regulatory function of the corpus striatum in motor control.

As expected in such a complex control system, this description is only part of the story and other areas of the brain and other neurotransmitters, including GABA and glutamate, are also intimately involved but not described here for simplicity's sake. However, an additional point relevant to the following discussion of PD treatment is that acetylcholine is also released in the corpus striatum, acting mainly on M_5 receptors. It has the opposite effect to dopamine, so that while dopamine release in the nigrostriatal pathway dampens skeletal muscle activity, ACh is excitatory. When the nigrostriatal pathway degenerates and dopamine levels fall, the excitatory action of ACh is allowed to predominate. This explains the use of anticholinergic drugs in the management of PD, especially in drug-induced parkinsonism.

Signs and Symptoms of Parkinson's Disease

PD is characterised by an inhibition of voluntary movement (bradykinesia), accompanied by increased muscle tone and rigidity. Once a movement sequence is initiated, the ability to alter or adjust is impaired: for example, once an individual has begun walking, changing speed or direction, or stopping altogether, may be difficult or impossible. Dystonias, involuntary and repetitive contraction of skeletal muscle, may occur, causing twisting of body parts, e.g. ankle inversion or toe curling, and abnormal body postures, e.g. trunk curling or the head turned to one side. They may be painful and significantly inhibit normal movement. A resting tremor is usually an early symptom, often unilateral in the early stages but becoming bilateral with disease progression. There is higher than average incidence of depression and Alzheimer's disease in people with PD.

DRUG TREATMENT IN PARKINSON'S DISEASE

No currently available drug treatment prevents or reverses the ongoing neurodegeneration in the nigrostriatal pathway. The main focus lies in replenishing dopamine

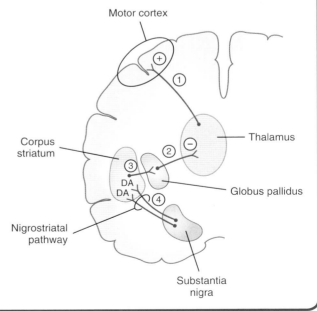

Fig 4.13 Coronal section of the brain showing the key structures involved in voluntary muscle control and in Parkinson's disease. 1. Neurones projecting from the thalamus to the motor cortex exert a constant excitatory stimulus. 2. Thalamic activity is restrained by inhibitory nerves from the globus pallidus. 3. The corpus striatum stimulates the globus pallidus, maintaining its inhibition of the thalamus. 4. The nigrostriatal pathway regulates the corpus striatum. When these nerves degenerate in Parkinson's disease, the striatum can no longer stimulate the globus pallidus and the train of inhibitory nerve signals (2) falls. The thalamus, released from inhibition by the globus pallidus, increases its stimulation of the motor cortex, leading to increased muscle tone and rigidity. DA, Dopamine.

Continued

levels in the corpus striatum. Although 75% of the brain's dopamine content is found in the nigrostriatal pathway, dopamine has key functions in other pathways, e.g. vomiting, that cause many of the adverse effects of dopamine replacement therapy.

Dopamine Receptor Agonists

Examples: ropinirole, pramipexole, rotigotine (newer agents), bromocriptine, apomorphine (older agents, now less frequently used)

The newer dopamine agonists are often first-line treatment, especially in younger patients, because although they are not the most effective treatment (which is **L-DOPA/levodopa**, see below), they are better tolerated and delay the onset of the troublesome side-effects associated with levodopa. Most are given orally, although **rotigotine** is available as a transdermal patch, which levels out the fluctuations in plasma levels associated with oral dosing, and **apomorphine**, which must be given by intravenous or intramuscular injection or by infusion. They are relatively selective for the D_2 receptors present in the corpus striatum, but through their action in other dopaminergic pathways in the brain, they cause nausea, vomiting, and sudden daytime sleepiness and can trigger impulsive and compulsive behaviours, such as gambling, shopping, and increased sexual interest. Patients and their families should be warned of this possibility. Hallucinations, confusion, and postural hypotension can also occur. **Apomorphine** can be used as a 'rescue' treatment in more advanced disease when the effectiveness of other treatments is diminishing, but because it is a powerful emetic, it usually needs to be used with the anti-emetic **domperidone**.

L-DOPA (Levodopa)

The discovery of the effectiveness of levodopa in the treatment of PD dramatically revolutionised the management of the disease, which till that point was essentially untreatable. Levodopa was isolated in 1913, but for 50 years after this the general belief was that dopamine was merely a stepping-stone in the synthesis of adrenaline, and little interest was taken in studying either dopamine or levodopa. Work in the early 1960s, however, showed that the corpus striatum of post-mortem brains from people who had died with PD contained much less dopamine than normal. Once the connection between PD and dopamine depletion was made, it was reasoned that supplying levodopa, the dopamine precursor, would increase dopamine synthesis in the brain and reverse the signs and symptoms of the disease. Dopamine itself cannot be used because it does not cross the blood–brain barrier, and because it is a precursor in NA and adrenaline synthesis, it produces extensive and unacceptable sympathetic side-effects including hypertension and tachycardia. Levodopa was licensed for use in 1970 and in the 50-plus years since, no more effective drug has been developed.

Levodopa is converted to dopamine by the enzyme DOPA decarboxylase (Fig. 4.11) and is further converted to NA and adrenaline in sympathetic nerves and in the adrenal medulla, respectively. This leads immediately to an obvious problem: of an oral dose of levodopa, only 1%–2% actually crosses the blood–brain barrier, and the remainder distributes in the periphery, where it is rapidly converted to dopamine and to NA and adrenaline in sympathetic nerves and the adrenal medulla, respectively. This gives intolerable and unacceptable side-effects. The solution is to block the conversion of dopamine in peripheral tissues with DOPA-decarboxylase inhibitors, but it is essential that these inhibitors do not cross the blood–brain barrier, otherwise the production of dopamine in the brain will also be blocked (Fig. 4.14). The main DOPA-decarboxylase inhibitors are **carbidopa** and **benserazide**, usually given in combination with levodopa. Using DOPA-decarboxylase inhibitors to reduce levodopa loss by peripheral conversion means that levodopa doses can be significantly reduced, which also helps to reduce side-effects.

On starting levodopa treatment, up to 80% of people report improvement, some of whom experience complete remission. With continued treatment, however, levodopa's efficacy declines, requiring increasing doses, and the incidence of side-effects rises. Managing symptoms for as long as possible on as low a dose as possible is important, and combining levodopa with other drugs, such as dopamine agonists, can help.

Levodopa has many side-effects. Nausea and vomiting are common because dopamine stimulates the chemosensitive trigger zone (CTZ) in the medulla oblongata, which lies outside the blood–brain barrier. It can be managed with **domperidone**, an anti-emetic that blocks the D_2 receptors in the CTZ but does not interfere with dopamine function in the brain because it does not cross the blood–brain barrier. With extended therapy, most patients eventually develop tardive dyskinesias

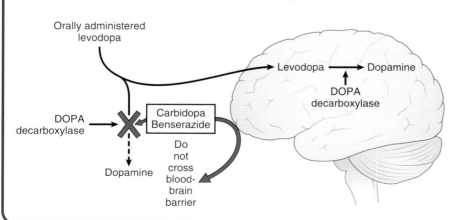

Fig 4.14 The use of DOPA-decarboxylase inhibitors to increase levodopa delivery into the brain.

(unwanted, repetitive, involuntary movements) usually of the face and limbs, including lip smacking, grimacing, or slow writhing movements, which can become severely disabling. Another feature of levodopa treatment is the 'on-off' phenomenon, in which the patient can become suddenly and completely immobilised. This seems to correlate with the dips in plasma concentrations of levodopa in between doses, and it can be helped by dividing the dose and giving smaller quantities more regularly to even out plasma concentrations. **Apomorphine** can be given to reverse the immobility of the 'off' state, and it can be spectacularly and immediately effective, restoring movement to a 'frozen' patient.

Monoamine Oxidase and Catechol-O-Methyl Transferase Inhibitors

MAO and COMT are responsible for dopamine destruction and termination of its action at healthy dopaminergic synapses. Blocking the activity of either or both the enzymes increases dopamine levels in the corpus striatum and improves motor function in PD. However, although these drugs reduce levodopa requirements, they are not effective enough treatments alone and are usually used in conjunction with levodopa.

Selegiline is a monoamine oxidase inhibitor relatively selective for MAO-B, the form of the enzyme found in the corpus striatum (for further explanation, see below and Fig. 4.17). Although its half-life is short (1–3 hours), it irreversibly inactivates MAO-B, so its action is long-lived and it is given only once daily. It can cause gastrointestinal side-effects including constipation,

dyspepsia, and nausea, and because it is metabolised in the liver to amphetamine-like substances, it can also cause hallucinations, strange dreams, confusion, agitation, and insomnia.

Entacapone inhibits COMT. COMT deactivates both levodopa and dopamine, so entacapone used in conjunction with levodopa preserves levodopa levels, increasing conversion to dopamine, and protects dopamine from destruction. It can reduce levodopa requirements by 30% but is also associated with dopaminergic side-effects such as increased sexual urges and compulsive and pleasurable behaviours like gambling.

Antimuscarinic Drugs

Examples: orphenadrine, procyclidine

Before levodopa was discovered, the only useful treatments for PD were anticholinergic drugs, mainly **atropine**. It is thought that as dopamine levels in the corpus striatum fall, the dopamine:ACh balance is tilted in favour of the excitatory ACh and contributes to disruption of motor control. Antimuscarinic drugs have significant and widespread side-effects, including tachycardia, sedation, dry mouth, and constipation (see Focus on: Antimuscarinic Side-Effects) because they block muscarinic receptors throughout the body. Nowadays their use is generally restricted to managing PD-like side-effects caused by antipsychotic drugs used in schizophrenia and other psychotic conditions, whose principal action is to block dopamine receptors.

Fig. 4.15 summarises the mechanisms of action of the main drugs used in PD.

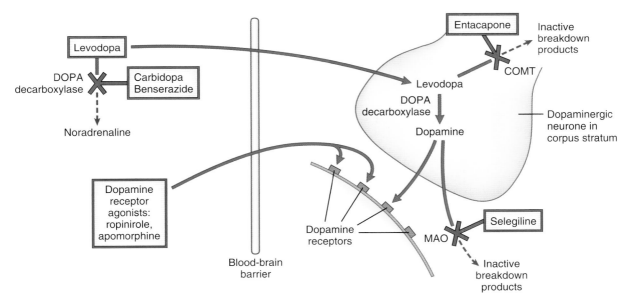

Fig 4.15 Mechanisms of action of the main drugs used in Parkinson's disease. COMT, Catechol-O-methyl transferase; MAO, monoamine oxidase.

Histamine and motion sickness. Motion sickness is believed to arise when information from the eyes and information from the vestibular apparatus (semi-circular canals and utricle) in the inner ear, reporting information on movement and balance, conflict. For example, when reading a book in a swaying ship, the eyes are not reporting movement, but the semi-circular canals are. The visual and sensory information relating to body movement, posture, and balance is received by the vestibular nuclei in the brainstem, which use a number of transmitters, including histamine acting on H_1 and H_3 receptors, ACh acting on muscarinic receptors, and serotonin. When the vestibular nuclei receive conflicting input, they activate various autonomic responses, including sweating, nausea, and vomiting. **Antihistamines** are widely used to treat the nausea and vomiting associated with motion sickness. Antimuscarinic drugs like **scopolamine** are also effective. Additionally, **ginger** is reported to suppress motion sickness, probably due to blockade of serotonin receptors.

Endorphins (Endogenous Opioids)

The term 'opioid' refers to any substance with a range of pharmacological effects similar to morphine. First isolated in 1975, endorphins represent a family of naturally occurring opioids produced in many body tissues. Their discovery was not by chance. Opioid receptors for **morphine** and morphine-like drugs had been isolated a few years earlier, and researchers reasoned that for these receptors to exist, they must be functional: that is, there must be a natural agent synthesised by the body that activates them. The endorphins are strongly associated with pain modulation, and their pharmacology and that of morphine and other opioids is discussed on p. 104.

Glutamate

Glutamate is an amino acid in widespread use in the CNS as an excitatory neurotransmitter.

There are several types of glutamate receptors, of which the N-methyl-D-aspartate (NMDA) receptor is the best studied. **Ketamine** is an antagonist at this receptor.

ANTIDEPRESSANTS, MOOD STABILISERS, AND ANXIOLYTICS

Changes in mood and anxiety levels are normal features of good mental health. Feelings of sadness, excitement, and anxiety are all normal emotional responses in a range of situations. However, some mental health conditions are associated with excessive, inappropriate, or distorted emotional states and/or inappropriate, sometimes disabling, anxiety levels. Disorders of mood are also referred to as affective disorders.

ANTIDEPRESSANT AND MOOD-REGULATING DRUGS

Depressive illness is common: the Global Burden of Disease collaboration (2018) estimates that more than 264 million people globally are affected. Women are more frequently affected than men, and depression is a major factor in mortality from a range of causes, including suicide and cancer. Depressive episodes requiring therapeutic intervention are usually associated with significant life events, e.g. bereavement, illness, or childbirth, but about 10% occur with no such obvious trigger. This is called endogenous depression, which often has a genetic component and may affect a susceptible individual several times over their lifetime. Depressive episodes are a feature of bipolar disorder.

Signs and Symptoms of Depression

A wide range of signs and symptoms of depression may be present, but feelings of sadness and negativity and persistent low mood that interfere with normal daily function or significantly affect enjoyment of normal activities are highly characteristic. There may be feelings of guilt, worthlessness, hopelessness, low self-esteem, and anxiety. There is loss of enjoyment in the company of friends and family, and in activities and hobbies that previously gave pleasure. The individual may withdraw from social contact, become irritable and intolerant of others, and become unwilling to leave the house for even necessary activity such as food shopping. There is often poor concentration, an inability to make decisions, loss of libido, and sleep disturbances. Loss of energy, motivation, and appetite contribute to the inability to engage with normal daily living. Severely depressed people can become completely unable to function. Depression is thought to contribute to up to 50% of all suicide attempts, and depression, particularly severe depression, increases the lifetime risk of suicide.

Treatment of Depression

Pharmacological management of depression is usually only part of a treatment package and is not necessarily the most effective option; up to 80% of people suffering from depression do not respond to standard antidepressants, emphasising the complex pathophysiology of this condition. Drug treatment of depression is generally most effective when combined with non-pharmacological approaches, including cognitive behavioural therapy and counselling. Mild to moderate depression generally responds poorly to standard antidepressant drugs, and all current antidepressant drugs show a time lag between beginning of treatment and the onset of a therapeutic effect. Most antidepressants increase the activity or concentrations of monoamine neurotransmitters, mainly norardenaline and 5-HT, in central synapses, and their mechanisms of action are summarised in Fig. 4.16. In general, SSRIs are first-line treatment. Tricyclic antidepressants and monoamine oxidase inhibitors are used much less frequently, but may be useful in some situations, and both classes of drugs are finding a place in the treatment of other conditions, e.g. **amitriptyline** is used in neuropathic pain, and **selegiline** is used in Parkinson's disease.

THE BIOLOGY OF DEPRESSION

Depressive illness is associated with changes in brain structure, metabolism, and neurotransmitter release, but there is as yet no overarching understanding of the underlying pathophysiology. There is strong evidence that depletion of key excitatory monoamine transmitters, mainly 5-HT and NA, as well as dopamine, can lead to depressive states. This is called the monoamine theory of depression and dates from the mid-1960s, but not all research in the area supports it; some supporting and contradictory evidence is summarised

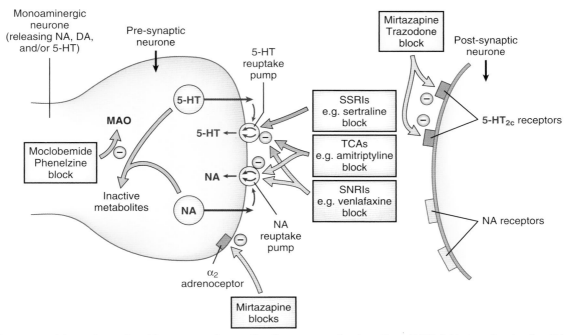

Fig 4.16   Summary of the actions of antidepressant drugs affecting monoamine function. 5-HT, 5-Hydroxytryptamine; DA, dopamine; NA, noradrenaline; SNRI, serotonin and noradrenaline re-uptake inhibitor; SSRI, selective serotonin re-uptake inhibitor; TCA, tricyclic antidepressant.

Table 4.3   Supporting and Inconsistent Evidence in the Monoamine Theory of Depression

Supporting evidence	Evidence inconsistent with the theory
Monoamine levels are reduced in the brain in depression and monoamine oxidase activity is higher in depressed individuals	Drugs that increase monoamine levels in the brain do so rapidly, but clinical improvement can take weeks
Depressive symptoms can be induced by drugs that reduce monoamine levels in the brain	Not all drugs that increase monoamine levels in the brain are antidepressants
Some drugs that increase monoamine levels in the brain have antidepressant activity	Not all drugs with antidepressant activity increase monoamine levels in the brain

in Table 4.3. In addition to the monoamines, links have been made between depression and abnormal glutamate neurotransmission, elevated plasma cortisol levels, neuroinflammatory conditions, and reduced neurogenesis and nerve–nerve communication, particularly in the hippocampus.

ANTIDEPRESSANTS THAT BLOCK MONOAMINE RE-UPTAKE

Re-uptake mechanisms (Fig. 4.2) clear transmitters from the synapse by actively transporting them back into nerve endings. Blocking re-uptake of monoamine transmitters is an important mechanism of action for several important groups of antidepressant drugs.

Tricyclic antidepressants (TCAs)

Examples: amitriptyline, nortriptyline, clomipramine

These are old drugs, first developed in the 1950s. Although they have multiple side-effects, a recent (2018) meta-analysis by Cipriani and colleagues showed that amitriptyline produced the most significant improvement in acute depression in adults when compared with 20 other commonly used antidepressants. These agents block re-uptake of NA and 5-HT from synapses (Fig. 4.16), thereby increasing neurotransmitter levels in the brain. Their efficacy in treating neuropathic pain is probably due to their additional ability to block Na^+ channels.

Pharmacokinetics

TCAs are all given orally, are well absorbed, and are metabolised mainly in the liver. They leave the bloodstream and bind to body tissues, which extends their half-life and increases the risk of accumulation and toxicity. Long half-lives are characteristic of these drugs. The half-life of amitriptyline is 24 hours, which lengthens even more in older people and those with liver impairment.

Adverse Effects

TCAs have multiple adverse effects and should always be used with great care. They sedate, particularly in elderly people. They interact with numerous other drug groups and can cause life-threatening respiratory depression when used with **alcohol**. They block muscarinic receptors, producing the characteristic range of antimuscarinic side-effects: dry mouth, constipation, urinary retention, tachycardia, etc. They cause cardiac arrhythmias and seizures, both common causes of death in TCA toxicity, because they block Na^+ channels in myocardial and nerve cell membranes, interfering with the generation and conduction of action potentials. There are characteristic electrocardiography (ECG) changes, including prolongation of the PR interval and wide QRS complexes. Excitation, agitation, confusion, delirium, and coma are all seen, especially in toxicity.

Serotonin-Selective Re-Uptake Inhibitors

Examples: fluoxetine, sertraline, citalopram

The first SSRI marketed for the treatment of depression was **fluoxetine** (Prozac), available from the late 1980s and by 1990 was the most prescribed drug in the USA. SSRIs selectively increase 5-HT levels in the brain by selectively blocking the serotonin re-uptake pump (Fig. 4.16). SSRIs are also used in panic disorder, some phobias, and obsessive-compulsive disorder.

Pharmacokinetics

SSRIs are taken orally, are well absorbed, and are metabolised in the liver. Many have long half-lives; for example, **fluoxetine**, **sertraline**, and **citalopram** have half-lives ranging from 23–75 hours. Even longer half-lives are seen in reduced liver function. **Fluoxetine** metabolism produces an active metabolite that has a half-life in the order of 6 days. The likelihood of accumulation and toxicity should therefore always be borne in mind with this group of drugs.

Adverse Effects

Largely because noradrenaline levels are relatively unaffected, SSRIs have a different spectrum of adverse effects and interactions to the TCAs. They are generally less toxic in overdose, less sedative, and do not cause the antimuscarinic side-effects of the TCAs. However, they commonly cause nausea and vomiting, and they can reduce libido and prevent orgasm, which are distressing side-effects in sexually active people. Serotonin syndrome is a rare but potentially life-threatening adverse effect associated with mania, confusion, hyperthermia, tachycardia, and muscle tremor and rigidity. Suicidal thoughts and behaviour have also been reported, especially in younger people. Hyponatraemia can occur, possibly due to reduced antidiuretic hormone secretion, which increases blood volume and dilutes plasma sodium.

Serotonin and Noradrenaline Re-Uptake Inhibitors

Examples: venlafaxine, duloxetine

Like the TCAs, serotonin and noradrenaline re-uptake inhibitors (SNRIs) block re-uptake of both NA and 5-HT (Fig. 4.16), but they have fewer side-effects, including antimuscarinic side-effects, and they do not cause cardiac arrhythmias. They may be used in other disorders: **venlafaxine** and **duloxetine** are used to treat anxiety, and **duloxetine** can be helpful in treating urinary incontinence. Both have long half-lives and can cause nausea and vomiting, sexual dysfunction, drowsiness, insomnia, and confusion. Venlafaxine can cause cardiac arrhythmias and should not be used in susceptible people.

DRUGS THAT BLOCK MONOAMINE BREAKDOWN

Examples: phenelzine, iproniazid

MAO is one of the main enzymes that degrades monoamine neurotransmitters, namely NA, 5-HT, and dopamine.

Inhibitors of this enzyme, the MAOIs, first introduced in the 1950s to treat depression, increase levels of these transmitters in the brain, and their antidepressant action is traditionally attributed to this activity. Because these neurotransmitters are widespread in both the central and peripheral nervous systems, MAO distribution is also widespread. Two main forms of the enzyme exist, MAO-A and MAO-B, with different substrate preferences (Fig. 4.17). MAO-A is found in neurones that release NA or 5-HT and is therefore more active in breaking down NA and 5-HT than dopamine. MAO-B is found in dopaminergic neurones and is more active in breaking down dopamine than NA or 5-HT. Most MAOIs block both forms of the enzyme and reduce breakdown of NA, 5-HT, and dopamine; an important exception is **selegiline**, which is relatively selective for MAO-B and is used in Parkinson's disease to increase dopamine levels in the corpus striatum. MAO is also found in the wall of the gastrointestinal tract, where it destroys tyramine and other related amines found in a wide range of common foodstuffs including cheese and red wine (see Key Point: The Cheese Reaction below).

Pharmacokinetics

MAOIs are given orally, are well absorbed, and are metabolised in the liver. Most bind irreversibly to MAO, permanently deactivating it. Because it may take 2 or 3 weeks to restore the depleted MAO levels to normal, the effects of these drugs are long lasting and not easily reversed in overdose. An exception is **moclobemide**, which inhibits MAO reversibly and has a half-life of 2 hours.

Adverse Effects

MAOIs have multiple adverse effects, mainly relating to their inhibition of NA, 5-HT, and dopamine breakdown. Counterintuitively for drugs that increase the levels of sympathetic neurotransmitters, a common side-effect is postural hypotension. This is thought to be due to increased levels of tyramine, which would normally be destroyed by MAO being taken up into sympathetic nerve endings and converted to an inactive 'false' transmitter which when released does not have sympathetic activity. There may be tremor, excitement, agitation, convulsions, and antimuscarinic side-effects.

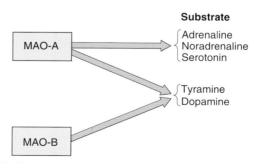

Fig 4.17   The two forms of monoamine oxidase and their main substrates. MAO, Monoamine oxidase. (From Waller DG, Sampson A, and Hitchings A (2022) Medical pharmacology and therapeutics, 6th ed, Fig. 22.3. Oxford: Elsevier.)

KEY POINT: THE CHEESE REACTION

The so-called 'cheese reaction' is potentially one of the most dangerous side-effects of monoamine oxidase inhibitor therapy. An individual taking monoamine oxidase inhibitors must avoid foods containing significant levels of tyramine, including many cheeses, red wine, cured and aged meats, and fermented foods including sauerkraut, beer, and concentrated yeast extracts like Marmite. In the presence of a monoamine oxidase inhibitor, tyramine in these foods cannot be metabolised in the wall of the gastrointestinal tract and is absorbed, taken up into sympathetic nerves, and causes noradrenaline release, leading to widespread sympathetic stimulation. This can cause hypertension, a crashing headache, tremors, excitement, cardiac failure, myocardial infarction, agitation, and increased appetite. This interaction (the 'cheese reaction') led to these drugs falling out of regular use when alternative agents (tricyclic antidepressants) became available in the 1960s.

Preparations containing **adrenaline** or other sympathomimetics (e.g. nasal decongestants) should not be taken with MAOIs.

MONOAMINE RECEPTOR BLOCKERS

It may seem counterintuitive that drugs that block monoamine receptors should have antidepressant activity, given that the major groups of antidepressant drugs enhance monoamine activity. It underlines the complexity of neurotransmitter function and communication in the pathogenesis of affective disorders.

Mirtazapine

This drug blocks several receptor types, including 5-HT$_{2C}$ and H$_1$ receptors (Fig. 4.16). Its main mechanism of action is thought to be by blocking pre-synaptic α_2 receptors. As explained earlier (Fig. 4.7), these receptors are part of the synaptic self-regulation system, and when they are strongly stimulated by rising transmitter levels, they shut down transmitter release at that synapse. Blocking them shuts down this feedback control and increases synaptic concentrations of NA and 5-HT. Mirtazapine is sedative, because of its antihistamine action, and can cause increased appetite and weight gain.

Trazodone

Trazodone blocks 5-HT$_{2C}$ receptors (Fig. 4.16), which indirectly leads to increased NA and dopamine activity in the brain, thought to underpin its antidepressant activity. It is sedative and may be used to treat insomnia. Unlike the TCAs and SSRIs, it has little antimuscarinic activity, and so may be useful in patients for whom antimuscarinic effects may be especially troublesome, e.g. in chronic constipation or benign prostatic hypertrophy.

OTHER ANTIDEPRESSANT DRUGS

St. John's wort is a popular herbal remedy taken to improve mood, although there is little evidence of any benefit in mild to moderate depression. It is important to be aware that it is an inducer of liver enzymes and therefore can increase the metabolism of other drugs, including antidepressants.

Agomelatine

Disruption of sleep patterns and poor sleep quality are frequently seen in depression and can significantly reduce quality of life and cause slow recovery. The suprachiasmatic nucleus (SCN) in the hypothalamus is the main driver of the circadian rhythms directing the body's internal 24-hour body clock. The SCN is linked to the pineal gland, which releases melatonin, and at night, the SCN stimulates melatonin release from the pineal gland, promoting sleep. SCN function is disrupted in depressive disorders, interrupting the sleep–wake cycle, and agomelatine, a melatonin analogue, is used to regulate sleep patterns in depression (and other conditions featuring sleep disorders). It promotes sleep by activating the body's natural melatonin receptors. Agomelatine also antagonises 5-HT$_{2C}$ receptors (see also **trazodone**), which may contribute to its usefulness in depression. It is generally well tolerated, although adverse effects include insomnia, gastrointestinal disturbances, increased sweating, headache, drowsiness, and dizziness.

Future Developments

Ketamine, introduced in the 1960s as an anaesthetic, has a history of illegal and recreational use. In the early 2000s, researchers trialled the closely related agent **esketamine** in severely depressed patients resistant to standard treatments, and not only did the drug relieve the signs and symptoms of depression, it did so rapidly, sometimes within hours of administration. This contrasts markedly with conventional treatments, all of which require weeks for achievement of full therapeutic effect. It is believed to act by increasing levels of the excitatory transmitter glutamate in the brain. It is not currently licensed for use in the UK because of safety concerns but research is ongoing in the search for analogues with fewer side-effects and less potential for addiction and abuse.

ANXIOLYTIC AND SEDATIVE DRUGS

Anxiety, and the fear reaction linked to it, is a normal emotional response to unfamiliar and potentially hazardous situations. It confers survival advantage, because it increases alertness and triggers a sympathetic flight or fight response, e.g. increased heart rate and raised blood glucose levels, to ensure a rapid and effective physical reaction to potential threats. Appropriate levels of anxiety reduce risk-taking behaviours and improve judgement associated with potentially dangerous situations. However, in psychiatric and psychological disorders with an anxiety component, the anxiety response is exaggerated, inappropriate, and detrimental to both physical and mental health. This in turn interferes with sleep, exacerbating mental health issues.

Anxiety Disorders

Anxiety disorders are common and include generalised anxiety disorder, phobic states, and panic disorder. They may co-exist with depression, and there is often a genetic component. The main neurotransmitters in the brain thought to be important in anxiety disorders include GABA, noradrenaline, serotonin, and dopamine, and structural changes in areas of the brain involved in emotional and anxiety responses, including the amygdala, hippocampus, and other limbic system structures, have been identified. The main anxiolytic drugs include the **benzodiazepines**, but other agents including the **SSRIs** (increasingly the first choice in treating anxiety disorders), **beta-blockers**, certain anticonvulsant drugs like **gabapentin**, and some atypical (second-generation) antipsychotics, e.g. **olanzapine**, have all proved useful in anxiety disorder management.

NON-BENZODIAZEPINE ANXIOLYTICS

BDZ-mediated sedation can be a significant disadvantage in treating anxiety disorders because daytime sleepiness interferes with normal daily living. In addition, the risk of dependence is high. The search for non-sedative agents with anxiolytic activity has led researchers to investigate medications acting at a range of other neurotransmitters, including glutamate.

Buspirone

Buspirone was initially developed as an antipsychotic agent, but its activity in this area was disappointing, and its anxiolytic activity was explored instead. It is most useful in generalised anxiety states and is usually tolerated better than BDZs because it is not sedative and does not interfere with motor control. Buspirone is an agonist at 5-HT receptors, although how this translates into its anxiolytic effect is uncertain. There is a delay of 2–3 weeks between starting treatment and improvement of symptoms, so it is believed that whatever its mode of action, buspirone must trigger some form of adaptation in the brain, particularly in the amygdala, which takes time to develop. It also activates a range of other receptors, including dopamine and noradrenaline receptors, but the relevance of this to its clinical action is unknown.

Pharmacokinetics

Buspirone is given orally and is well absorbed, with a half-life of 2–4 hours. Much of an oral dose is destroyed by the liver in first-pass metabolism, and its bioavailability is therefore low. Because of this, it is important to consider hepatic function when prescribing. Reduced liver function can increase the proportion of an oral dose reaching the bloodstream several fold, causing potentially toxic plasma levels.

Adverse Effects

Buspirone commonly causes dizziness, reported by over 10% of patients. Other side-effects include nausea, diarrhoea, headache, confusion, drowsiness or excitement, mood changes, and nervousness. It is not associated with tolerance or dependence and does not interfere with sexual desire or performance, unlike **SSRIs**.

HYPNOTICS

Hypnotics, drugs that induce sleep, are used to treat insomnia. Insomnia is a persistent inability to fall asleep or stay asleep despite appropriate time and opportunity, leading to daytime fatigue, irritability, poor concentration and memory, and impairment of normal daily function, and it is experienced by nearly everybody at some point in their lives. Insomnia is frequently short-term, e.g. related to jet lag or the stress of an upcoming examination. More prolonged periods of insomnia may follow bereavement or other personal stressors. Chronic insomnia may be caused by psychiatric or physical illness, e.g. in chronic obstructive pulmonary disease, dyspnoea can interrupt sleep. Pain, acute or chronic, and snoring can also cause poor sleep. Chronic insomnia is associated with increased rates of depression and poor quality of life and requires careful investigation. The initial approach to treatment should attempt to identify the cause of the insomnia through taking of sleep history, a general medical and psychiatric history, a review of the patient's current social and personal situation, and a review of all medications, including **caffeine**, **tobacco**, and **alcohol** use. Following good sleep hygiene practices, e.g. avoiding stimulants and screen use prior to bedtime, following a regular bedtime routine, and ensuring a comfortable and quiet sleep environment, often improve or resolve sleep problems. Hypnotics may provide a temporary improvement in sleep times and sleep quality, but they disrupt the normal sleep cycle (described below) and can reduce the length of time spent in deep sleep or in rapid-eye movement (REM) sleep.

The Physiology of Sleep

Sleep is a physiologically active condition essential for health and indeed for life itself. In fatal familial insomnia, a rare degenerative brain disorder, progressive insomnia is the characteristic symptom, and the sleep deficiency leads to physical and mental deterioration and eventual death. Sleep–wake cycles are a key feature of the body's circadian rhythm and are governed by the suprachiasmic nucleus, a group of neurones in the hypothalamus. Light-sensitive ganglion cells in the retina send constant input to the suprachiasmic nucleus so that the circadian sleep–wake rhythm synchronises with light–dark cycles. During waking periods, the hypothalamus maintains arousal pathways in the brain (see also **histamine** above), and when dark, these pathways are silent, allowing the brain to sleep.

Rapid-Eye Movement and Non-Rapid-Eye Movement Sleep. Recording electrical activity in the brain during sleep shows two distinct phases, which cycle during an average night's sleep: REM sleep and non-REM (NREM) sleep. The first phase of sleep entered when falling asleep is NREM sleep, which accounts for 75%–80% of total sleep. Sleep in the initial stages of NREM activity is light, moving into the deepest phases of sleep after about 15 minutes, and is thought to be induced by increased activity in GABAergic neurones. Metabolic activity falls, growth hormone secretion is increased, skeletal muscle is deeply relaxed, and blood flow to the brain is significantly reduced. From NREM sleep, the sleeper moves into REM sleep. Dreaming occurs during REM sleep, and metabolic activity and cerebral blood flow are equivalent to those seen when awake. Heart rate and respiratory rate rise, blood pressure increases, and there may be sexual arousal. REM sleep episodes in the early part of the night are short, likely about 10 minutes long, and they get longer in the later parts of the sleep period. The final REM period may be up to an hour long. There are generally four to five such cycles in a good night's sleep.

Benzodiazepines

BDZs, discussed in detail in the Focus Box below, all have hypnotic activity. Their action in enhancing GABA activity promotes the onset of sleep, and they are widely used in sleep complaints. However, they predispose to dependence; reduce the length of time spend in deep sleep; cause hangover effects the next day because of their long half-lives; increase the risk of accident, injury, and falls, especially in elderly people; and cause cognitive and memory impairment.

Focus on: Benzodiazepine Pharmacology

Examples: diazepam, clonazepam, midazolam, lorazepam

Prior to the 1960s, **barbiturates** were the main drugs used to manage anxiety (anxiolytics), to calm and soothe (tranquillisers/sedatives), and to induce sleep (hypnotics). These were not ideal from a clinical point of view because they strongly induced dependence, caused multiple side-effects including respiratory depression, and overdose was difficult to manage. The first benzodiazepine (BDZ), **chlordiazepoxide** (Librium), was marketed in 1960, with a number of related BDZs, including **diazepam** (Valium), **clonazepam**, and **lorazepam**, following within the next 15 years. Initial excitement in the medical community for these new, safer tranquillisers and hypnotics led to widespread prescribing and, although it is now firmly established that BDZs cause significant dependence and potentially dangerous withdrawal syndromes, they remain globally in the top three most frequently prescribed drugs. **Diazepam, lorazepam**, and **midazolam** are on the World Health Organisation's list of essential drugs, but most healthcare systems regulate BDZ prescribing, recognising the challenges presented by their use, and they are no longer considered first-line treatment in anxiety disorders.

Mechanism of Action

BDZs modulate the activity of GABA$_A$ receptors, which are widespread in the CNS. GABA is the most common inhibitory neurotransmitter in the CNS, and when it is released by a pre-synaptic nerve and binds to its receptors on the post-synaptic nerve, the post-synaptic nerve is hyperpolarised, i.e. inhibited.

GABA$_A$ receptors are a structural component of CNS Cl⁻ ion channels (Fig. 4.18). When GABA binds to its receptor, the Cl⁻ channel opens, allowing Cl⁻ to flow into the neurone, which hyperpolarises and desensitises it (Fig. 4.18A). BDZs enhance this effect, i.e. they potentiate GABA-mediated nerve inhibition. In the presence of a BDZ, the Cl⁻ channels spend more time in the open state, increasing Cl⁻ entry and deepening nerve inhibition (Fig. 4.18B).

Pharmacodynamics

Because GABA-mediated inhibitory control of neurones is widespread in the brain, the dampening of neuronal activity by BDZs gives wide-ranging clinical effects. BDZs are sedative, anxiolytic, anticonvulsant, hypnotic, and reduce skeletal muscle tone. They impair short-term memory, causing amnesia, which may be useful when used in patients undergoing potentially stressful procedures such as dental extractions, but which has been exploited by individuals using them for criminal purposes, e.g. as date-rape drugs. The main clinical uses of the BDZs are listed in Box 4.1.

Pharmacokinetics

The pharmacokinetics of the various members of the BDZ family are similar in many respects, and the choice of drug usually depends on its half-life and duration of action. They are highly fat soluble, so they are rapidly and completely absorbed following oral administration and are taken up into fat stores. This leads to accumulation, especially in older people, and increases the risk of toxicity. Some may be given intravenously; shorter-acting agents like **midazolam** and **lorazepam** are used as preoperative medication or for conscious sedation in procedures like endoscopy. **Midazolam** may be given buccally to control seizures if intravenous access is difficult, and **diazepam** is available in rectal formulations for the same purpose. The spectrum of half-lives is wide and often long. Most are highly plasma protein-bound, so there is significant reservoir of drug circulating in the

---

Box 4.1 The Main Clinical Uses of Benzodiazepines

Anxiety
Acute panic attacks
Insomnia
Prevention of seizures
Emergency treatment of status epilepticus/febrile convulsions/seizures caused by poisoning
Adjunct to anaesthesia/conscious sedation
Muscle relaxant: useful in reducing physical tension in anxiety, when used as an adjunct to anaesthesia, and in conditions featuring muscle spasm
Alcohol withdrawal

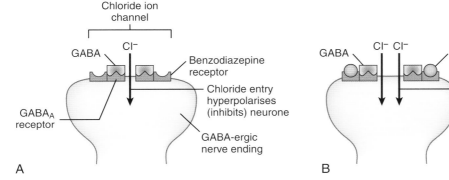

Fig 4.18   GABA$_A$ and benzodiazepine receptors and chloride ion channels on brain neurones. GABA, Gamma-aminobutyric acid. (Modified from Stevens V, Redwood S, Neel J, et al. (2007) Rapid review behavioral science, 2nd ed, Fig. 10.2. Philadelphia: Mosby.)

Continued

bloodstream, which contributes to the long half-lives of many BDZs. Several are metabolised to active products, extending the effects of the drug even further. Consideration of a BDZ's half-life is a significant factor in choosing a specific agent for a particular clinical situation. For example, **midazolam** is favoured in conscious sedation because it has a relatively short half-life and minimises recovery times after a procedure. **Diazepam** has a half-life of around 40 hours and is an active metabolite, so when used regularly as, for example, as a night-time sedative or as an anticonvulsant, the incidence of accumulation and daytime sleepiness is high. **Clonazepam** is used as prophylactic treatment in epilepsy because of its long duration of action. **Temazepam** is used as a night-time hypnotic because its relatively short half-life and absence of active metabolites reduce the likelihood of a morning 'hangover' effect on waking. Half-lives and metabolite activities for some key BDZs are summarised in Table 4.4.

Adverse Effects

BDZs cause sedation, impaired memory, confusion, and cognitive impairment, especially in elderly people. They cause skeletal muscle weakness and ataxia, and impair co-ordination and fine motor control, increasing the risk of accidents, falls (especially in elderly people), and injury, e.g. from operating machinery. They potentiate the effects of other CNS depressants, including **alcohol** and **opioids**, and in combination with these agents can cause life-threatening respiratory depression. Tolerance develops rapidly, requiring steady increase in dosing when used in the medium to long term. Dependence is common in medium- to long-term treatment, and it is recommended that treatment should not exceed 4 weeks. Both physiological and psychological dependence develop, with well-defined withdrawal syndromes. The likelihood of dependence increases with the duration of treatment, with higher doses, and with shorter-acting

Table 4.4 Half-Lives and Metabolite Activity of Some Key Benzodiazepines

Drug	Average half-life	Metabolites
Diazepam	20–40 h, often longer in older people and in liver insufficiency	Diazepam is metabolised to temazepam and oxazepam, both active agents in their own right, and N-desmethyldiazepam, which has a half-life of 100 h
Temazepam	10 h, often longer in older people	No active metabolites
Midazolam	2 h	Active metabolite produced, with half-life of about 2 h
Lorazepam	10–20 h	No active metabolites
Clonazepam	30–40 h	No active metabolites

agents such as **lorazepam**. Withdrawal symptoms include anxiety, insomnia, irritability, depression, and sometimes convulsions.

Benzodiazepine Toxicity

BDZs are safer in overdose than older anxiolytic and hypnotic agents like the **barbiturates**, and if taken alone in excessive doses generally produce extended sleep from which the person eventually wakes naturally. However, if overdose reversal is required, for example if other CNS depressants such as **opioids** or **alcohol** have also been taken, the BDZ antagonist **flumazenil** is given. Flumazenil binds to and blocks the BDZ receptor, but its half-life is only about 1 hour, considerably shorter than that of the BDZs it is being used to reverse, so is usually given by infusion rather than as a one-off dose.

The Z-Drugs: Zolpidem, Zaleplon, and Zopiclone

Like the BDZs, these drugs bind to the Cl⁻ channel associated with the GABA$_A$ receptor, increase its opening time, and increase Cl⁻ flow into the nerve. This hyperpolarises the cell, enhancing the inhibitory action of GABA. They are not chemically similar to BDZs, however, and do not bind to the same site on the Cl⁻ channel. They have no anxiolytic activity.

Pharmacokinetics

These drugs are given orally, are well absorbed, and are metabolised in the liver to inactive metabolites. One advantage over the BDZs is their shorter half-life, usually no longer than 5 hours, reducing the incidence of accumulation and hangover effects in the morning.

Adverse Effects

The Z-drugs cause dependence, cognitive impairment, and hangover effects despite their relatively short half-life.

Other Hypnotic Drugs

Melatonin, a hormone naturally released by the pineal gland to shift the brain into sleep mode (see above), is given to manage short-term insomnia, for example, in jet lag. Some antihistamines, e.g. **diphenhydramine** and **doxepin**, are used clinically as sedatives and hypnotics. They are effective here because histamine is an important neurotransmitter in arousal pathways (see above). **Chlormethiazole (clomethiazole)** is used in severe insomnia, especially in older people. It binds to the GABA$_A$ receptor, although at a site different from the BDZs or the Z-drugs, and facilitates GABA's action, causing hyperpolarisation and inhibition of nerve activity.

MOOD-STABILISING DRUGS

The main mood-stabilising agent is **lithium**, but the range of drugs used for this purpose is expanding and includes certain anticonvulsant drugs, e.g. **lamotrigine** and **sodium valproate**, and some atypical antipsychotics, e.g. **risperidone** and **olanzapine**. Mood stabilisers prevent mood swings in bipolar disorder.

Bipolar Disorder

This condition has a strong heritable component and usually manifests in young adulthood. It is characterised by fluctuating and alternating episodes of depression, episodes of mania (elevated mood), and periods of euthymia (normal mood). The depressive component is usually more marked than the manic condition and is treated with standard antidepressant therapy. The manic episodes feature euphoria, reckless and impulsive behaviour, loss of inhibition and increased libido, and even psychotic symptoms such as delusions and hallucinations. The risk of suicide is significantly increased in bipolar disorder. **Lithium** or **sodium valproate** (p. 75) are the mainstays of treatment, with **antidepressants**, **antipsychotics**, and **anticonvulsants** used as supplementary agents.

Lithium

Lithium is usually effective in regulating mood and preventing relapse, but it has significant side-effects and toxicity, and controlling plasma levels is challenging. It is given as lithium carbonate, which dissociates to release lithium ion (Li^+), the active agent. The mechanism by which lithium stabilises mood is not known, although it has been shown to have multiple effects on enzyme activity, gene expression, and nerve excitability in the brain, and accumulates inside body cells because it passes through Na^+ channels.

Pharmacokinetics

Lithium is given orally and is excreted by the kidney. Because it is not metabolised, clearance of lithium from the body depends entirely on renal function, so care must be taken in individuals with any degree of renal compromise. Lithium has a long half-life, partly because so much of it collects within cells via Na^+ channel uptake. Initiating lithium treatment must therefore be done gradually, with regular measurements of plasma levels, because it takes 2 weeks or more to achieve steady state, and reversing toxic levels is slow because excretion is slow. The therapeutic plasma range is narrow, only 0.4–1 mmol/L, making safe lithium management even harder.

Adverse Effects

Lithium's side-effects are common and significant and contribute to the declining use of this drug despite its well-documented efficacy in stabilising mood. It causes nausea in up to 20% of patients, diarrhoea in up to 10% of patients, and vomiting. Up to 70% of patients experience excessive thirst (polydipsia) and production of large volumes of dilute urine (polyuria). Polyuria is due to lithium's interference with the kidney's ability to respond to anti-diuretic hormone, which acts on the distal tubules and collecting ducts, increasing water reabsorption and concentrating the urine. Lithium blocks this action, leading to the production of large quantities of dilute urine, and triggering thirst. Tremor is seen in about 25% of patients and can be severe or inconvenient enough to require additional management, usually with a β-blocker. Weight gain is common and frequently a reason for the patient failing to comply with treatment or wishing to discontinue. The reasons for lithium-induced weight gain are not known, but it is thought that the drug interferes in some way with fundamental control mechanisms in the brain that regulate bodyweight, metabolism, or appetite. Lithium accumulates in the thyroid gland and can impair thyroid hormone synthesis and release, causing goitre and hypothyroidism.

ANTIPSYCHOTIC DRUGS

Psychotic illness is characterised by a loss of contact with reality. It features hallucinations (experiencing events that are not happening), delusions (false and abnormal beliefs), and emotional blunting and disordered thinking, and the person has no insight into their condition. Although psychotic episodes may be caused by a range of situations, e.g. alcohol withdrawal, recreational drug use (e.g. **cocaine**, **amphetamines**, **cannabis**), childbirth (post-puerperal psychosis), and some therapeutic drugs (e.g. **vigabatrin**), it may manifest itself as part of a chronic psychiatric illness, notably schizophrenia. The term 'antipsychotic agent' is generally taken to mean a drug used to treat schizophrenia.

SCHIZOPHRENIA

This is a common and serious psychiatric condition, affecting 20 million people worldwide, and is more common in men than women. It generally manifests early in life, has a strong heritable component, and increases the risk of premature death, partly because of higher suicide rates. The signs and symptoms of schizophrenia are classified into four groups: positive symptoms, negative symptoms, cognitive symptoms, and mood symptoms, shown in Box 4.2. Positive symptoms are 'add-ons' to normal behaviour, whereas negative symptoms are elements of behaviour and emotional responses that are missing or depressed compared to normal. Individuals whose schizophrenia displays predominantly positive symptoms tend to respond better to drug treatment than those whose illness features mainly negative symptoms.

Box 4.2 Clinical Features of Schizophrenia

Positive symptoms	Negative symptoms	Cognitive symptoms	Mood symptoms
Hallucinations, often auditory	Poverty of speech	Poor memory and attention span	Inappropriate mood
Delusions, often paranoid	Social withdrawal	Poor organisational and planning skills	Depression common
Thought disorder, with jumbled and incoherent thinking processes, often reflected in garbled and irrational speech	Flattened emotional range and inability to enjoy pleasurable activities or situations	Lacking in empathy and inability to 'read' other people and their social cues	Guilt
Behavioural abnormalities, sometimes stereotyped movements	Loss of interests and motivation; general apathy and inertia		Anxiety
Catatonia			

Neurophysiology of Schizophrenia

The underlying neurophysiology is not fully understood, but in schizophrenia there are abnormalities in brain structure and volume and neurotransmitter activity. The most clearly implicated neurotransmitter is dopamine, and all known antipsychotic drugs block dopamine receptors, particularly D_2 receptors, emphasising the role of dopamine in the aetiology of schizophrenia. Dopamine is released at nerve endings in four main pathways in the brain, three of which are shown in Fig. 4.19. The nigrostriatal pathway is essential to skeletal muscle control, and its degeneration is the cause of Parkinson's disease. The fourth important pathway releasing dopamine, not shown here, is the tuberoinfundibular pathway, which controls prolactin release and therefore breast growth and lactation. Release of dopamine here inhibits prolactin release (see Fig. 5.2).

The Mesocortical Pathway and D_1 Receptors

The mesocortical pathway links the ventral tegmental area in the midbrain to the cerebral cortex and is thought to be important in cognitive functions, motivation and reward, and emotional responses. Dopamine released by these nerves acts mainly through D_1 receptors in the cortex. It is thought that decreased function in this pathway is responsible for the negative and cognitive features of schizophrenia.

The Mesolimbic Pathway and D_2 Receptors

The mesolimbic pathway links the ventral tegmental area to structures of the limbic system, including the amygdala, hippocampus, and nucleus accumbens. It is strongly associated with memory formation, reward, and emotional responses, and it is believed that overactivity in this pathway is responsible for the positive symptoms in schizophrenia. Dopamine released by these nerves acts mainly through D_2 receptors.

Serotonin and Glutamate in Schizophrenia

Although abnormalities of dopamine transmission are undoubtedly involved in schizophrenia, other neurotransmitters may also play a part. It is interesting that **clozapine**, possibly the most effective antipsychotic agent, is actually

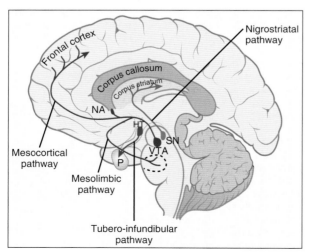

Fig 4.19 Dopamine pathways in the brain. (From Satoskar RS, Rege N, Bhandarkar SD. (2021) Pharmacology and pharmacotherapeutics, 26th ed, Fig. 5.1. New Delhi: RELX India Pvt Ltd.)

a fairly weak dopamine receptor blocker. It does, however, block a range of other receptors, including histamine receptors, α receptors, muscarinic receptors, and 5-HT receptors, although how this contributes to the clinical activity of the drug is not understood. There is also more recent evidence that activity of the excitatory transmitter glutamate is abnormal in schizophrenia, although this research is still in its early stages and has not produced any useful antipsychotic drugs.

ANTIPSYCHOTIC DRUGS

These are generally considered under two main headings: the older, typical antipsychotics, including **chlorpromazine**, **haloperidol**, and **flupentixol**, and the newer atypical antipsychotics, sometimes also called second-generation antipsychotics, including **clozapine** and **risperidone**. The distinction between the two groups is not clear-cut, but in general, typical antipsychotics are fairly selective antagonists for D_2 receptors, whereas the atypical agents have a wider spectrum of receptor-blocking activity, including at 5-HT and histamine receptors.

Actions of the Antipsychotics

Because all antipsychotic drugs block dopamine receptors, particularly D_2 receptors, they all produce adverse effects related to dopamine blockade. Most block other receptor types as well, giving several significant unwanted effects.

Extrapyramidal Adverse Effects

Antipsychotic drugs block D_2 receptors in the nigrostriatal pathway, an integral part of motor control. As a result, they cause motor disturbances including Parkinson's-like symptoms such as bradykinesia, tremor and dystonias, and tardive dyskinesias. Dystonias, sustained muscular spasms, are most likely to occur in the first weeks of starting treatment and may affect any body part: for example, there may be contraction of muscles in the neck and shoulder causing torticollis (Fig. 4.20). Severe dystonia in the head and neck area may threaten the airway. Dystonias disappear when the drug is withdrawn. Tardive dyskinesias, similar to those seen with **L-DOPA** treatment in Parkinson's disease, develop in up to 40% of patients taking antipsychotic medication and are a major reason for non-compliance with treatment. Dyskinesias generally persist after the drug is withdrawn, suggesting that the drug has induced a long-term change in dopamine signalling in the brain, perhaps by altering the population of dopamine receptors. Akathisia is also seen: this is a feeling of needing to jump out of one's skin, leading to agitation, restlessness, and an inability to sit quietly. The incidence of extrapyramidal side-effects may be less with atypical than typical agents, but studies looking at this do not agree on this point.

Endocrine Effects

The release of dopamine in the tuberoinfundibular pathway switches off prolactin secretion via D_2 receptors (see Fig. 5.2). Dopamine antagonists release the hypothalamus and the posterior pituitary from its suppression, and prolactin is secreted into the bloodstream. This can cause swelling of the breasts and lactation in both men and women.

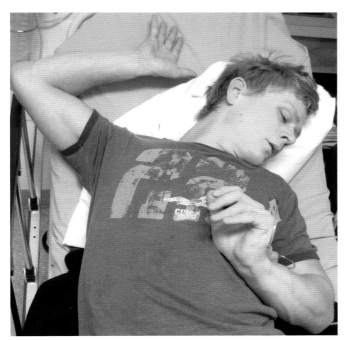

Fig 4.20 Torticollis: an example of an acute antipsychotic-induced dystonia. (From Wikipedia: James Heilman, MD)

Anti-Emetic Activity

Dopamine is a transmitter in the chemosensitive trigger zone and stimulates vomiting. Antipsychotic drugs including **metoclopramide** and **domperidone** are therefore anti-emetic (see p. 194).

Blockade of Other (Non-Dopamine) Receptors

Most antipsychotic drugs, particularly the newer atypical agents, block a range of receptors in the brain and in peripheral tissues, leading to related side-effects. H_1 receptor blockade (an antihistamine-like action) in the brain causes sedation. Many block muscarinic receptors throughout the body, giving rise to the usual range of antimuscarinic side-effects: dry mouth, constipation, blurred vision, tachycardia, and urinary retention. It is thought, however, that the antimuscarinic side-effects may help to alleviate the Parkinson's-like symptoms (for a fuller explanation, see Parkinson's disease). There may be loss of libido and other sexual dysfunction, thought to be due to blockade of a combination of dopamine, muscarinic, and α receptors, and an important reason for non-compliance.

Other Adverse Effects

Many antipsychotic drugs are cardiotoxic and increase the risk of sudden cardiac death, probably by blocking ion channels in the membranes of heart muscle cells and inducing life-threatening arrhythmias. For example, they extend the QT interval on the ECG, delaying repolarisation of the ventricular muscle. This increases the chance that abnormal ectopic foci may begin to fire, interrupting normal ventricular function and precipitating ventricular fibrillation. It is therefore important to assess cardiac risk before commencing treatment. Weight gain is a common side-effect, distressing for the patient and increasing the risk of diabetes and cardiovascular disease. Hypotension is also seen because

antipsychotics block sympathetic receptors in the peripheral nervous system.

TYPICAL (FIRST-GENERATION) ANTIPSYCHOTICS

Examples: chlorpromazine, haloperidol, flupentixol

The typical antipsychotics are highly effective in the control of the positive symptoms of schizophrenia, thought to be directly linked to their blockade of D_2 receptors in the mesolimbic pathway. However, their use is often limited by the appearance of movement disorders due to blockade of D_2 receptors in the nigrostriatal pathway.

Chlorpromazine

This was the first drug introduced to clinical medicine specifically as an antipsychotic and was in widespread use by the late 1950s. Structurally, it belongs to the same family as the **antihistamines**, and like the antihistamines it is very sedative; this led researchers to investigate the possibility of its being useful as a premedication before surgery, and from there its usefulness in psychotic disorders was quickly recognised. It is sometimes used for intractable hiccups and tics, and in nausea and vomiting in serious illness when other anti-emetics have failed.

Pharmacokinetics

Chlorpromazine is well absorbed orally and is highly plasma protein-bound. It is heavily metabolised in the liver and has a half-life of around 30 hours. It should not be taken with alcohol, and it can be an irritant in the gastrointestinal tract, so taking with food is recommended.

Haloperidol

Haloperidol is one of the most potent antipsychotic drugs and can be given orally or as a depot preparation given as a deep intramuscular injection, giving effective plasma levels over an extended period. This smooths out plasma levels and eliminates the possibility of the patient forgetting to take a dose. It is sometimes used as an anti-emetic in serious illness, and to calm and sedate in a range of conditions associated with agitated, aggressive, or hyperactive behaviour, e.g. Tourette's syndrome and acute psychotic episodes.

Flupentixol

Flupentixol is absorbed slowly and incompletely after oral administration and is often used as a depot preparation. It is highly bound to plasma proteins, and its half-life generally falls between 19 and 39 hours. It is sometimes also used in depression.

ATYPICAL (SECOND-GENERATION) ANTIPSYCHOTICS

Examples: clozapine, risperidone, aripiprazole

The atypical antipsychotics may give better results in treatment-resistant disease and in patients with a higher incidence of negative symptoms, and they tend to give fewer extrapyramidal side-effects, but there is no evidence that they are more effective overall than the typical antipsychotic drugs.

Clozapine

Clozapine and the related agent **olanzapine** bind to a wide range of receptors in the brain, and their dopamine receptor blockade is actually fairly weak, which probably accounts for their relative lack of extrapyramidal symptoms. They bind strongly to H$_1$ receptors and so are sedative, although less so than the typical antipsychotics. They also bind strongly to 5-HT receptors and muscarinic receptors. Clozapine is especially useful in patients whose psychosis has not responded to other treatments. However, it can cause dangerous intestinal obstruction, fatal agranulocytosis, and potentially fatal myocarditis.

Pharmacokinetics

Clozapine is rapidly and almost completely absorbed following oral administration and is very highly plasma protein-bound. Its average half-life is about 8 hours, and it is metabolised in the liver.

Risperidone

Risperidone is used in a range of psychotic disorders and to treat mania. It is associated with a higher incidence of extrapyramidal side-effects than clozapine, but less than the typical antipsychotic agents. It is well absorbed from an oral dose, is highly plasma protein-bound, and its half-life can range from 3 to 20 hours. It is metabolised in the liver to the active metabolite paliperidone and cleared by the kidney.

Aripiprazole

Aripiprazole is also used in bipolar disorder. It is associated with fewer side-effects than other atypical antipsychotics, possibly because it has an unusual interaction with dopamine receptors. It has partial agonist activity, so that even though it occupies the receptor and prevents dopamine from attaching, it causes a minor degree of receptor stimulation. The incidence of extrapyramidal symptoms is reduced and prolactin levels do not increase. In addition, weight gain is not usually a problem. It also has few antimuscarinic side-effects.

Pharmacokinetics

Aripiprazole is well absorbed orally, although if taken with a fatty meal, absorption is delayed. It is almost 100% plasma protein-bound and has a very long half-life of 75 hours. It is metabolised in the liver to an active product which has an even longer half-life. This extended half-life means that aripiprazole can be useful in maintenance treatment.

ANAESTHETICS

'Anaesthesia' means 'absence of sensation'. **General anaesthetics** (GAs) depress nerve function in the CNS and produce controlled unconsciousness associated with analgesia and amnesia. **Local anaesthetics (LAs)** interrupt the conduction of action potentials in peripheral sensory nerves and cause loss of sensation in the tissues served by these nerves; clinically, eliminating pain signals is the primary aim, but temperature and pressure sensation is also lost or impaired. In high enough concentrations, LAs block conduction in all electrically excitable cells, and therefore also silence motor nerves, central nerves, and muscle cells.

GENERAL ANAESTHETICS

Before the introduction of the first successful inhalational anaesthetic, **ether**, used in 1846 for a dental extraction, surgical procedures had to be fast and crude, and the unfortunate patient physically restrained. Many patients died of shock from the pain or from infection. **Alcohol** and **opioids** could be given beforehand, but doses that achieved adequate sedation were in themselves life-threatening. The horrors and dangers of pre-anaesthetic surgery were such that people tolerated intensely painful or debilitating conditions rather than present themselves for treatment. The introduction of general anaesthesia transformed surgery, giving surgeons time to perform increasingly complex and precise procedures. Early anaesthetics included ether, hazardous because of its high flammability, and **chloroform**, which was associated with a high death rate because of cardiovascular and hepatic toxicity. Both have been superseded with newer, safer agents, and both inhalational and intravenous drugs are available.

Chemically speaking, GAs are a diverse group of substances. The inert gas **xenon** and **nitrous oxide** (N$_2$O), both simple structures, induce anaesthesia. Other agents have much more complex molecular structures. However, they do have one important property in common: they are all highly lipid-soluble and on administration are rapidly and extensively taken up into tissues, including the CNS. Anaesthetic potency therefore increases with lipid solubility.

Mechanism of Action of Anaesthetic Agents

There is no single, tidy, and well-established explanation for the anaesthetic action of this structurally diverse group of drugs. It is currently thought that GAs affect ion channels at synapses, regulating the entry of ions into nerves, which in turn controls the excitability of the nerve. Several are believed to act at GABA$_A$ receptors, enhancing opening of the associated Cl$^-$ channels, allowing Cl$^-$ entry into the nerve and inhibiting it (Fig. 4.18). There is also evidence that some inhibit the action of excitatory transmitters, e.g. glutamate acting at NMDA receptors.

Drugs Used as Adjuncts in Anaesthesia

Premedication, often with a **benzodiazepine**, sedates and reduces pre-operative anxiety. GAs may have analgesic and muscle relaxant properties, in addition to their anaesthetic actions, but they are not all equally potent in each respect (Table 4.5). The use of preoperative sedatives and additional analgesics and muscle-relaxant agents supports anaesthesia and reduces the dose of anaesthetic required. For example, although GAs cause muscle relaxation, some surgical procedures, e.g. abdominal surgery, require complete paralysis of skeletal muscle not achievable at safe anaesthetic concentrations with anaesthetic alone. Neuromuscular blocking drugs, e.g. **pancuronium**, are therefore used as adjuncts. Other drugs frequently used include anti-emetics, e.g. **metoclopramide**, because many inhalational anaesthetics, as well as **opioid analgesics**, trigger nausea and vomiting by acting on the chemosensitive trigger zone in the medulla oblongata. Antimuscarinic agents, e.g. **hyoscine**, are sometimes used to dry up respiratory and salivary secretions, which can be stimulated by intubation and the irritant action of some inhalational anaesthetics, e.g. **isoflurane**, and which threaten the airway and increase the risk of aspiration.

The Stages of Anaesthesia

Depth of anaesthesia is assessed according to four named stages, I–IV (Table 4.6). The higher centres of the brain in

Table 4.5 Pharmacological Actions of Some General Anaesthetics

Drug	Analgesic	Muscle relaxant	Hangover effect	Amnesia
Desflurane	No	Potent		Potent
Etomidate	No	Weak	Some	Potent
Isoflurane	No	Potent		Potent
Ketamine	Potent	Weak	No	No
Nitrous oxide	Potent	Weak		No
Propofol	No	Weak	Some	Potent
Thiopental	No	Weak	Yes	Potent

Table 4.6 The Four Stages of Anaesthesia

Stage	Physiological events
I: Analgesia	Sedation, disorientation, confusion but not unconsciousness Analgesia
II: Excitation. Safe anaesthetic practice should minimise this stage	Airway reflexes including coughing are intact and laryngeal spasm may occur if intubation attempted Hypertension, tachycardia Disinhibition, delirium and may physically struggle or fight Vomiting, which can threaten the airway Amnesia
III: Surgical anaesthesia	There are four planes, I–IV, representing deepening anaesthesia. Loss of consciousness; loss of protective reflexes, e.g. corneal, pupillary, and laryngeal reflexes; progressive loss of muscle tone; progressive respiratory depression which becomes severe in plane IV with diaphragmatic paralysis and apnoea
IV: Medullary depression	Loss of spontaneous respiratory effort Loss of cardiovascular control: hypotension and reduced cardiac contractility Cardiorespiratory support essential to maintain life Skeletal muscle flaccidity

the cortex, limbic system, and hypothalamus are most sensitive to the inhibiting action of GAs and are suppressed first, with unconsciousness, analgesia, and amnesia. Higher anaesthetic concentrations are needed to suppress the neural circuits used to maintain involuntary activity, including withdrawal and laryngeal reflexes and autonomic nervous system function that must be inhibited for surgical-level anaesthesia. Even higher concentrations eventually suppress the basic life-support functions of cardiovascular and respiratory control and threaten life.

Progression through these stages correlates with anaesthetic concentration and is affected by other drugs given before and during anaesthesia. For example, effective analgesia during anaesthesia is important because even in an anaesthetised state, painful stimuli from the surgical procedure trigger various stress responses, including increased sympathetic activity, e.g. increased heart rate and blood pressure. This increases the risk to the patient, and although it can be suppressed by increasing the dose of the anaesthetic, this exposes the patient to the greater risks of very profound anaesthesia. Most anaesthetics have no inherent analgesic activity (Table 4.5), so administering adequate analgesia, usually with **opioids**, during surgery reduces this pain-evoked sympathetic stimulation and allows anaesthetic doses to be reduced.

Induction and Maintenance of Anaesthesia

Rapid induction of anaesthesia, i.e. getting the patient from full consciousness to surgical anaesthesia as quickly as possible, is desirable because it reduces the time spent in stage II. Inhalational anaesthetics induce anaesthesia relatively slowly because of the time needed for the drug to equilibrate between the alveoli and the bloodstream and then between the bloodstream and the CNS. A bolus dose of intravenous anaesthetic can be used for rapid induction, with anaesthesia then maintained with an inhalational agent. Total intravenous anaesthesia, in which anaesthesia is both induced and maintained using intravenous agents, can be performed in some short procedures.

INHALATIONAL ANAESTHETICS

These are low-molecular-weight gases or volatile liquids (i.e. liquids that release gas). They are inhaled into the alveoli of the lungs, from where they rapidly diffuse into the bloodstream. Because they are so lipid-soluble, they dissolve poorly in the water-based medium of the blood and are rapidly taken up into the CNS because of its rich blood supply and relatively high lipid content.

The Minimum Alveolar Concentration of an Inhaled Anaesthetic

Anaesthetic potency is measured as the minimum alveolar concentration (MAC) of the drug required to achieve anaesthesia.

KEY POINT: ANAESTHETIC POTENCY AND MINIMUM ALVEOLAR CONCENTRATION

Potent anaesthetic agents achieve anaesthesia at lower minimum alveolar concentrations, whereas less potent anaesthetics require higher alveolar concentrations to induce anaesthesia.

The MAC decreases with age and is reduced in certain situations, e.g. anaemia, hypoxia, pregnancy, and alcoholic intoxication. It is increased in chronic alcohol use and in people with (naturally) red hair.

Pharmacokinetics

Achieving MAC depends on the concentration of inhaled anaesthetic, the rate and depth of respiration, and the presence of certain pathologies, e.g. emphysema. The higher the anaesthetic concentration and the deeper and faster the respiratory effort of the patient, the faster the MAC is reached. In emphysema, total lung volume is increased, although the number of functional alveoli is reduced, so the anaesthetic concentration in functional alveoli is diluted and it takes longer to achieve MAC. With continued administration, the drug equilibrates between the alveoli, the bloodstream, and the tissues, including the CNS (Fig. 4.21A). Blood flow to an organ is an important determinant of equilibration; well-perfused tissues receive higher quantities of drug and equilibrate quickly, whereas tissues with a lower blood supply, e.g. adipose tissue, equilibrate more slowly. Termination of action (reversal) of an inhaled anaesthetic relies almost entirely on pulmonary excretion. On withdrawal of the anaesthetic, its alveolar concentration immediately falls, meaning that it is no longer in equilibrium between alveolar air and the bloodstream, and the drug transfers down its concentration gradient into the alveoli and is excreted in the breath (Fig. 4.21B). As blood levels fall, the drug transfers from tissues into the bloodstream, reducing levels in the CNS and initiating recovery. The 'hangover' effect seen with some inhalational anaesthetics is due to the accumulation of the drug in body fat stores. Because adipose tissue has a poor blood supply, anaesthetics are taken up relatively slowly despite their high fat solubility, but for the same reason, they are released slowly after reversal and can lead to drowsiness and impaired motor function for up to 24 hours. In recovery, the patient passes through the four stages of anaesthesia (Table 4.6) in reverse, including the excitation stage. An ideal inhaled anaesthetic therefore reverses very quickly, minimising time spent in this potentially dangerous period. Factors that depress respiration, e.g. **opioid** administration, slow down recovery.

Modified Ethers

Examples: desflurane, isoflurane, sevoflurane

These are simple molecules based on the chemical structure of ether. They target multiple channels and molecular sites in the CNS, inhibiting synaptic transmission and reducing nerve activity. **Sevoflurane** and **desflurane** give faster induction and recovery than **isoflurane**. They all suppress respiration by reducing the sensitivity of the respiratory centres in the brainstem to carbon dioxide, an important stimulant to the inherent rate and rhythm of breathing. They relax smooth muscle, including in blood vessel walls, causing vasodilation and hypotension. This reduces perfusion of key organs including the heart and the liver. In addition, they may directly depress myocardial contractility, worsening any hypotension. They relax the uterus, which can slow labour and increase the risk of haemorrhage, because the contracting uterus normally compresses blood vessels that are damaged as the placenta separates during the third stage of labour. They induce postoperative nausea and vomiting

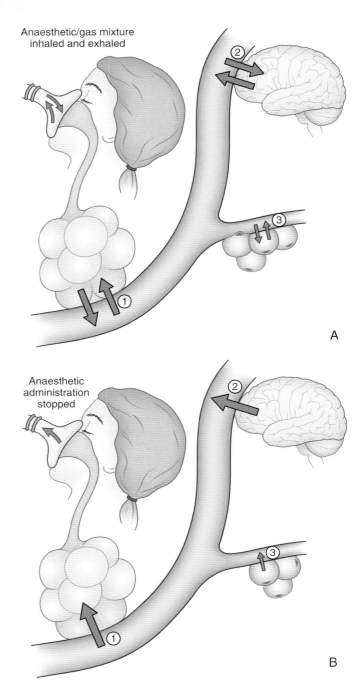

Fig 4.21 Equilibration of inhaled anaesthetic between lungs, tissues, and blood. A. Induction and maintenance. 1: The anaesthetic equilibrates between alveolar air and arterial blood. Provided the minimum alveolar concentration (MAC) has been reached, this means that blood levels are high enough to achieve anaesthesia. 2: Well-perfused tissues, e.g. the central nervous system (CNS), liver, and other organs, rapidly equilibrate. Provided arterial drug levels remain high enough, anaesthesia is induced and maintained. 3: Poorly perfused tissues, e.g. adipose tissue, also equilibrate but more slowly. B. Reversal. 1: When administration stops, alveolar anaesthetic concentration rapidly drops. The drug diffuses rapidly out of the bloodstream into the alveoli and is excreted in the breath. 2: As blood levels fall, anaesthetic diffuses rapidly down its concentration gradient from the tissues, including the CNS, into the blood. Well-perfused tissues clear the drug very quickly. 3: Anaesthetic levels fall more slowly in poorly perfused tissues, which may still contain measurable levels of anaesthetic for hours after administration has stopped.

because they stimulate the chemosensitive trigger zone of the medulla oblongata, and they may irritate the respiratory tract, causing coughing and laryngospasm. **Sevoflurane** is the least irritant in this group.

Nitrous Oxide

N_2O induces anaesthesia rapidly and is pleasant to use because it is odourless and non-irritant. Its mechanism of action has not been clearly explained, but it is known to interact with a range of neurotransmitter receptors in the brain, including inhibition of the excitatory NMDA receptor family. It also releases endogenous opioids in the brainstem, activating endogenous pain-modulating pathways in the spinal cord, and presumably contributing at least in part to its excellent analgesic activity. It is less cardiodepressant and less emetic than the modified ethers, but it does not achieve high enough alveolar concentrations to give full anaesthesia on its own. It is often used with other inhaled anaesthetics, which allows the concentration of the second agent to be reduced, and it is used as an analgesic in labour and other situations where short-term or emergency pain relief may be needed, e.g. after fracture or burns.

INTRAVENOUS ANAESTHETICS

Examples: thiopental, propofol, etomidate, ketamine

These may be used as a bolus to induce anaesthesia or by infusion to maintain anaesthesia in shorter procedures.

Pharmacokinetics

These lipid-soluble drugs enter the CNS within seconds following intravenous injection, giving fast onset of anaesthesia. If given as a single bolus, anaesthesia is short-lived, because although the drug is initially taken up into the CNS due to its rich blood supply, it then steadily distributes throughout body tissues and CNS levels quickly fall. Reversal therefore depends upon drug distribution. If the anaesthetic is infused over a period of time, it equilibrates throughout body tissues, and reversal becomes dependent upon metabolism.

Thiopental

Thiopental is a barbiturate, a class of drugs largely abandoned in clinical medicine because of dangerous side-effects. It is very lipid-soluble and gives a very fast induction, but it has significant depressant activity on cardiovascular

and respiratory function. Thiopental induces anaesthesia by enhancing GABA activity.

Propofol

Propofol potentiates the inhibitory action of GABA at $GABA_A$ receptors. It is mainly used as an induction agent and in lower doses for conscious sedation. It depresses cardiovascular and respiratory function and can cause pain on injection because it has very low solubility in water and is formulated as an oil-in-water suspension. However, it causes little nausea or vomiting, reverses rapidly with little hangover, and its amnesiac action is useful for patients undergoing short procedures with conscious sedation.

Etomidate

Etomidate potentiates the inhibitory action of GABA at $GABA_A$ receptors, but it is not chemically related either to the **benzodiazepines** or the **barbiturates**. It is very rapid acting and has a short plasma half-life of 6–10 minutes, because it is rapidly degraded by plasma and liver esterases to inactive products. It causes less cardiovascular depression than **propofol**, but it can be painful on injection and causes postoperative nausea and vomiting. It is not used for maintenance of anaesthesia because it causes adrenal suppression. Adrenal steroids, e.g. cortisol, are essential for an effective stress response, essential to supporting physiological function in illness and trauma, including surgery. Adrenal suppression therefore increases risk, especially in severely ill patients.

Ketamine

Ketamine affects the function of a range of receptors in the brain, including blockade of excitatory NMDA receptors. Its analgesic properties are probably due to activation of internal opioid pain modulation mechanisms. It gives slow induction and slow recovery, and causes hangover effects and postoperative nausea and vomiting. It induces a state called 'dissociative anaesthesia', in which the patient appears awake, with eye opening, good muscle tone, and preserved laryngeal reflexes, but with excellent analgesia. It stimulates the sympathetic nervous system, supporting cardiovascular and respiratory function, and has a significant psychotropic effect—people report hallucinations, vivid dreams, and detachment from reality.

Focus on: Local Anaesthetics

Examples: cocaine, lidocaine, tetracaine, benzocaine, bupivacaine

LAs are used to deaden sensation in a well-defined body part. The original LA, **cocaine**, is found in the leaves of the coca bush, whose natural habitat is the tropical areas of South America, particularly the Peruvian Andes. The psychostimulant properties of the plant were well known to the local people, who had chewed the leaves as part of their religious, medicinal, and social practices for thousands of years prior to the arrival of European explorers in the 16th century. The numbing of the mouth, tongue, and throat that accompanied chewing was a

well-recognised consequence of the habit. Because the leaves did not travel well, it was some time before coca extracts became common outside its native lands, but by the 19th century, cocaine was used in a range of products, including wines, tablets, medicinal formulations, and Coca-Cola, which were in widespread use and available for general sale. In the early 20th century, legislation and restrictions were introduced in the sale and use of cocaine (it was removed from Coca-Cola in 1904, although the company fought a successful battle to retain the name and a cocaine-free extract of the coca leaf is still used in the recipe). Although cocaine is still used as a local anaesthetic in some specialities, e.g. ophthalmic surgery, its use is restricted due to its psychotropic, addictive,

Continued

and cardiotoxic properties. Newer agents, e.g. **lidocaine** and **benzocaine**, are amides, structurally different from cocaine, and other than their local anaesthetic action, behave differently from cocaine.

Mechanism of Action

LAs block Na^+ channels in the membranes of excitable tissues, mainly muscle and nerve (Fig. 4.22). LA molecules are generally weak bases and diffuse through nerve cell membranes into the neurone in an uncharged form, from where they enter Na^+ channels and block them. This prevents the nerve from conducting action potentials (Fig. 4.23). If the Na^+ channel is in its closed state, as in a resting nerve, the LA cannot enter.

Factors Affecting Local Anaesthetic Efficacy

The effectiveness of LAs is changed in the following situations:

Blood Flow

LA action is terminated when the drug distributes away from the site, and the primary route for this is via the bloodstream. The drug is therefore lost faster from well-perfused tissues. In addition, most LAs cause vasodilation because they block Na^+ channels in vascular smooth muscle, relaxing it. Vasodilation increases blood flow and accelerates drug loss from the site of administration. To counteract this, a vasoconstrictor, usually **adrenaline**, is combined with the anaesthetic. Care must be taken, however, to avoid ischaemia, and it should not be used in areas with a restricted blood supply, e.g. the fingers. Additionally, great care must be taken not to deliver the combination into a blood vessel because of adrenaline's cardiovascular actions.

Inflamed or Infected Tissues

The pH of injured or infected tissues falls, i.e. becomes acidic, because microbial and tissue metabolic products are generally acidic. In addition, blood flow through these tissues is usually reduced, and these waste products are not washed away. This affects the ability of LA molecules to cross the nerve cell membrane. Because LA molecules are weak bases, they attract and attach excess hydrogen ions in the acidic medium of infected or inflamed tissues. This positive charge impedes the ability of the molecules to diffuse into the nerve, and since they can only block Na^+ channels from the nerve interior, their anaesthetic activity is lost. This presents a practical problem when trying to achieve anaesthesia in, for example, dental surgery, where there may be infection or inflammation present.

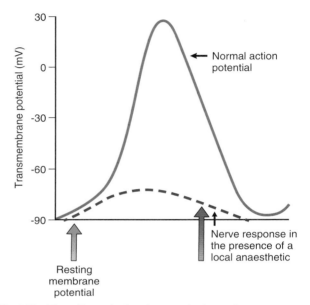

Fig 4.23 The effect of a local anaesthetic on the nerve membrane potential. By blocking sodium channels, the threshold potential is not reached and the action potential is prevented. (Modified from Stoelting RK and Miller RD (1994) Basics of anesthesia, 3rd ed. New York: Churchill Livingstone.)

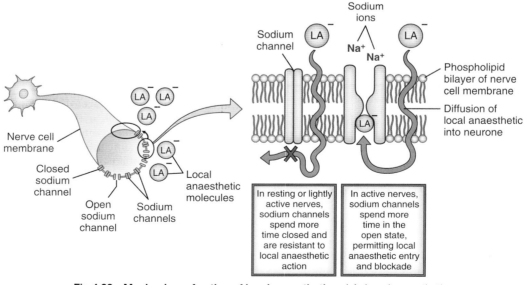

Fig 4.22   Mechanism of action of local anaesthetics. LA, Local anaesthetic.

It may be necessary to pre-treat with antibiotics before surgical intervention can be attempted under LA.

Neuronal Factors

Small-diameter neurones are more susceptible to LA action than larger ones. This is fortunate, because pain neurones are small-diameter free nerve endings, whereas other sensory and motor nerves are larger and require higher drug concentrations before their conductance is impaired. Additionally, a myelin sheath presents an extra barrier to LA penetration, so that non-myelinated nerves are more susceptible than myelinated ones. This too is clinically advantageous, because sensory pain fibres are non-myelinated. In addition, the duration of the action potential affects tissue susceptibility. Pain neurones and cardiac muscle cells both have longer than average action potentials, meaning their Na^+ channels stay open for longer. This is beneficial when abolishing pain signals and explains why LAs can significantly depress heart function if they achieve high enough levels in the bloodstream. Sensory modalities are lost in a predictable order as LA concentration rises, reflecting the sensitivity of sensory and motor nerves to LA: pain sensation is lost first, followed by temperature, then touch, then deep pressure, and finally motor function.

Use-dependence

Neurones with high rates of firing, e.g. pain fibres, are highly susceptible to LA action because their Na^+ channels spend more time in the open state. This is clearly clinically useful. High rates of firing are also characteristic of other electrically active tissues, including ectopic foci in the heart. This is the reason why LAs, e.g. **lidocaine**, are used to treat some arrhythmias.

Pharmacodynamics

LAs are lipid-soluble, allowing them to diffuse across nerve cell membranes, and the more lipid-soluble they are, the more potent they are. The degree to which they bind to tissue proteins determines their duration of action; strong protein binding helps the drug to be retained at its site of administration and prolongs its action. **Cocaine** and **tetracaine** have a very short plasma half-life (less than 3 minutes), because they are metabolised by plasma enzymes, but the amides, e.g. **lidocaine** and **benzocaine,** are metabolised in the liver and have plasma half-lives ranging from 1 to 3 hours. The key properties of some important LAs are given in Table 4.7.

Side-Effects

There may be a localised allergic reaction, but the most dangerous side-effects of LAs occur when they escape into the circulation in high enough concentrations to inhibit excitable tissues elsewhere. They reduce myocardial contractility and can interfere with the heart's internal pacemaker activity and impulse conduction. This cardiodepressant activity along with their hypotensive action can lead to cardiovascular collapse and death. **Cocaine** is an exception to the general pattern of hypotension and cardiac depression because it causes vasoconstriction, stimulates the heart, and increases blood pressure. Local anaesthetic toxicity in the CNS shows a biphasic pattern, with initial excitation followed by depression. Excitation might seem counterintuitive, since these drugs inhibit neural function, but it occurs because the first nerves to be blocked are inhibitory neurones that suppress excitatory pathways. With their inhibitory neurones silenced by the anaesthetic, overactivity of these excitatory pathways leads to a spectrum of effects ranging from mild excitement to convulsions. With increasing doses, a generalised depression of CNS function follows, including shutting down of basic life-support mechanisms in the cardiovascular and respiratory centres in the brainstem, coma, and death.

Table 4.7   Key Properties of Some Important Local Anaesthetics

Drug	Onset of action	Duration of action	Protein binding
Lidocaine	Fast	Medium (0.5–1.5 h)	65%
Prilocaine	Medium	Medium (0.5–1.5 h)	55%
Bupivacaine	Slow	Long (2–4 h)	60%–80%
Tetracaine	Very slow	Long (2–4 h)	80%

ANTICONVULSANTS

A seizure is caused by a sudden and uncontrolled episode of electrical disturbance in the brain, originating in a group of hyperexcitable neurones called the epileptogenic focus. Epilepsy, sometimes called seizure disorder, is a chronic condition characterised by recurrent, unprovoked seizures, but not all seizures are associated with epilepsy. The aim of anticonvulsant therapy is, whenever possible, to prevent seizures from occurring, or at least to reduce their frequency and severity as much as possible.

CAUSES OF SEIZURES

A wide range of diseases and disorders, not necessarily neuropathological in origin, can trigger seizures. The most common cause of seizures is epilepsy, but one-off seizures may be caused by infection, hyponatraemia (e.g. in poorly monitored diuretic therapy), high fever (especially in young children), hypoglycaemia, recreational drug use (e.g. **cocaine**), or during **alcohol** withdrawal. Traditionally, epilepsy has been considered to be caused by an imbalance between excitatory and inhibitory nerve activity, permitting episodic dominance of excitatory neurotransmission.

A range of brain abnormalities have been associated with epilepsy, including neurodegeneration, inflammation, and structural and functional changes in excitatory and inhibitory neurotransmitters and their receptors and associated ion channels. Epilepsy can be caused by congenital brain malformations, cerebral hypoxia, scarring following brain injury, a tumour, haemorrhage, or stroke. In other people, epilepsy can arise with no obvious underlying cause. Some forms of epilepsy have a strong hereditable component, and there is an increasing list of 'epilepsy genes', an important area of research in the aetiology of epilepsy.

TYPES OF SEIZURE

Seizures are classified according to the location of the epileptogenic focus in the brain, their duration, and the characteristic features of the event, which is determined by which part(s) of the brain are affected. For example, if the abnormal neuronal discharge occurs in the motor cortex, the seizure will involve involuntary activity in skeletal muscle.

Focal Seizures

If the abnormal electrical discharge remains localised within one cerebral hemisphere, it causes a focal seizure. The patient may remain aware throughout the seizure and have full memory afterwards (focal aware seizure) or may lose awareness with limited recall (focal impaired awareness seizure). There may be a range of involuntary activities called automatisms, including hand rubbing and lip smacking. Drugs with a range of modes of action, including Na$^+$-channel blockers, e.g. **carbamazepine** and **phenytoin**, drugs that increase the activity of GABA, e.g. the **benzodiazepines** and **vigabatrin**, and drugs that reduce the activity of glutamate, e.g. **lamotrigine**, are effective in treating focal seizures.

Generalised Seizures

In generalised seizures, the abnormal electrical activity occurs in both cerebral hemispheres, and may either evolve from a focal seizure or begin as a generalised seizure. Consciousness is almost always lost. Two important forms of seizure in this category are tonic-clonic convulsions and absence seizures.

Tonic-Clonic Seizures

In tonic-clonic seizures (formerly called grand mal), there is an initial sudden and widespread stiffening of skeletal muscle, causing respiratory arrest and often incontinence. This is followed by the clonic phase, in which skeletal muscles alternately contract and relax, causing violent jerking of the limbs. Afterwards, the patient is generally sleepy, confused, irritable, and disoriented. Drugs that block Na$^+$ channels in nerve axons, e.g. **phenytoin**, or that increase the levels of GABA, e.g. **vigabatrin**, are effective in controlling tonic-clonic seizures.

Absence Seizures

In absence seizures, (previously called petit mal epilepsy) which are usually seen in children, there are few motor symptoms. The child abruptly stops whatever they were doing, including talking, and appears to be daydreaming, with no awareness of their surroundings. Return of full awareness is also abrupt, and the child is not aware that the seizure has occurred. The aetiology of absence seizures is not understood, but they seem to be associated with a particular pattern of electrical discharge in a neuronal circuit between the thalamus and the cortex. Abnormalities in Ca^{2+} channels and in GABA activity have both been demonstrated in this circuit, reflected in the agents used to treat absence seizures. The most effective drugs include **sodium valproate** and **ethosuximide**, which block the abnormal Ca^{2+} channels. Agents that increase GABA activity, e.g. **vigabatrin**, can make absence seizures worse, as can Na$^+$-channel blockers such as **phenytoin**.

Status Epilepticus

This is either a single extended seizure or a continuous series of seizures with no recovery between them persisting for over half an hour. It carries a mortality of up to 15%, and there is high risk of permanent hypoxic brain damage following recovery. If the seizure involves convulsions, skeletal muscle damage (rhabdomyolysis) can release significant quantities of myoglobin into the bloodstream, which may cause acute kidney injury. Benzodiazepines e.g. **diazepam** and **midazolam**, intravenous anticonvulsants, e.g. **phenytoin,** and general anaesthetics, e.g. **propofol** or **thiopental,** are used to terminate status epilepticus.

PHARMACOLOGICAL MANAGEMENT OF SEIZURES

For most people with epilepsy, drug treatment can either completely prevent or at least control their seizures, but anticonvulsant agents are often themselves quite toxic with multiple interactions. They are a disparate group of drugs, associated with a range of mechanisms of action, and are used to reduce or eliminate the abnormal neuronal discharge causing the seizure rather than addressing any underlying pathology that may be causing it.

It is important to realise that there is not one single electrical abnormality underpinning all types of epilepsy. Neuronal function in the brain is controlled by a range of ionic gradients and ion movements controlled by specific ion channels. The role of Na$^+$ and K$^+$ in action potential conduction is a fundamental neurophysiological mechanism and is described above, but the movement of other ions, including Ca^{2+} and Cl$^-$, also generate localised currents essential to the electrical circuitry of the brain. In addition, fine control of neuronal function involves both excitatory (e.g. glutamate) and inhibitory (e.g. GABA) neurotransmitters. An understanding of any molecular abnormality and the role of relevant neurotransmitters in an epileptic condition is therefore essential in choosing the best drug to manage it, especially as in some cases an inappropriate drug choice can actually worsen the disorder.

The first documented use of a drug to control convulsions dates from 1857, when Locock began treating epileptic patients with **potassium bromide**. This remained the mainstay until 1912 when the barbiturate **phenobarbital** was introduced, followed by **phenytoin** in 1938. Since then, the range of drugs available has expanded considerably, advanced by huge improvements in the understanding of the neurochemistry underlying seizure pathophysiology, which has allowed for rational drug design and much improved tailoring of treatment for individual patients. In particular, the introduction of newer drugs such as **sodium valproate** and **carbamazepine** in the 1970s increased the proportion of patients who could be successfully treated with a single anticonvulsant (monotherapy).

Monotherapy is preferred whenever possible over treatment with two or more drugs, which increases the incidence and severity of side-effects and introduces the possibility of drug interactions. Many anticonvulsants are strongly associated with fetal abnormalities, and the management of epilepsy in pregnancy needs specialist care.

Many anticonvulsant drugs affect multiple sites in the brain and probably work through more than one mechanism of action. They are described here under the heading thought to represent their main therapeutic activity, and some key drugs and their targets are illustrated in Fig. 4.24.

ANTICONVULSANTS THAT BLOCK SODIUM CHANNELS

Conduction of action potentials along nerve axons depends upon the opening of Na^+ channels in the neuronal membrane, allowing Na^+ to flood into the nerve. Blockade of these Na^+ channels therefore reduces their capacity to conduct electrical signals and reduces their excitability. The hyperexcitable nerves of an epileptogenic focus are more susceptible to the inhibitory action of these drugs because their Na^+ channels spend more time in the open state. Good seizure control with these drugs therefore depends upon getting the dose just right: high enough to selectively inhibit the hyperactive epileptogenic nerves but not so high that normally functioning neurones are depressed.

Phenytoin

Phenytoin is used in all types of epilepsy except absence seizures.

Pharmacokinetics

Phenytoin is completely absorbed after oral dosing, and is 90% bound to plasma proteins, giving a substantial reservoir of drug in the bloodstream. Its metabolism is complex because it induces a range of liver enzymes, including those that catalyse its own breakdown. This means that in the initial stages of treatment, phenytoin has a long half-life (36 hours) which falls to 12–18 hours with continued use. It increases the breakdown of a range of other drugs, including **anticoagulants**, an important cause of interactions.

Phenytoin's metabolism is not straightforward. As plasma levels rise, its metabolism shifts from linear to saturation kinetics (p. 19 and Fig. 2.21). Fig. 2.21 shows plasma levels in three individuals receiving phenytoin treatment. For all individuals, the transition between linear kinetics and saturation kinetics, i.e. the point at which the metabolising enzymes are working at full capacity and any additional drug simply accumulates in the bloodstream, is seen at subtherapeutic levels. In addition, this figure demonstrates the significant variability between individuals in the ability to metabolise phenytoin, an additional complicating factor in safe management of phenytoin treatment. The daily dose of phenytoin required to achieve mid-therapeutic levels for the patient whose plasma levels are represented by the red curve is three times lower than the patient results shown by the green curve. It also reinforces the point that even small changes in daily dose can have significant effects on plasma levels, which would impact on seizure control and the likelihood of side-effects. Therapeutic drug monitoring is important to ensure that plasma levels remain in the therapeutic range, especially when adjusting drug dose or introducing other drugs.

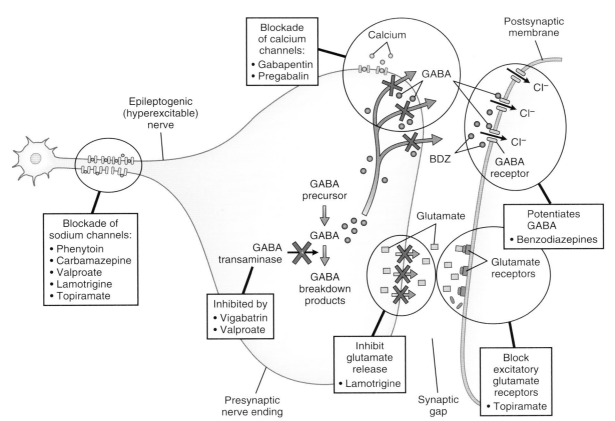

Fig 4.24 **Summary of the mechanism of action of some important anticonvulsant drugs.** BDZ, Benzodiazepine; GABA, gamma-aminobutyric acid.

Adverse Effects

Phenytoin has a narrow therapeutic index, and a range of dose-dependent adverse effects caused by its interference with CNS function appear at the upper end of its therapeutic dose range. Ataxia, tremor, and vertigo are common, and in higher doses the drug is sedative and causes confusion and reduced intellectual function. Allergy occurs in a small number of patients and may manifest as a mild skin rash or can involve life-threatening desquamation reactions, including Stevens–Johnson syndrome (Fig. 3.13). Phenytoin stimulates connective tissue growth, particularly affecting the gums, and causes acne and hirsutism, probably through a stimulation of testosterone release. It increases the risk of fetal and facial and digital malformations when used in pregnancy. It can also cause blood disorders because it interferes with the metabolism of folic acid, an essential factor in blood cell synthesis.

Carbamazepine

Carbamazepine is used in most types of epilepsy except absence seizures. It is also sometimes used in neuropathic pain, e.g. trigeminal neuralgia and diabetic neuropathy, because it silences the pain signals generated by abnormal or injured neurones and can also be effective in bipolar disorder.

Pharmacokinetics

Carbamazepine is well absorbed when given orally and is up to 80% plasma protein-bound. Like phenytoin, carbamazepine induces liver metabolic enzymes, including its own. Its half-life in the initial stages of treatment is about 36 hours, but with continued administration and autoinduction of metabolism, this falls to 12–17 hours. It induces the metabolism of other drugs, notably **oestrogens** in contraceptive preparations, leading to rapid clearance of oestrogen and possible contraception failure. Carbamazepine metabolites are inactive and are mainly excreted in the urine.

Adverse Effects

Carbamazepine causes a range of dose-dependent neurological side-effects related to its depressant activity on the CNS; they include ataxia, headache, and drowsiness. There may be hypersensitivity reactions, mainly skin rashes, but occasionally severe allergy is seen, including Stevens–Johnson syndrome (Fig. 3.13). It can cause water retention and oedema because it antagonises the effects of antidiuretic hormone, and the increased fluid load dilutes blood Na^+ levels and causes hyponatremia.

ANTICONVULSANTS THAT ENHANCE GAMMA-AMINOBUTYRIC ACID

As discussed above, GABA is a key inhibitory neurotransmitter widespread in the brain. It is thought that deficiency in GABA function is a factor in the pathophysiology of some epilepsies, and enhancing its levels or activity has been an important focus in the development of anticonvulsant agents.

Benzodiazepines

All BDZs have anticonvulsant activity, but because they are sedative and induce dependence and tolerance, their usefulness in long-term therapy is limited. The main agents used in maintenance treatment are **clobazam** and **clonazepam**. However, BDZs are the drugs of choice in controlling status epilepticus and are given rectally or intravenously. **Diazepam**, **lorazepam**, and **midazolam** are the main agents used. The pharmacology of the BDZs is described above.

Vigabatrin

Vigabatrin irreversibly blocks GABA transaminase, the enzyme that destroys GABA. Reducing its enzymatic destruction elevates GABA levels in the brain and enhances its inhibitory action. It is an example of rational drug design, having been formulated specifically to act against this specific enzyme. It is a second-line agent used in combination with other anticonvulsants to improve control when the primary agent is not fully effective. Vigabatrin is highly effective in some forms of childhood epilepsy and in most adult epilepsies, but its use is restricted because it causes permanent peripheral vision loss in up to 40% of patients.

Pharmacokinetics

Vigabatrin is well absorbed from an oral dose, does not bind significantly to plasma proteins, and is not metabolised. Its plasma half-life is about 10 hours, but because it irreversibly deactivates GABA transaminase, its duration of action depends on how quickly the brain synthesises new enzyme rather than how long the drug persists there. This also means that plasma levels of the drug do not correlate with its therapeutic activity and measuring them is not useful.

Adverse Effects

The most significant side-effect of vigabatrin is permanent impairment of peripheral vision because the drug damages retinal neurones and causes them to atrophy. The risk is greater in males than females and increases with the duration of treatment, but it has been reported after only 4 weeks of using the drug. It is common, with up to 40% of patients developing constriction of their visual field. Although central vision is unaffected, restricted peripheral vision can have a range of negative effects, including reducing one's ability to play sports requiring awareness of players or a ball approaching from the side, or limiting a driver's ability to see pedestrians stepping onto the road (Fig. 4.25). Regular vision tests are therefore essential for patients taking this drug, especially in children who are likely to be unaware of their gradual vision loss. A wide range of other side-effects, including dizziness, drowsiness, memory loss, and paraesthesias, have also been reported.

Tiagabine

Tiagabine is a GABA analogue: that is, its chemical structure is very similar to GABA, and once it enters the brain, it competes with GABA for the GABA transporter that removes GABA from the synapse. This preserves GABA levels in the synapse and prolongs its inhibitory activity. It is used in conjunction with other anti-epileptic drugs to improve seizure control when a single drug is not effective enough on its own.

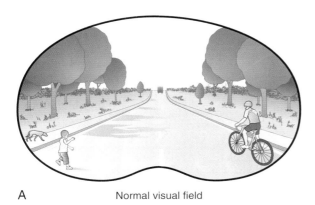

A   Normal visual field

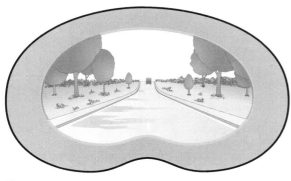

B   Vigabatrin reduces peripheral vision

Fig 4.25   Reduction of peripheral visual fields by vigabatrin. A. Normal field of view. B. Vigabatrin treatment reduces peripheral vision.

ANTICONVULSANTS THAT BLOCK CALCIUM CHANNELS

Ca^{2+} movement through Ca^{2+} channels in nerve cell membranes generates local electrical currents that regulate and modify a range of nerve functions in the brain. For example, Ca^{2+} entry into nerve endings is essential for neurotransmitter release. Another example of Ca^{2+} function is in certain circuits between the thalamus and cortex, important in the maintenance of arousal, and which is dysfunctional in absence seizures.

Gabapentin and Pregabalin

Gabapentin is so-called because it was originally designed in 1975 as a GABA analogue, but its anti-epileptic activity, and that of the similar drug pregabalin, is thought to be mainly through blocking Ca^{2+} channels and inhibiting the release of excitatory neurotransmitters like glutamate. Pregabalin is better absorbed after oral dosing than gabapentin. Both drugs are excreted largely unchanged by the kidney, so it is important to be aware of any renal impairment. With normal renal function, their half-lives are 5–7 hours, but these are significantly extended if renal function is poor. Both are also used in neuropathic pain. Adverse effects are generally less severe than those of the older anticonvulsants: they include arthralgia, malaise, and tremor.

Ethosuximide

This anticonvulsant is used mainly in absence seizures in children (see above). It is well absorbed when taken orally and has a half-life of around 60 hours in adults, although this is shorter in children (30 hours) because of increased hepatic metabolism.

Sodium Valproate

This drug was discovered by accident in a series of experiments in 1962, during which valproic acid was used to dissolve several experimental compounds undergoing a range of pre-clinical tests, including seizure tests. As part of the standard experimental design, valproic acid was used alone as a control and its anticonvulsant effect was immediately obvious. It is now one of the most prescribed anticonvulsants worldwide, used in most types of epilepsy including absence seizures. It is included here with drugs that block Ca^{2+} channels in the brain, but this is thought to be only one of its mechanisms of action. It also blocks Na^+ channels in axon membranes, and it inhibits GABA transaminase, the enzyme that degrades GABA, so it is likely that both action potential inhibition and increasing GABA levels in central synapses contribute to its anticonvulsant action. It may also increase GABA synthesis, and it suppresses the action of pro-epileptic genes. Its full spectrum of action is clearly wide and not yet fully understood. It is also used in bipolar disease and to prevent migraine.

Pharmacokinetics

Valproate is well absorbed after oral administration, has a plasma half-life of about 15 hours, and is metabolised in the liver.

Adverse Effects

Valproate is strongly teratogenic, causing spina bifida and other neural tube defects, and it should not be used in sexually active women without effective contraception. It may also cause potentially fatal hepatitis, but fortunately this is rare. It is a potent enzyme inhibitor, reducing the metabolism and increasing the plasma levels of a range of other drugs, including other anticonvulsants: this is an important cause of valproate-mediated drug interactions. It has a range of other adverse effects, including hair loss (not permanent, and the regrowth may be curly), confusion, memory loss, and tremor.

ANTICONVULSANTS THAT REDUCE GLUTAMATE ACTIVITY

As discussed above, glutamate is a key excitatory transmitter widespread in the brain. Drugs that reduce glutamate levels and activity have effective anticonvulsant activity.

Lamotrigine

Lamotrigine blocks glutamate release from excitatory neurones, which reduces the levels of glutamate in the synapse and reduces excitatory transmission. Lamotrigine also has appreciable Na^+-channel blockade activity. It is used in many types of seizure disorders either as monotherapy or in combination with other anticonvulsants and in maintaining mood stability in bipolar disorder.

Pharmacokinetics

Lamotrigine is well absorbed after an oral dose, and its bioavailability is almost 100% because there is almost no first-pass metabolism. It is metabolised in the liver and mainly excreted in the urine. Its half-life is long and variable between individuals, ranging from 22 to 37 hours. It is often used with **valproate**, a potent enzyme inhibitor, in which case its half-life can increase to 60 hours.

Adverse Effects

Lamotrigine can cause headache, drowsiness, nausea and vomiting, and tremor, among others. It is sometimes associated with serious skin conditions, including Stevens–Johnson syndrome (Fig. 3.13).

Topiramate

Topiramate was discovered by accident by researchers looking for antidiabetic agents. It blocks glutamate receptors on the post-synaptic membrane. This reduces the excitability of the nerve by inhibiting its ability to respond to this excitatory neurotransmitter. This drug also blocks Na^+ channels and probably Ca^{2+} channels, so its mechanism of action in seizure control is probably complex. It is also used in migraine.

Pharmacokinetics

Topiramate is well absorbed orally and is not strongly bound to plasma proteins. Up to 70% is excreted unchanged by the kidney, so care must be taken in people with any degree of renal impairment. Its half-life is usually within 19–23 hours.

Adverse Effects

This drug can cause hair loss, confusion, gastrointestinal upset, nausea, and tremor. It is strongly associated with congenital malformations, especially cleft palate.

REFERENCES

Atkin, T., Comai, S., Gobbi, G., 2018. Drugs for insomnia beyond benzodiazepines: pharmacology, clinical applications and discovery. Pharmacol. Rev 70 (2), 197–245.

Becker, D.E., Reed, K.L., 2006. Essentials of local anaesthetic pharmacology. Anesth. Prog 53 (3), 98–109.

Cipriani, A., Furukawa, T.A., Salanti, G., et al., 2018. Comparative efficacy and acceptability of 21 antidepressant drugs for the acute treatment of adults with major depressive disorder: a systematic review and network meta-analysis. Lancet 391 (10128), 1357–1366.

Egan, T.D., 2019. Are opioids indispensable for general anaesthesia? Br. J. Anaesth 122 (6), e127–e135.

GBD 2017 Disease and Injury Incidence and Prevalence Collaborators, 2018. Global, regional and national incidence, prevalence and years lived with disability for 354 diseases and injuries for 195 countries and territories, 1990-2017: a systematic analysis for the Global Burden of Disease study 2017. Lancet 392 (10159), 1789–1858.

Gitlin, M., 2016. Lithium side-effects and toxicity: prevalence and management strategies. Int. J. Bipolar. Disord 4, 27.

Guardiola-Lemaitre, B., De Bodinat, C., Delagrange, P., Millan, M.J., Munoz, C., Mocaër, E., 2014. Agomelatine: mechanism of action and pharmacological profile in relation to antidepressant properties. Br. J. Pharmacol 171 (15), 3604–3619.

Guzman, F., 2019. The four dopamine pathways relevant to antipsychotics pharmacology. Available at: https://psychopharmacologyinstitute.com/publication/the-four-dopamine-pathways-relevant-to-antipsychotics-pharmacology-2096.

Jesulola, E., Micalos, P., Baguley, I.J., 2018. Understanding the pathophysiology of depression: from monoamines to the neurogenesis model-are we there yet? Behav. Brain Res 341, 79–90.

Scammell, T.E., Jackson, A.C., Franks, N.P., Wisden, W., Dauvilliers, Y., 2019. Histamine: neural circuits and new medications. Sleep 42 (1), 1–8.

Wick, J.Y., 2013. The history of benzodiazepines. Consult. Pharm 28 (9), 538–548.

Wilson, T.K., Tripp, J., 2020. Buspirone. In: StatPearls [Internet]. StatPearls Publishing, Treasure Island (FL). Available from: https://www.ncbi.nlm.nih.gov/books/NBK531477/.

Drugs and Endocrine Function

5

INTRODUCTION

The endocrine system comprises a collection of glands and tissues dispersed around the body and the hormones they produce and release. Many hormones are released into local blood vessels and are carried to distant target tissues in the bloodstream. This is called endocrine control. Other hormones act locally, in the tissues close to their site of release, and regulate the activity and behaviour of cells in their immediate environment. This is called paracrine control. Paracrine substances are referred to as mediators and regulate local responses such as inflammation. They include growth factors; inflammatory mediators including **prostaglandins**, **histamine**, and bradykinin; and cytokines, a broad group of small peptides involved in inflammation, immunity, and the production of blood cells. Mediators are increasingly important as drug targets in

the treatment of inflammatory, malignant, and immune disease and will be discussed, as appropriate, in other chapters.

KEY POINT: ENDOCRINE VS. NERVOUS CONTROL

In conjunction with the nervous system, endocrine regulation provides the internal communication system essential for integrated control of body function. Hormonal control is generally of slow onset and is sustained over extended periods of time, whereas nervous control can be adjusted within fractions of a second and provides moment-to-moment regulation. The endocrine system therefore is the main regulator of continuous, ongoing physiological processes like growth and reproduction, and the nervous system is the primary controller of factors that require finely controlled and rapid adjustments, such as cardiovascular control.

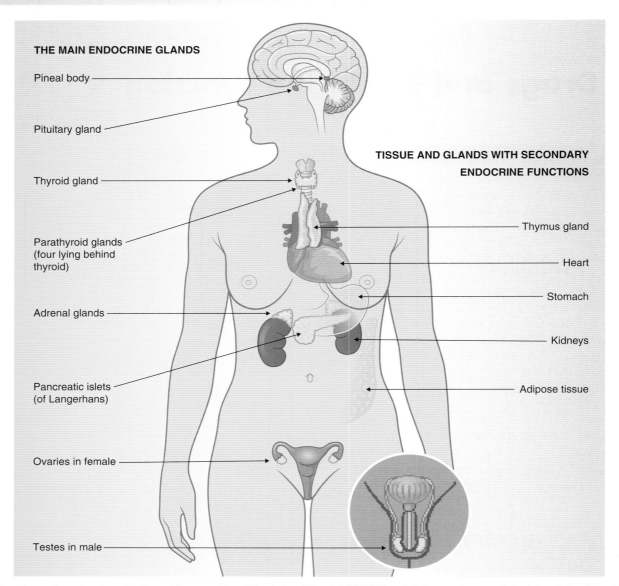

THE MAIN ENDOCRINE GLANDS

Pineal body

Pituitary gland

Thyroid gland

Parathyroid glands
(four lying behind
thyroid)

Adrenal glands

Pancreatic islets
(of Langerhans)

Ovaries in female

Testes in male

TISSUE AND GLANDS WITH SECONDARY
ENDOCRINE FUNCTIONS

Thymus gland

Heart

Stomach

Kidneys

Adipose tissue

Fig. 5.1   The main endocrine glands and tissues. (From Waugh A and Grant A (2020) Ross & Wilson anatomy and physiology in health and illness, 14th ed, Fig 9.1. Oxford: Elsevier.)

The main endocrine glands and tissues are shown in Fig. 5.1. Endocrine disorders usually involve under- or over-secretion of hormones; thus, pharmacological management generally involves hormone replacement or the use of hormone antagonists or drugs that suppress hormone synthesis or release.

HORMONE LEVELS AND NEGATIVE FEEDBACK

Hormone levels in the blood are usually kept within a preset normal range, and secretion of the hormone is constantly adjusted, upwards or downwards, to maintain this. Some endocrine glands autonomously control the level of their own hormone product: for example, the pancreas, which produces insulin, constantly measures blood glucose levels and regulates insulin secretion into the bloodstream accordingly. When blood glucose levels rise, the pancreas increases insulin release, and when blood glucose levels fall, it reduces it. This is an example of direct negative feedback control. Indirect negative feedback, in which hormone secretion by one gland is controlled by another gland, is a feature of the hypothalamic–pituitary axis, described below.

THE HYPOTHALAMIC–PITUITARY AXIS

Certain key endocrine glands, including the thyroid and adrenal glands and the gonads, are regulated by the hypothalamus and the pituitary gland: this control mechanism is called the hypothalamic–pituitary axis. The hypothalamus has multiple roles in the control of autonomic and endocrine function, one of which is control of hormone release by the pituitary gland. In this respect, it functions as an endocrine gland, releasing a range of hormones that govern hormone release by the pituitary. The pituitary gland is directly linked to the hypothalamus via a stalk of tissue called the infundibulum, and has two lobes, the anterior and the posterior. The hypothalamus communicates with the anterior pituitary via a network of blood capillaries and with the posterior pituitary via a tract of nerves that originate in the hypothalamus and terminate in the gland below.

Hypothalamus–Anterior Pituitary Communication

Glandular cells in the hypothalamus secrete a number of hormones into the capillary network linking it to the

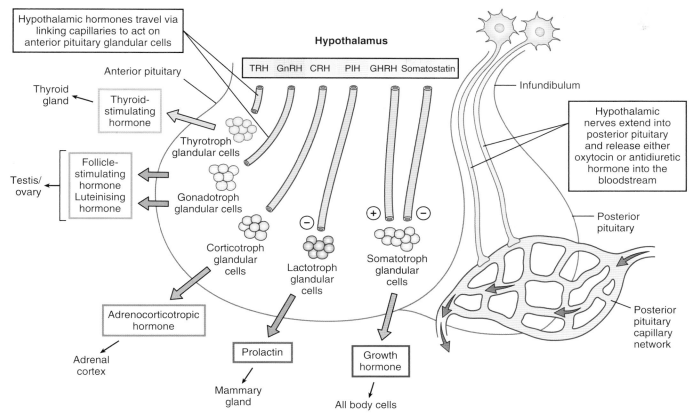

Fig. 5.2   The hormones of the hypothalamic–pituitary axis. CRH, Corticotropin-releasing hormone; GHRH, growth hormone-releasing hormone; GnRH, gonadotropin-releasing hormone; PIH, prolactin inhibitory factor (dopamine); TRH, thyrotropin-releasing hormone.

anterior pituitary. Each hypothalamic hormone acts on specific glandular cells in the anterior pituitary. Hypothalamic hormones are mainly stimulatory, i.e. trigger release of a pituitary hormone, but some are inhibitory and suppress pituitary secretion. The hypothalamic hormones and the pituitary hormones they control are shown in Fig. 5.2.

- Thyrotropin-releasing hormone (TRH) from the hypothalamus stimulates thyrotroph glandular cells in the anterior pituitary to release thyroid-stimulating hormone (TSH), which in turn stimulates the thyroid gland to release thyroxine.
- Gonadotropin-releasing hormone (GnRH) from the hypothalamus stimulates gonadotroph glandular cells in the pituitary to release follicle-stimulating hormone (FSH) and luteinising hormone (LH). These hormones act on the gonads (the male testis and the female ovary) to regulate the release of sex hormones, mainly oestrogen, progesterone, and testosterone.
- Corticotropin-releasing hormone (CRH) from the hypothalamus stimulates pituitary corticotroph glandular cells to release adrenocorticotropic hormone (ACTH), which regulates steroid release from the adrenal glands.
- Growth hormone–releasing hormone (GHRH) from the hypothalamus stimulates pituitary somatotroph glandular cells in the pituitary to release growth hormone (GH), and somatostatin (SST) which blocks GH release. SST is also released by δ-cells of the pancreatic islets.
- Prolactin inhibitory factor. This is **dopamine** (see also Chapter 4). It is released by the hypothalamus and inhibits release of pituitary prolactin.

Hypothalamus–Posterior Pituitary Communication

Glandular cells in the hypothalamus secrete two hormones, antidiuretic hormone (ADH) and oxytocin, which travel by axonal transport down the nerves linking the hypothalamus and the posterior pituitary and are released from there.

CONTROL OF HORMONE LEVELS BY THE HYPOTHALAMIC–ANTERIOR PITUITARY AXIS

As shown in Fig. 5.2, hypothalamic and pituitary hormones in turn control hormone release by a range of other glands. Blood levels of these final hormones, including thyroid hormones, oestrogen and progesterone from the ovary, and cortisol from the adrenal cortex, are continuously measured by the hypothalamus and pituitary gland, not by the gland responsible for their secretion. Rising levels of the final hormone suppress release of the relevant hypothalamic and pituitary releasing hormones, switching off the stimulus for their release and allowing blood levels to fall. When blood levels fall below the normal range, this is detected by the hypothalamus and pituitary, which resume their production of the relevant releasing hormones. This is called indirect negative feedback control because the gland secreting the final hormone is not in direct control of its own secretion, and it is illustrated in Fig. 5.3, using the thyroid gland as an example. The hypothalamus releases TRH, which stimulates the pituitary gland to release TSH. TSH stimulates the thyroid to release tri-iodothyronine (T_3) and thyroxine (T_4). Thyroid hormone levels in the blood therefore increase, and when they exceed the normal range, the hypothalamus reduces TRH production and the pituitary reduces TSH

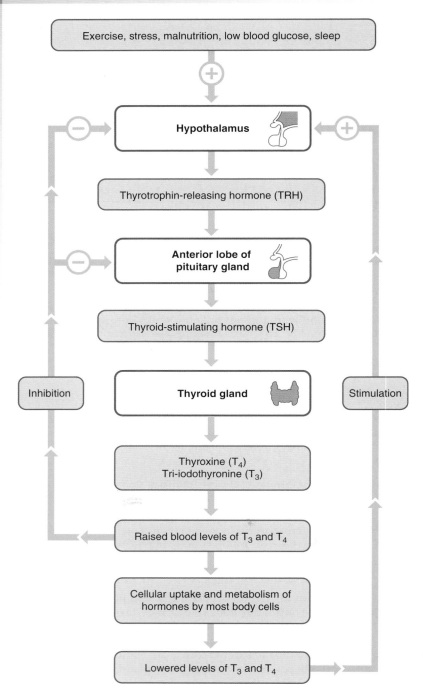

Fig. 5.3   Indirect negative feedback control of thyroid hormone secretion. (From Waugh A and Grant A (2020) Ross & Wilson anatomy and physiology in health and illness, 14th ed, Fig 9.1. Oxford: Elsevier.)

production. Hormone release by the thyroid gland is therefore reduced and decreases until T_3 and T_4 levels dip below the minimum of the normal range, at which point TRH and TSH release resumes.

HYPOTHALAMIC AND PITUITARY HORMONES IN THERAPEUTICS

Hormones of the hypothalamic–pituitary axis (Fig. 5.2) can be used therapeutically to replace hormone deficiency in disorders that involve hypothalamic or pituitary failure.

Additionally, drugs that antagonise hormone synthesis, release, or activity can be used in conditions associated with over-activity of these glands. Conditions disrupting hypothalamic and/or pituitary function, e.g. malignant disease, trauma, or infection, can affect secretion of more than one hormone if more than one type of secretory cell is affected. Because the hypothalamic–pituitary axis is a complex physiological mechanism, and normal control of any of its final hormones depends upon healthy function of at least two glandular tissues, there are multiple opportunities to intervene with therapeutic drugs. Fig. 5.4 summarises the main drugs relating to the hypothalamic–pituitary axis.

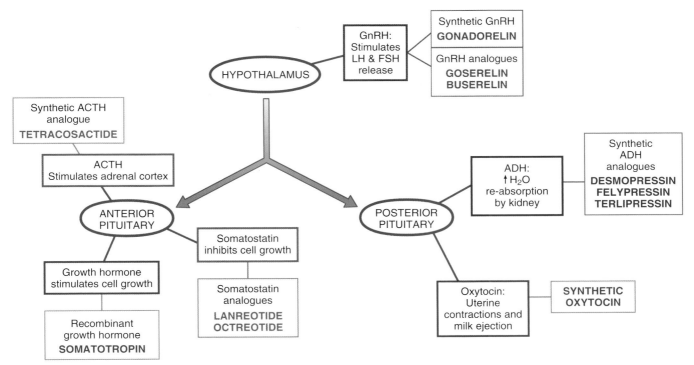

Fig. 5.4   Drugs related to the hypothalamic–pituitary axis.

ANTERIOR PITUITARY HORMONES

TSH and TRH are considered in the section discussing drugs and thyroid function.

ADRENOCORTICOTROPHIC HORMONE

The synthetic ACTH analogue **tetracosactide** is used to test adrenal cortex function. It is given by injection, and the adrenal cortex response is measured by measuring plasma steroid levels. In adrenocortical insufficiency, the adrenal cortex cannot respond adequately to the stimulus, and steroid levels remain low.

GROWTH HORMONE

Growth rates are controlled by GH from the anterior pituitary, which affects all body tissues, stimulating cell division and increasing body mass, including skeletal muscle. It promotes cartilage cell division in the growth plates of bones, and so it is essential for increasing height in a growing child and young person. It increases blood glucose levels by stimulating gluconeogenesis (glucose synthesis from non-carbohydrate nutrients, e.g. amino acids) and increases blood fatty-acid levels, ensuring that nutrient supply to growing tissues is adequate. GH deficiency is rare and can be due to hypothalamic failure causing a lack of GHRH, or pituitary failure causing GH deficiency. It may be congenital, a consequence of a traumatic head injury, meningitis or other central nervous system infection, or irradiation. In children, it retards growth and reduces height (dwarfism), and even though GH levels fall naturally with age, this hormone seems to be important for normal metabolism and maintenance of body mass in adults. Excessive GH release in childhood leads to gigantism, with long limbs and unusually tall adult stature. In adults, however, in whom the growth plates of the limb bones have closed, growing taller is not possible, and excess GH thickens and enlarges bone and other connective tissues, a condition called acromegaly. Coarsening of facial features is characteristic of this disorder, with enlargement of the nose, jaw, hands, and feet.

Somatropin: Recombinant Growth Hormone

GH used in medicine is produced by recombinant DNA technology and is called **somatropin**. It is given by injection to treat GH deficiency in children or adults. Adverse effects include carpal tunnel syndrome, painful joints and muscles, and localised loss of adipose tissue, all of which are caused by the hormone mobilising nutrient stores and stimulating tissue growth.

SOMATOSTATIN

SST inhibits GH release, and therefore reduces cell division and tissue growth. It also suppresses the secretion of a range of digestive enzymes and hormones, including insulin, gastrin, and pancreatic enzymes, which enhance its anti-growth activity.

Somatostatin Analogues

Lanerotide and **octreotide** are synthetic analogues of SST given by subcutaneous or intramuscular injection to treat conditions associated with excessive GH activity, e.g. acromegaly. They are also used in a range of conditions featuring excessive secretion of gastrointestinal (GI) hormones, including GI tumours. Unsurprisingly, their main adverse effects involve the GI tract and metabolic function, and include nausea, vomiting, abdominal pain, diarrhoea, and impaired glucose tolerance. They also increase the risk of gallstones because they reduce the release of cholecystokinin, which triggers gallbladder contraction. In its absence, the gallbladder empties more slowly and less frequently, allowing bile to stagnate and increasing the risk of stone formation.

GONADOTROPIN-RELEASING HORMONE, LUTEINISING HORMONE, AND FOLLICLE-STIMULATING HORMONE

GnRH stimulates pituitary release of LH and FSH in both males and females. It is secreted in pulses rather than continuously, allowing blood levels to regularly fall, which preserves the responsiveness of its receptors on the pituitary gland. LH and FSH control the synthesis and release of male and female sex steroids (mainly testosterone in men and oestrogen in women). The role of LH and FSH in female fertility and the drugs used in contraception, fertility treatment, and the management of menopausal symptoms are discussed below.

Gonadorelin

Gonadorelin is a synthetic preparation of GnRH used to test pituitary function. It is administered by either intravenous or subcutaneous injection and the pituitary response assessed by measuring plasma LH levels at set time intervals over the following 2 hours.

Gonadotropin-Releasing Hormone Analogues

This group of drugs includes **goserelin** and **buserelin**. They are structurally very similar to GnRH and initially stimulate pituitary release of LH and FSH, which in turn causes a short-lived surge of sex steroids. However, once steady-state drug levels are achieved in the plasma, the GnRH receptors on the pituitary gland are rapidly desensitised, because they are now being continually stimulated. This is unlike the natural pulsatile secretion pattern, which allows plasma levels to fall in between peak levels. The pituitary therefore stops responding, LH and FSH levels fall, and in turn, testosterone and oestrogen levels fall. This is useful in conditions associated with unwanted effects of these hormones: for example, many prostate cancers are testosterone-dependent, and reducing testosterone levels is therapeutically beneficial. Similarly, in oestrogen-dependent breast cancer, these drugs reduce oestrogen levels, inhibit tumour growth, delay recurrence, and increase survival times. In general, these drugs have short half-lives and are often given as depot formulations, which provide slow and steady drug release that can maintain blood levels for several months, depending on the preparation. Adverse effects are mainly due to the loss of sex hormones. Both sexes may experience reduced libido; women develop menopausal symptoms, and men may develop feminisation characteristics, e.g. gynaecomastia.

POSTERIOR PITUITARY HORMONES

ADH (vasopressin) and oxytocin are almost identical small peptides composed of nine amino acids, whose structures differ by a single amino acid. This explains the overlap in their pharmacological effects: for example, both cause smooth muscle contraction.

ANTIDIURETIC HORMONE

ADH increases water re-absorption by the kidney, which increases blood volume and blood pressure. The stimulus for ADH release is a rise in plasma osmolarity, i.e. an increase in the plasma concentration, or a reduction in plasma volume. ADH's target tissues are the proximal convoluted tubule and collecting ducts of the renal nephron, the regions of the tubule mainly responsible for water re-absorption. ADH increases the number of water channels in the wall of the nephron, increasing water re-absorption into the bloodstream. The plasma osmolarity therefore falls as the plasma becomes more dilute, the blood volume rises, and a smaller, more concentrated volume of urine is passed. ADH also causes vasoconstriction, increasing blood pressure. It also reduces bleeding time by activating platelets and stimulating clotting. ADH itself is sometimes used to treat diabetes insipidus, a condition characterised by inadequate ADH secretion.

Synthetic Antidiuretic Analogues

Examples: desmopressin, terlipressin, felypressin

Desmopressin is more potent than ADH and is given by nasal spray to reduce overnight urine production in children or adults who experience nocturnal enuresis (bedwetting). It is also used in diabetes insipidus. **Terlipressin** has less ADH activity than desmopressin but has more vasoconstrictor and pro-coagulant activity. It is used intravenously to stop bleeding and prevent hypotension in bleeding oesophageal varices. **Felypressin** is an effective and short-acting vasoconstrictor co-injected with local anaesthetic to reduce loss of the anaesthetic from the site and prolong its action.

OXYTOCIN

Oxytocin stimulates uterine contractions during childbirth and milk ejection during lactation and is important in a range of behaviours including eating, social interactions, and developing relationships, including establishing the parent-child bond. Synthetic oxytocin is given by intravenous infusion to induce and speed up labour when medically indicated and to prevent and treat post-partum haemorrhage. It can cause fluid retention because of its ADH-like activity, which can dilute body fluids and cause hyponatraemia.

DRUGS AND THYROID FUNCTION

The thyroid gland secretes two structurally closely related hormones: T_4 and T_3, which have essentially the same function. T_4 accounts for about 93% of the gland's output, but once released most of it is converted in the tissues to T_3, which is metabolically much more active. The thyroid gland is composed of large storage areas called follicles, each full of a high-molecular-weight substance called thyroglobulin, which is produced by linking together molecules of the amino acid tyrosine. Specialised iodide pumps in the membranes of the cells forming the walls of the follicles actively extract iodine from the bloodstream. The iodine is then added to tyrosine by the enzyme thyroid peroxidase (Fig. 5.5). If a tyrosine molecule has one iodide unit attached, it is called mono-iodotyrosine, and if it has two, it is called di-iodotyrosine. To release T_3 and T_4 from the thyroglobulin superstructure, enzymes clip off the tyrosine residues in pairs. If the released molecule is made of two di-iodotyrosine units, the resulting molecule, with four iodine atoms, is T_4; if it is made of a di-iodotyrosine unit and a mono-iodotyrosine unit, it is T_3.

In addition, C-cells embedded in the thyroid gland release calcitonin.

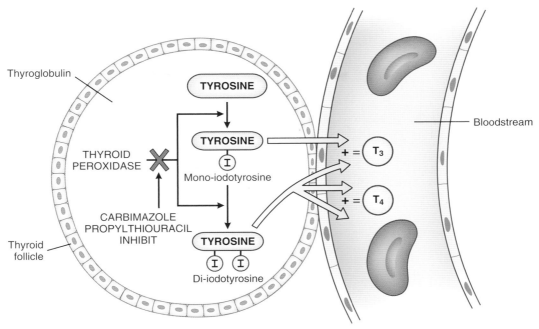

Fig. 5.5   The synthesis of thyroid hormones.

Functions of Tri-Iodothyronine and Thyroxine

These hormones increase protein synthesis and metabolic activity in nearly all body cells. They cross the plasma membrane, enter the cell nucleus, bind to specific genes within the cell's DNA, and activate them. This leads to the production of structural proteins, enzymes, growth factors, and other substances required for cellular activity. T_3 and T_4 are therefore essential for growth and metabolism in all body tissues.

KEY POINTS: PHYSIOLOGICAL EFFECTS OF THYROID HORMONES

Thyroid hormones increase heart rate, cardiac contractility, and blood pressure; stimulate respiration; and are essential for normal libido and sexual function. They increase cell division, basal metabolic rate, blood glucose levels, and the body's requirement for nutrients and oxygen; they trigger weight loss and increase gastrointestinal activity. Deficiency during fetal development, infancy, or childhood causes significant growth retardation and disrupts normal neurological development, including impairment of cognitive development.

The plasma half-life of thyroxine is 5–7 days, but T_3's half-life is 24 hours.

Functions of Calcitonin

Calcitonin reduces plasma calcium levels, opposing the effects of parathormone from the parathyroid glands. Its influence on plasma calcium levels is, however, thought to be relatively minor.

HYPOTHYROIDISM

Underactivity of the thyroid gland, hypothyroidism, is common. The most common cause, Hashimoto's disease, is an autoimmune disorder in which autoantibodies are produced to thyroid gland TSH receptors. The autoantibodies bind to and block the receptor, meaning that the thyroid gland cannot respond to TSH from the anterior pituitary, and thyroid hormone release falls. Other causes include a diet low in iodine, reversible with iodine supplements, and congenital hypothyroidism. Hypothyroidism also often follows antithyroid treatment for hyperthyroidism. In hypothyroid states caused by thyroid failure, plasma T_4 levels are low, but TRH and TSH levels can be significantly elevated because the hypothalamus and pituitary try to stimulate the failing thyroid to secrete additional T_4. Characteristic signs and symptoms of an underactive thyroid are listed in Box 5.1.

DRUG TREATMENT IN HYPOTHYROIDISM

The standard treatment for hypothyroidism is thyroid hormone replacement. Care must be taken in patients with cardiovascular disease or cardiovascular risk factors because thyroid hormones increase cardiac workload and blood pressure. In these people, treatment is started at a lower dose than normal and titrated upwards with care and regular cardiovascular monitoring. Care must also be taken in diabetes because the increased metabolic rate associated with T_4 is accompanied by hyperglycaemia; any antidiabetic medications, including insulin, may need to be increased.

Levothyroxine

This is the standard treatment for hypothyroidism. It is a synthetic drug, prepared as the sodium salt of the natural hormone and converted to T_3 in peripheral tissues.

Box 5.1 Characteristic Signs and Symptoms of Underactive and Overactive Thyroid

Underactive Thyroid	Overactive Thyroid
Decreased metabolic rate and weight gain	Increased metabolic rate and weight loss
Cold intolerance	Heat intolerance
Lethargy, fatigue, and apathy	Irritability, fatigue, and inability to sit still
Excessive sleepiness and sleep	Insomnia
Mental impairment	Inability to concentrate
Reduced libido and menorrhagia	Reduced libido and amenorrhoea
Bradycardia and hypotension	Tachycardia, palpitations, and hypertension
Slow speech and hoarse, deep voice	Tremor
Myxoedema (thickening of the skin)	Exophthalmos (protrusion of the eyeballs)
Dry skin and hair loss	Excessive sweating and hair loss
Constipation	Diarrhoea

Pharmacokinetics

Levothyroxine is given orally and moderately well absorbed. Absorption is reduced or slowed in the presence of food and when gastric pH is higher than normal, e.g. in people taking antacid medications. Levothyroxine has a long half-life, usually over a week in hypothyroid patients, so it equilibrates slowly and can take several weeks to reach a stable steady state. It is almost completely bound to T_4-binding globulin, the plasma protein responsible for transporting it in the bloodstream, which contributes to its long half-life. It is metabolised in body tissues to T_3 by removal of an iodine atom and from there to inactive products.

Liothyronine

Synthetic T_3 is available, also as a sodium salt, as the drug **liothyronine**. It has a much shorter half-life than levothyroxine, usually less than 24 hours, and its onset of action is faster. These properties mean that it is preferred to levothyroxine in acute or severe hypothyroid states.

ADVERSE EFFECTS

Excessive doses of levothyroxine or liothyronine give the same physiological effects as the natural hormone. Cardiovascular stimulation can cause tachycardia, palpitations, arrhythmias, and hypertension. There may be diarrhoea, weight loss, heat intolerance, sweating, insomnia, tremor, and menstrual disturbances. Levothyroxine crosses the placenta and can affect the fetus, so should be used very cautiously in pregnancy.

HYPERTHYROIDISM

Overactivity of the thyroid gland, hyperthyroidism (thyrotoxicosis), is common. The most common cause, Graves' disease, is an autoimmune disorder in which autoantibodies are produced to the TSH receptor on the thyroid gland. These autoantibodies bind to and stimulate the TSH receptor, triggering thyroid hormone production. Exophthalmos, protrusion of the eyeballs due to deposition of extracellular matrix at the back of the eye sockets, is a characteristic of Graves' disease. Other causes of hyperthyroidism include toxic nodular goitre caused by a benign functional thyroid tumour, which releases large quantities of thyroid hormone. Some drugs can also cause hyperthyroidism; e.g. the antiarrhythmic agent **amiodarone** (p. 137) is structurally similar to T_4 and contains significant quantities of iodine: a 200 mg tablet (the usual daily maintenance dose) delivers 75 mg of iodine. For reference, the daily recommended iodine intake is only 0.14 mg/day.

DRUG TREATMENT IN HYPERTHYROIDISM

Pharmacological treatment of hyperthyroidism may be used to reduce the size of an enlarged gland (goitre) in preparation for surgery. Because the gland is very vascular, shrinking it reduces the risk of bleeding during the procedure. It may also be used as maintenance therapy.

Carbimazole

Like the similar agent **propylthiouracil**, carbimazole inhibits the enzyme thyroid peroxidase, which catalyses the addition of iodine to tyrosine in thyroglobulin (Fig. 5.5), blocking the production of thyroid hormone. There is also evidence that these drugs reduce levels of the anti-TSH receptor antibody that stimulates T_4 production in Graves' disease. They are taken orally and metabolised in the liver.

Pharmacokinetics

Carbimazole is a pro-drug, converted in the bloodstream to the active agent **thiamazole.** Both thiamazole and **propylthiouracil** are taken up and concentrated in the thyroid gland. This means that although their plasma half-lives are relatively short—carbimazole has a half-life of around 5 hours and propylthiouracil's half-life is even shorter—their effective duration of action is much longer. It can take several weeks of treatment with carbimazole for thyroid hormone levels to fall to normal (become euthyroid) because the half-life of T_4 is so long, and there are usually substantial T_4 stores in the thyroid follicles that take some time to be used up.

Adverse Effects

The most significant adverse effect of these agents is bone marrow suppression, more commonly with propylthiouracil than carbimazole. Although this is rare, it can cause a rapid fall in white blood cell numbers with significant immunocompromise. Patients must be warned to report any signs of infection, e.g. fever or sore throat. Bone marrow function usually returns if the drug is stopped.

Radioactive Iodine

The radioactive isotope of iodine, ^{131}I, given orally, is treated by the thyroid in exactly the same way as the stable form: that is, it is rapidly and actively extracted by iodide pumps in cell membranes of the thyroid cells, and built into thyroglobulin to form mono-iodotyrosine and di-iodotyrosine. It emits radiation in the form of β particles, which have a very short range, so that although over time they kill the thyroid gland cells, they do not damage other local tissues. Because this agent permanently destroys the glandular function of the thyroid, individuals invariably become hypothyroid and need T$_4$ replacement therapy.

DRUGS AND PANCREATIC FUNCTION

The pancreas is mainly composed of exocrine tissue, which produces digestive enzymes that are secreted into the duodenum to digest fats, carbohydrates, and proteins. Additionally, scattered throughout the pancreatic tissue are nests of cells called islets, which are endocrine in function and produce insulin and glucagon, hormones essential for the body's metabolic use and storage of nutrients, especially glucose. Islets comprise only 2% of the mass of the gland but are richly supplied with blood vessels to carry their hormone products away, and with autonomic nerves to regulate hormone production.

INSULIN

Insulin is an anabolic hormone; its overarching function in metabolism is in conservation and storage of energy-rich nutrients. It stimulates body cells to remove glucose, fats, and amino acids from the bloodstream to use in energy production; promotes the storage of excess fuel molecules as glycogen or fat; and increases protein synthesis. It is a small-molecular-weight peptide composed of 52 amino acids, synthesised in β-cells within pancreatic islets. The main stimulus for its release is rising blood glucose, but an increase in blood levels of fatty acids and/or amino acids has the same effect. Insulin therefore reduces circulating blood glucose—a hypoglycaemic effect—and levels of other nutrients. Liver, skeletal muscle, and fat are the most insulin-responsive tissues.

GLUCAGON

Glucagon is synthesised by α-cells in the pancreatic islets, and the main stimulus for its release is falling blood glucose levels. Falling blood fatty-acid levels also increase glucagon secretion. It stimulates glycogen breakdown in the liver, releasing glucose, and breakdown of adipose and muscle tissue, releasing fatty acids and amino acids, respectively. Its metabolic actions therefore oppose those of insulin, and it is given subcutaneously, intravenously, or intramuscularly to increase blood glucose levels in insulin-induced hypoglycaemia. Glucagon also has an adrenaline-like effect on the heart and is used to improve cardiac function in shock caused by β-blocker overdose. It can cause vomiting, so it is important to protect the airway in unconscious patients treated with glucagon.

DIABETES MELLITUS

Diabetes mellitus (DM) is a very common condition characterised by high blood glucose levels, as well as an inability of body cells to respond appropriately to insulin (insulin resistance) and/or an absolute insulin deficiency. Without insulin, cells cannot import glucose no matter how much is available in the blood and are forced to rely on other energy molecules such as fats and amino acids. This is tolerable in the short term but unsustainable in the long term. The discovery that the pancreas is the source of the agent that prevents diabetes was made in 1890 when the pancreas was removed from a dog, which rapidly developed diabetes and died. It was over 30 years following that important discovery before the first clinical use of insulin. Prior to this, type 1 diabetes (T1D), usually presenting in childhood, invariably led to a slow, miserable, wasting death within a year or two of diagnosis. In 1922, a team of researchers in Toronto, led by Frederick Banting, Charles Best, and John MacLeod, treated a ward of seriously ill diabetic children with pancreatic extracts, with dramatic and immediate success: comatose children were restored to full consciousness, and children facing imminent and inevitable death were, to all intents and purposes, cured. Fig. 5.6 shows the dramatic

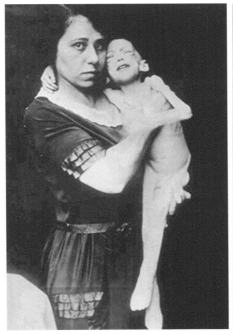
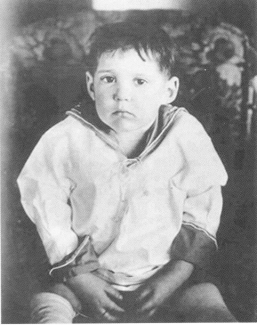

Fig. 5.6 An early insulin success story. The anabolic effects of insulin are clearly seen in a diabetic child pre-treatment (left image) and following treatment (right image). (Reproduced with permission from Eli Lilly and Company archives.)

difference in a diabetic child before and after starting treatment with insulin. Although life expectancy in DM is shorter than average, continuing improvements in management, including better pharmacological treatment, is slowly closing the gap.

The Action of Insulin on Body Cells

Glucose is the cells' preferred fuel molecule, and without insulin, they cannot extract it from the bloodstream and so are deprived of their main energy source. Most body cells express insulin receptors on their plasma membrane, although brain neurones take up glucose using an insulin-independent mechanism. Insulin binding to its receptor triggers a range of cellular effects, including an increased number of glucose transporters (GLUTs) at the cell surface, through which the cell then actively imports glucose from the extracellular fluid surrounding it. In addition to ensuring that all body cells can import the glucose and other nutrients they need, insulin allows liver and muscle cells to extract excess glucose from the bloodstream and convert it to glycogen for storage. Glycogen storage capacity is limited, and when glycogen stores are full, insulin allows cells to convert glucose to fat for storage in adipose tissue. Insulin increases the uptake of amino acids into muscle, converts them into protein, and promotes the storage of fats in adipose tissue. In liver cells, insulin prevents gluconeogenesis, the conversion of non-carbohydrate molecules, mainly fats and amino acids, into glucose.

Control of Insulin Secretion

The β-cells in the pancreas constantly monitor blood glucose levels. Their plasma membranes contain a large number of GLUT-2 glucose transporters which permit glucose to enter the cell (Fig. 5.7). The higher the blood glucose level, the more glucose enters the β-cell, where it is used to generate ATP. ATP in turn shuts potassium channels in the β-cell membrane, so that potassium cannot leave the cell, and potassium levels in the cell rise. This activates (depolarises) the cell membrane, which in turn opens membrane calcium channels and allows calcium to enter. Rising intracellular calcium triggers fusion of insulin storage vesicles with the cell membrane and secretion of insulin into the bloodstream. Some antidiabetic drugs enhance insulin release by interfering with one or more components of this mechanism: for example, **sulphonylureas** (e.g. **glibenclamide**) directly block potassium channels in the β-cell membrane, depolarising the cell and stimulating insulin release.

Basal blood insulin levels are low in the fasting state but rapidly increase up to 10-fold in the minutes following a nutrient-rich meal. This initial peak is stimulated most strongly by rising blood glucose, but fatty acids and amino acids also trigger it. It represents release of stored insulin, which is quickly depleted. However, after an initial fall, insulin levels rapidly rise again as the pancreas produces and releases new insulin, and they remain high until blood glucose levels are brought back within the normal range (Fig. 5.8). Autonomic nervous system activity also influences insulin release. Physiological stress, rising blood glucocorticoids, and sympathetic nervous system activity inhibit insulin release; this allows blood glucose levels to rise, ensuring that body cells have an adequate glucose supply to meet potentially

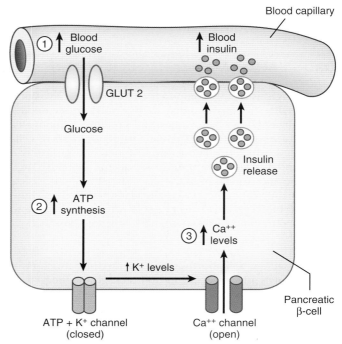

Fig. 5.7 Mechanism of insulin release by pancreatic β-cells. 1, Rising blood glucose increases glucose entry into the β-cell. 2, This generates large quantities of ATP, closes potassium channels, and depolarises the cell. 3: Depolarisation of the cell opens calcium channels, increasing calcium entry and stimulating insulin release. (Modified from Vaz M, Kurpad A, and Raj T (2020) Guyton and Hall textbook of medical physiology, 3rd SAE ed, Fig. 93.6. New Delhi: Elsevier India.)

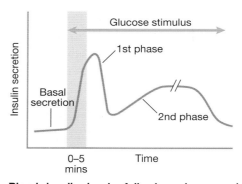

Fig. 5.8 Blood insulin levels following glucose administration. First phase represents release of pre-formed insulin, and second phase represents release of newly synthesised insulin. (Modified from Penman ID, Ralston SH, Strachan MWJ, et al. (2023) Davidson's principles and practice of medicine, 24th ed, Fig. 21.4. Edinburgh: Elsevier.)

increased requirements. Parasympathetic nervous system activity, associated with rest, low physical activity, and low physiological stress levels, increases insulin levels and promotes the packaging away of blood-borne nutrients into storage areas.

Insulin release is also stimulated by hormones released by the GI tract during eating. This explains the perhaps unexpected observation that consuming glucose by mouth raises blood insulin levels faster than an intravenous glucose infusion. GI hormones that increase insulin release are collectively called incretins and include glucagon-like peptide 1 (GLP-1). Their blood levels rise when foodstuffs enter the GI tract and stimulate insulin release in anticipation of rising blood sugar levels as the products of digestion are absorbed (Fig. 5.9). Some antidiabetic drugs, e.g. **liraglutide**, stimulate insulin release by mimicking the action of incretins, i.e. act as incretin agonists. Following their release, incretins are rapidly destroyed by the enzyme dipeptidyl peptidase (DPP-4). The **gliptins**, including **linagliptin** and **vildagliptin**, inhibit DPP-4, protecting incretins from destruction and therefore increasing insulin release.

Fig. 5.10 summarises the main factors controlling blood insulin levels.

Energy Metabolism in Diabetes

In the absence of insulin, cellular metabolism is forced to switch from using glucose as an energy source to using fats instead. Adipose tissue is broken down, and the individual loses weight. Blood lipid levels rise, contributing significantly to the increased risk of cardiovascular disease associated with DM. To release the energy they require, cells deprived of glucose metabolise fats, producing ketone bodies (acetoacetic

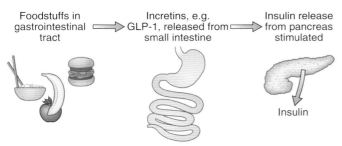

Fig. 5.9 The role of incretins in insulin release.

acid, β-hydroxybutyric acid, and acetone), which body cells can use for fuel. This is the normal route by which fats are broken down: for example, in a low-calorie diet for weight loss, stored body fat is burned this way for energy. In non-diabetic people, the body's energy balance is maintained using both fats and carbohydrates as energy sources, but in DM, fat breakdown becomes disproportionately important because the cells have no access to glucose. Large quantities of ketone bodies are manufactured, causing ketosis and a metabolic acidosis. Acute ketoacidosis is a medical emergency and can be fatal unless rapidly treated.

Signs and Symptoms of Diabetes

Hyperglycaemia is characteristic. Glucose appears in the urine (glycosuria) because the renal threshold for glucose is exceeded. Glucose is a small molecule that is filtered out of the blood as it flows through the glomerulus and appears in the filtrate. Provided glucose levels are not excessive, GLUTs in the nephron re-absorb it all back into the bloodstream, and none appears in the urine. However, in DM, there is so much glucose in the blood that the glucose load appearing in the filtrate is excessive. The GLUTs in the kidney tubule are saturated, and their capacity to re-absorb glucose is exceeded, leading to glycosuria. Glucose in the urine increases its osmolarity, drawing water with it and causing dehydration and thirst. Body fat and protein stores are broken down to release alternative fuel molecules to glucose, so there is weight loss and muscle wasting. Over time, hyperglycaemia damages small blood vessels, partly because structural components within their walls, e.g. collagen, take up glucose and form advanced glycation end-products. The tiny blood vessels of the renal glomerulus are particularly susceptible, and renal disease is very common in diabetes. Retinal capillaries and the tiny blood vessels supplying nerves are also commonly affected, causing diabetic neuropathy. In

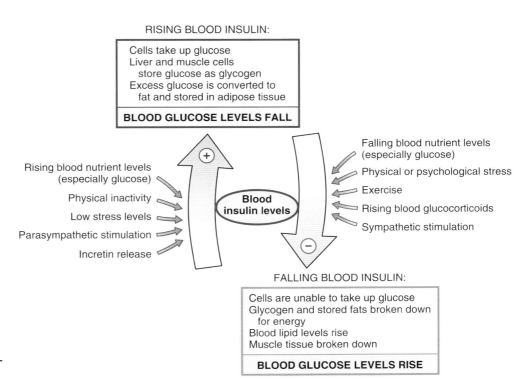

Fig. 5.10 The main factors controlling blood insulin levels.

addition to these microvascular changes, large blood vessels are progressively damaged by the hyperlipidaemia associated with diabetes, with atherosclerosis, hypertension, and increased risk of thrombosis. The risk of myocardial infarction and stroke are consequently increased. There are a few different forms of DM, but the two most common are type 1 and type 2.

TYPE 1 DIABETES

This form usually manifests in childhood. The pancreatic islets are progressively destroyed, usually by an autoimmune reaction, and so the child's pancreas stops producing insulin. This is called absolute insulin deficiency, and the cornerstone of treatment is insulin replacement. The aim of treatment is to stabilise blood glucose levels, minimising hyperglycaemia and therefore reducing long-term cardiovascular risk, but also avoiding potentially dangerous hypoglycaemia.

TYPE 2 DIABETES

This is associated with adult-age onset and obesity, and although the individual usually continues to produce some insulin of their own (so-called relative insulin deficiency), the cellular response to insulin is abnormal. Overeating and obesity are associated with sustained elevated blood insulin levels, because constantly high blood nutrient levels stimulate insulin release (Fig. 5.10). Over time, it is thought that the continual exposure of insulin receptors on body cells to elevated insulin levels desensitises them and disrupts the normal biochemistry of the cellular response to insulin. This is called insulin resistance. Although type 2 diabetes (T2D) is treated with a range of drugs to increase pancreatic release of insulin or to improve the cellular response to insulin, many people eventually require supplementary insulin treatment too. Because these patients usually produce at least some insulin, hypoglycaemic episodes are much less likely than in T1D, and the main management goal is to minimise postprandial hyperglycaemia to minimise long-term cardiovascular risk.

INSULIN

Insulin cannot be given orally because it is a small peptide and is rapidly digested in the stomach. It is generally given subcutaneously in maintenance treatment but can be given intravenously or intramuscularly if a faster effect is needed. Its plasma half-life is short—about 10 minutes—and it is metabolised in the liver to inactive products which are excreted in the urine. The molecular action of insulin is described above, but there is now a range of modified insulins which vary in their onset and duration of action, and which can be combined in individualised and flexible treatment regimes. Insulin molecules tend to assemble themselves into stable hexamers (six insulin molecules grouped around zinc ions); they are found in this formation in pancreatic islets and assemble into hexamers in the tissues following injection. The onset of action of injected insulin then depends upon how quickly individual insulin molecules are released from the hexamer structure. Insulin analogues are chemically modified to alter the speed at which insulin dissociates from the hexamers; rapidly acting insulins dissociate the fastest and long-acting insulins dissociate much more slowly. Pre-mixed insulins are available, for example combining an intermediate-acting insulin with a short-acting insulin, which reduce the number of daily injections required.

Short-Acting Insulins

Examples: soluble insulin, insulin aspart, insulin lispro

Short-acting insulins include **soluble insulin**, which can be used by regular injections or by infusion. Insulin is absorbed slowly from its injection site due to the assemblage of insulin hexamers in the tissue. **Insulin aspart** and **insulin lispro** are modified insulins, in which very minor alterations to the structure of the insulin molecule increase its release from the hexamers without reducing its pharmacological activity. They therefore act more quickly than soluble insulin but have a shorter duration of action.

Intermediate Insulins

Examples: isophane insulin

Isophane insulin is produced by treating soluble insulin with zinc and protamine. This reduces its solubility at physiological pH and slows its release into the bloodstream, avoiding a peak, and prolongs its action; it can be effective for up to 24 hours. Biphasic insulin is produced by combining **soluble insulin** with **isophane insulin**, giving a pre-mixed preparation that provides both short- and medium-term blood glucose control.

Long-Acting Insulins

Examples: insulin glargine, insulin detemir, insulin degludec

Long-acting insulins are insulin analogues with very minor alterations to the amino-acid structure. These structural changes reduce solubility, slow absorption from the injection site, and extend their duration of action: this avoids a peak. **Insulin glargine** is soluble at pH 4, and when injected into the tissues, which are pH-neutral, it loses solubility and precipitates out as microcrystals from which it is slowly released into the bloodstream. It takes over an hour before onset of action, but it is active for 24 hours, providing the equivalent of naturally secreted basal insulin. **Insulin detemir** has fatty-acid residues bound to the peptide structure, which promote hexamer formation and slow its absorption, and increase its binding to plasma proteins, both of which extend its duration of action. **Insulin degludec** also has a fatty-acid residue attached, which causes it to precipitate out in the tissues after injection and slows its release into the bloodstream.

Basal Bolus Regimes

Traditional insulin treatment plans involve regular insulin injections prior to mealtimes, with insulin dose based on blood glucose readings. Once the insulin is administered, the planned meal must be eaten, or hypoglycaemia will ensue. This is inflexible and does not give optimal control. Basal bolus therapy is designed to mimic the body's natural insulin release patterns. A long- or intermediate-acting insulin is injected once a day to deliver basal levels and ensure that there is always insulin in the bloodstream, and fast-acting insulins are used just before, during, or just after meals to deal with rising blood nutrient levels. Although it requires good patient education and motivation and multiple injections, when used well, it optimises blood glucose control and minimises the hyperglycaemia that causes long-term vascular damage.

Adverse Effects

The most frequent and most dangerous side-effect of insulin treatment, especially hazardous at night, is hypoglycaemia, which may be caused by insulin overdose, unexpected exercise, or inadequate food intake. Because the brain is highly dependent on glucose for fuel, hypoglycaemia causes confusion, impaired cognitive function, reduced conscious levels, and coma, and is potentially lethal. Falling blood glucose activates a sympathetic nervous system response and adrenaline release, which usually acts as an early warning of an impending hypoglycaemic episode, although not all people experience this and hypoglycaemia can develop without warning. Regular injections at the same site can cause a local accumulation of subcutaneous fat because of the anabolic action of insulin. Occasionally, adipose tissue can break down (lipoatrophy) around a site that is overused for injection, thought to be due to an immunologically mediated tissue damage. Using a range of injection sites (usually the abdomen and thigh) and not using the same site repeatedly helps to prevent these permanent tissue changes. Although initial management of T2D does not include insulin because most people with this form of diabetes produce some insulin of their own, about 50% of people eventually require insulin treatment. Insulin in T2D causes weight gain and increases cardiovascular risk, and its benefits should be weighed against this when deciding whether to add insulin to a treatment regimen.

Inhaled Insulin

The discomfort and inconvenience of multiple daily injections drove the search for alternative routes of insulin administration, and most work has been done in inhaled insulin. The alveoli of the lungs are very thin-walled and richly supplied with blood vessels and offer a very large surface area for drug absorption. Inhalable insulin is formulated as a powder to be delivered as an aerosol via an inhaler device. It was first licensed in the USA in 2006 by Pfizer, but it did not sell well mainly because of its cost. Although it acts more rapidly than even the fastest-acting injected insulin, which could in theory increase a patient's ability to control post-prandial hyperglycaemia, it is difficult to achieve precise dosing because pulmonary absorption may be unpredictable, and repeated dosing may be needed to control post-prandial hyperglycaemia. Inhaled insulin is not currently available on the National Health Service in the UK.

NON-INSULIN ANTIDIABETIC DRUGS

The mechanisms of action of the main groups of non-insulin antidiabetic drugs are summarised in Fig. 5.11. Note that some drugs have more than one antidiabetic action.

Metformin

Chemically, metformin is a biguanide, derived from a chemical found in French lilac, extracts of which were used in mediaeval Europe to treat diabetes. A range of biguanides was developed in the 1920s, but metformin is the only survivor in clinical use, the others having been discarded because they caused lactic acidosis. Metformin is frequently the first choice of treatment in newly diagnosed T2D, and globally is the most common oral antidiabetic drug. It has a range of actions that contribute to its hypoglycaemic action (Fig. 5.11). It is an insulin sensitiser: that is, it enhances the effects of insulin and so it is ineffective unless there

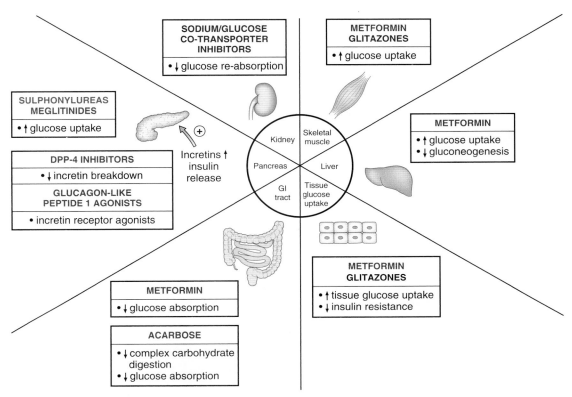

Fig. 5.11 Mechanism of action of non-insulin antidiabetic drugs.

is some circulating insulin present. It reduces glucose absorption from the GI tract, inhibits glucose re-absorption in the kidneys, reduces glucose production in the liver, and increases the uptake of glucose in body tissues, including skeletal muscle. It enters body cells and accumulates in mitochondria, the organelles responsible for energy metabolism, where it interferes with energy pathways, leading to the effects described above. Unlike some other antidiabetic drugs, metformin does not cause weight gain, so is particularly useful in overweight and obese patients, and does not cause hypoglycaemia. There is also evidence that metformin reduces total plasma cholesterol and low-density lipoprotein (LDL) cholesterol, both risk factors for cardiovascular disease. Such an improvement in blood lipid profiles is likely to be significantly beneficial in diabetes because of the increased risk of cardiovascular disease. In many patients, metformin used as monotherapy gives good glycaemic control, especially in milder disease. It can also be usefully combined with other antidiabetic agents if required; with time and progressive deterioration of islet function, second-line agents frequently need to be added to maintain good blood glucose control.

Pharmacokinetics

The half-life of metformin is about 5 hours, and there are modified-release preparations that extend this up to 8 hours. It is not metabolised in the liver, and is excreted largely unchanged in the urine, so renal function must be assessed regularly to ensure that the drug is not accumulating. In severely reduced renal function, it should be avoided altogether.

Adverse Effects

Metformin reduces the uptake of the waste product lactate from the bloodstream by liver cells. This can significantly increase blood lactate levels and precipitate lactic acidosis, most commonly in older adults and in those with poor renal function. Poor cardiac function also increases risk because it leads to hypoxia, and without adequate oxygen, cells respire anaerobically, producing excess lactate. Liver disease can also increase blood lactate and the drug should be avoided in severe liver impairment. Lactic acidosis is fortunately a rare side-effect, but it can be fatal. Most other side-effects of metformin are relatively mild and usually improve with time: they include a metallic taste in the mouth, nausea, and diarrhoea, which may be reduced by taking with food.

Sulphonylureas

Examples: glibenclamide, gliclazide, glipizide
The sulphonylureas are chemically related to the **sulphonamides**, a group of antimicrobial agents introduced in 1935 which caused hypoglycaemia as an unexpected side-effect: this led to the development and introduction of **tolbutamide**, the first sulphonylurea, in the 1950s. Tolbutamide remains in current use, although newer agents like **glibenclamide** are more potent. Sulphonylureas increase insulin release by the pancreas by blocking potassium channels in islet β-cells (Fig. 5.7). They are therefore only effective if there are functioning β-cells in the pancreatic islets, and they enhance both phases of insulin release: that is, the initial spike of pre-formed insulin and release of newly

synthesised insulin. Although they have traditionally been considered the first choice when supplementation of metformin treatment is needed and are generally well tolerated, **DPP-4 inhibitors** are now considered a superior option because they have fewer side-effects.

Pharmacokinetics

Sulphonylureas are taken orally and absorbed well, although food in the GI tract slows absorption. They bind extensively to plasma proteins and compete with other highly bound drugs (e.g. **warfarin**, **aspirin**) for binding sites, and this is an important cause of sulphonylurea-mediated interactions. Dose adjustment may therefore be necessary when such drug combinations are used. Different drugs in this class have different half-lives and duration of action, and increasing either increases the likelihood of hypoglycaemia. For example, **glibenclamide** has a long half-life of over 10 hours and produces an active metabolite, so it is particularly long-acting (sometimes more than 24 hours) and is prone to causing hypoglycaemia, especially at night and in older people. **Glimepiride** has a shorter half-life (5–8 hours), but because it too produces an active metabolite, its duration of action is 12–24 hours. **Glipizide** has a half-life of only 2–4 hours, produces no active metabolites, and is one of the shorter-acting agents in this group. Although **tolbutamide** is the oldest and least potent drug in this group, it has a short half-life (4 hours), meaning that there is little or no risk of hypoglycaemia. Most sulphonylureas are excreted by the kidney, so they must be used with caution if there is any degree of renal compromise.

When sulphonylureas are used with a number of other drugs, including **alcohol**, some **antifungals**, some **antibiotics**, and **non-steroidal anti-inflammatory** drugs, severe hypoglycaemia can occur. The basis of this interaction is probably caused by inhibition of metabolising enzymes, meaning that metabolism and clearance of the sulphonylurea is reduced and so its hypoglycaemic effect is enhanced.

Adverse Effects

Most sulphonylureas cross the placenta and appear in breast milk and should not be used in pregnancy or by breast-feeding mothers. They usually cause weight gain, so they must be used cautiously in overweight or obese people. Hypoglycaemia is a common side-effect, especially with longer-acting agents. Long-term use may increase the risk of cardiovascular disease, particularly concerning in DM. Less severe, although still troublesome, side-effects include allergic rashes and GI upset.

Meglitinides

Examples: nateglinide, repaglinide
This group of drugs is chemically closely related to the **sulphonylureas** and work in the same way, i.e. they block potassium channels in the β-cell membrane and increase insulin release from the pancreas. They are faster acting and have a shorter duration of action than the sulphonylureas, with a half-life of less than 2 hours, so they are less likely to cause hypoglycaemia. Because they are short-acting, they can be used to reduce post-prandial hyperglycaemia when **metformin** or the sulphonylureas are not adequate. Other than hypoglycaemia, their main side-effects include diarrhoea and abdominal discomfort.

Glitazones

Examples: pioglitazone, rosiglitazone

These are also called thiazolidinediones and are classed as insulin sensitisers because they increase cells' ability to respond to insulin. They reduce blood glucose levels by increasing its uptake into body cells, particularly skeletal muscle and fat. **Pioglitazone** is the only member of this group currently used in the UK, other glitazones having been discontinued due to significant side-effects.

Pharmacokinetics

The onset of action is slow and maximal hypoglycaemic effects may not be seen for up to 8 weeks. Pioglitazone is over 99% bound to plasma proteins and is extensively metabolised in the liver, producing active metabolites. Its plasma half-life is between 5 and 7 hours, but the active metabolites can significantly extend its duration of action. It is mainly excreted in the faeces (less than 30% is excreted in the urine). It has a beneficial effect on blood lipids, increasing levels of 'good' high-density lipoprotein (HDL) cholesterol and reducing levels of 'bad' very-low-density lipoprotein. It also reduces other cardiovascular risk factors and inflammatory markers, which in turn reduces cardiovascular disease in T2D.

Adverse Effects

The side-effects of pioglitazone can be significant. Common adverse effects include weight gain, caused partly by fat deposition, but it is also likely that fluid retention, another of its side-effects, contributes. Fluid retention causes oedema and increases circulating blood volume. Because of this, pioglitazone can precipitate heart failure, particularly in older patients and people with pre-existing cardiovascular disease, and when used in conjunction with insulin. There is also evidence that pioglitazone slightly increases the risk of bladder cancer, especially in high doses and long-term treatment, and it should be avoided in patients with risk factors for this tumour.

Dipeptidyl Peptidase Inhibitors (Gliptins)

Examples: linagliptin, saxagliptin

The gliptins were first approved in 2009 in the USA for the treatment of T2D. They work by blocking the breakdown of incretins by the enzyme DPP-4, and because incretins increase insulin release, when incretin destruction is blocked and incretin levels rise, insulin secretion is enhanced (Fig. 5.12). They may be used as monotherapy or in combination with other antidiabetic agents.

Pharmacokinetics

The gliptins have a long duration of action because they bind strongly to DPP-4, inhibiting it over a prolonged period; they are generally given only once daily. For example, **saxagliptin** has a plasma half-life of only 2.5 hours, and its active metabolite has a half-life of about 3 hours, but its hypoglycaemic action lasts for 24 hours.

Side-Effects

The gliptins can cause headaches, nausea, and abdominal pain. There may be an increased risk of infections, e.g. urinary tract and upper respiratory tract infection, but the evidence for this is mixed.

Incretin (Glucagon-Like Peptide 1) Agonists

Examples: exenatide, liraglutide

Incretins, including GLP-1, increase insulin release from the pancreatic β-cells, slow down gastric emptying, and inhibit glucagon release. Through these actions they reduce blood glucose levels. GLP-1 itself cannot be used to treat T2D because it is too rapidly destroyed by DPP-4 to be effective. However, synthetic drugs that bind to and activate GLP-1 receptors on β-cells, the GLP-1 agonists, mimic this action (Fig. 5.12) and are used as second-line therapy in combination with other oral antidiabetic drugs and/or insulin. GLP agonists are associated with a range of beneficial effects, not all of which are seen with the gliptins, including delayed gastric emptying and reduced appetite (Fig. 5.13).

KEY POINT: DISCOVERY OF THE GLUCAGON-LIKE PEPTIDE 1 AGONISTS

The history of these drugs is interesting. The Gila monster is one of the world's two venomous lizards; its bite is extremely painful and produces a range of metabolic and pro-inflammatory effects in the victim. Analysis of the salivary toxin isolated a hypoglycaemic agent called exendin-4, chemically and biologically very similar to glucagon-like peptide 1. From this, the first glucagon-like peptide 1 agonist, **exenatide**, was synthesised, becoming clinically available in 2005.

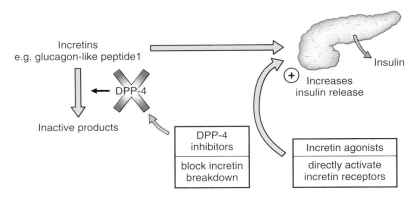

Fig. 5.12   Mechanism of action of the DPP-4 inhibitors and incretin agonists. DPP-4, Dipeptidyl peptidase.

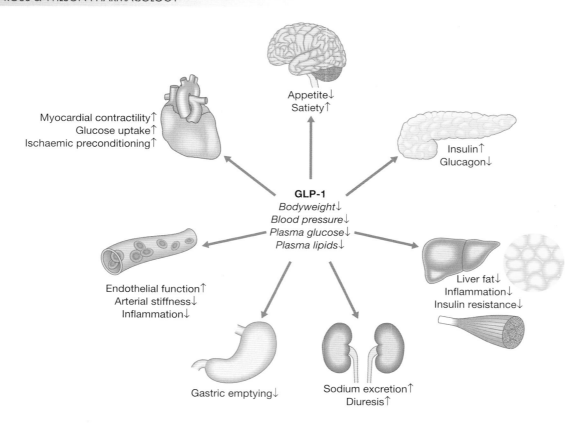

Fig. 5.13 Actions of the GLP-1 agonists. GLP-1, glucagon-like peptide 1 (From Penman ID, Ralston SH, Strachan MWJ, et al. (2023) Davidson's principles and practice of medicine, 24th ed, Fig. 21.4. Edinburgh: Elsevier.)

Pharmacokinetics

GLP-1 agonists are given by subcutaneous injection, not by mouth, because they are proteins and are digested in the stomach. The drugs in this group vary significantly in their duration of action; **dulaglutide** has a long half-life of approximately 5 days and is given only once a week, whereas **exenatide** and **liraglutide** are given daily.

Adverse Effects

These drugs tend not to cause weight gain because they do not stimulate appetite and can even help patients lose a little weight. Rarely, they can cause acute pancreatitis, and patients must be warned to report any relevant signs and symptoms. Commonly, they cause GI side-effects including abdominal pain, nausea/vomiting, and constipation or diarrhoea.

Sodium/Glucose Co-Transporter Inhibitors

Examples: canagliflozin, empagliflozin

These drugs reduce blood glucose levels by inhibiting the GLUTs in the renal tubule, reducing glucose re-absorption from the filtrate into the bloodstream, and therefore increasing glycosuria (Fig. 5.14). They are very recent additions to the armoury of antidiabetic agents; the first, **dapagliflozin**, was first approved in 2012. They are unlikely to cause hypoglycaemia, and glucose loss in the urine can help weight control.

Pharmacokinetics

Because they have long half-lives, drugs in this group are given once daily.

Adverse Effects

Glycosuria increases the risk of urinary tract and genital infections, and because the osmotic pressure of the urine is increased, it draws water with it, causing thirst and dehydration. There is evidence that some sodium/glucose co-transporter 2 inhibitors (**canagliflozin, dapagliflozin,** and **empagliflozin**) can sometimes cause serious ketoacidosis, and patients taking these agents should be taught to recognise warning signs, e.g. deep and rapid respiration, sudden weight loss, or a sweet odour to the breath. This class of drug has also very recently (2017) been associated with an increased risk of lower-limb amputation, particularly of the toes. The reason for this is not yet known, but one study has suggested that they decrease blood volume, thickening the blood and increasing the risk of blood clots. This would reduce tissue perfusion, especially in the periphery, already likely compromised in T2D.

Acarbose

Acarbose inhibits the enzyme glucosidase, which in the intestine breaks down larger carbohydrate molecules into glucose for absorption. This delays (but does not prevent)

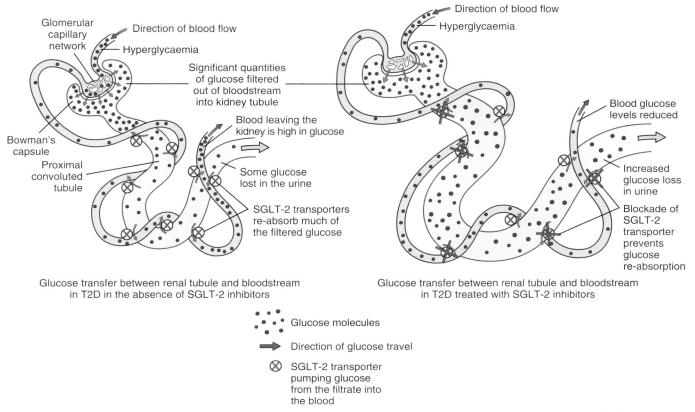

Glucose transfer between renal tubule and bloodstream
in T2D in the absence of SGLT-2 inhibitors

Glucose transfer between renal tubule and bloodstream
in T2D treated with SGLT-2 inhibitors

• • •   Glucose molecules

⟶   Direction of glucose travel

⊗   SGLT-2 transporter
pumping glucose
from the filtrate into
the blood

Fig. 5.14   Mechanism of action of SGLT-2 inhibitors in type 2 diabetes. SGLT-2, sodium/glucose co-transporter 2; T2D, Type 2 diabetes.

carbohydrate digestion following eating, so glucose levels in the intestinal brush border rise more slowly than normal, glucose absorption into the bloodstream is slowed, and the rapid post-prandial rise in blood sugar levels is flattened. Hyperglycaemic peaks are therefore reduced or avoided. It is generally used in conjunction with other antidiabetic agents because it is less effective at controlling blood glucose than other oral antidiabetic drugs and is usually insufficient on its own. Very little of an oral dose is absorbed into the bloodstream; most is excreted in the faeces, and the main side-effects include diarrhoea, abdominal bloating and discomfort, and flatulence. Its blood glucose-lowering action is not usually profound enough to significantly increase the risk of hypoglycaemia, but it does increase the overall risk when used with other hypoglycaemic agents.

PHARMACOLOGICAL CONTROL OF REPRODUCTIVE FUNCTION

Both male and female reproductive function is regulated by key hormones. The main male sex hormone is testosterone, produced by the Leydig cells in the testis, and the main female sex hormones are the oestrogens and progesterone, produced mainly by the ovary. Insufficient or excessive sex hormones can significantly disrupt sexual desire and activity, and reduce or eliminate fertility, and hormone treatment is used in the treatment of infertility and to treat conditions associated with hormone deficiency. Drugs that block sex hormone synthesis or function are used to treat cancers whose growth is sex hormone–dependent: for example, **tamoxifen**, an oestrogen receptor blocker, is a mainstay drug in the treatment of oestrogen-responsive breast cancer.

KEY POINT: PROGESTERONE OR PROGESTOGEN?

In this text, progesterone refers to the natural hormone. A progestogen is a synthetic drug with progesterone-like properties.

It is worth noting that the sex hormones are not sex-specific: testosterone plays a role in female physiology, and oestrogens play a role in male physiology.

Focus on: Sex Hormone Pharmacology

Structure of the Sex Hormones

The sex hormones are all steroid hormones derived from cholesterol. Because of their lipid-based structure, they travel easily across biological membranes, including cell membranes, and so they are generally well absorbed and distribute widely. Their biosynthetic pathways are interlinked (Fig. 5.15). The steps catalysed by aromatase and 5α-reductase are shown because these enzymes are important therapeutic targets. Aromatase inhibitors such as **anastrozole** are used to block oestrogen production in women with oestrogen-dependent breast cancer, and 5α-reductase inhibitors such as **finasteride** are used to inhibit growth of the prostate gland in benign prostatic hyperplasia.

Mechanism of Action of the Sex Hormones

Being highly lipid-soluble, these hormones readily diffuse across cell membranes and enter the cell cytoplasm, where they bind to a receptor protein. There are about 60 of these steroid binding proteins, some of which bind oestrogen (oestrogen receptors, ERs), some that bind progesterone, and some that bind testosterone (androgen receptors, ARs). These hormone-receptor complexes then travel to the nucleus, where they bind to specific genes, either activating or deactivating them. Target genes include those involved in cell growth and division, and the sex steroids are important in growth and proliferation of a range of body tissues.

Oestrogens

The ovary secretes three main oestrogens: oestradiol (the principal and most potent oestrogen), oestrone, and oestriol (Fig. 5.15). Oestrogens promote the development of the secondary sexual characteristics, e.g. growth of axillary and pubic hair and breast development, initiated at puberty. They stimulate cell growth and division in tissues that express oestrogen receptors, e.g. breast and uterine lining. This mitogenic property may be associated with the development of cancer in these tissues and offers a key therapeutic target in treat-

ment. Oestrogens regulate the reproductive cycle as described below, and additionally have a wide range of metabolic and physiological activities; they promote bone growth and maintain bone density and strength, they promote fat deposition, and they enhance sodium and water retention by the kidney. They increase coagulability of the blood, making thromboembolism more likely, but they also improve the blood lipid profile, reducing the risk of atheroma forming in blood vessels. This protective, anti-atherogenic lipid profile includes reduced total blood cholesterol and LDL cholesterol, and increased levels of HDL cholesterol, which is protective for blood vessels. Oestrogens dilate coronary arteries and protect blood vessels from atherogenic changes, reducing the risk of ischaemic heart disease in women compared with that in men.

Pharmacokinetics

Oestrogens are well absorbed from a range of sites, extensively metabolised in the intestinal lining and the liver, and excreted in the urine. Oestradiol metabolism produces several active metabolites, which extend its duration of action and half-life to up to 16 hours.

Oestrogen Receptors

ERs are found in the cytoplasm of oestrogen-responsive cells, including breast, vagina, and uterus, where they mediate the reproductive functions of oestrogens. However, ERs are found in a range of other tissues, including the bone, skin, heart and blood vessels, and brain. There are two types of ER: ERα and ERβ. Distribution of these receptor types differs between tissues, e.g. ERα is the main receptor type in the breast and is often overexpressed in breast cancer, whereas ERβ is the main type found in the brain.

Progesterone

Progesterone regulates the female reproductive cycle as described below and is essential in the maintenance of pregnancy, including breast growth and development in preparation for lactation. Synthetic progestogens, e.g. norethisterone and gestodene, are more potent than natural hormones. Some progestogens are androgenic (i.e. have masculinising action) because they are chemically

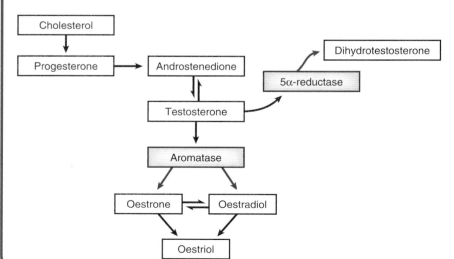

Fig. 5.15 Simplified diagram showing the biosynthesis of the main sex hormones, including key enzymes. (Modified from Aggarwal NR and Wood MJ (2021) Sex differences in cardiac diseases, Fig. 2. St. Louis: Elsevier.)

very similar to testosterone, bind to ARs, and can cause testosterone-related side-effects like acne and hirsutism. Newer synthetic progestogens have less androgenic activity because they do not bind to ARs. There is evidence that synthetic progestogens slightly increase the risk of breast cancer, especially when combined with an oestrogen. The reason for this is not clear, because while some studies show that progesterone stimulates cell division in breast epithelial cells, other studies show inhibition. It is likely to be due to the interaction of several factors, including oestrogen levels, duration of exposure, and the woman's age.

Pharmacokinetics

Progesterone is well absorbed from a range of sites, including the GI tract, but when given orally it distributes rapidly from the bloodstream and is extensively metabolised, with a plasma half-life of only 5 minutes. Peak plasma levels are reached in about 2 hours post-dose, but then fall rapidly, which can compromise contraceptive cover (see below). Progesterone metabolites are mainly excreted by the kidney.

Testosterone

Testosterone is the main androgenic hormone in humans, but it is converted in most tissues to the more active agent dihydrotestosterone. At puberty in the males, it promotes the development of secondary sexual characteristics, e.g. the growth of axillary and pubic hair and deepening of the voice, and maturation of the male sexual organs. It activates genes that produce muscle proteins and increases the bulk and strength of skeletal muscle. It increases libido and physical vigour and promotes sperm production in the testis. At puberty, rising levels of testosterone convert the cartilage growth plates at the ends of long bones to bone tissue, terminating any further increase in height. Testosterone and certain synthetic variants, e.g. **nandrolone** and **trenbolone acetate**, are sometimes used to increase muscle mass and power and athletic performance in professional and amateur sport or for occupational or cosmetic reasons. These agents are called anabolic steroids and can cause significant long-term harm, including infertility, acne, masculinisation in females, and increased risk of prostate cancer.

Pharmacokinetics

Testosterone is well absorbed from a range of sites, and its plasma half-life is very short (10–20 minutes) because it is rapidly metabolised by the liver. Synthetic analogues usually have longer half-lives.

FEMALE REPRODUCTIVE FUNCTION

The female reproductive years begin at puberty, with the development of secondary sexual characteristics and the onset of cyclical ovarian activity essential for fertility. They end at menopause, after which time the ovary stops releasing oocytes and the menstrual cycle ceases. **Oestrogens** and **progestogens** are used therapeutically if the ovarian cycle fails to establish naturally, causing a failure of puberty and primary infertility (infertility in a woman who has never been pregnant). They are used as contraceptives, to initiate and regulate the reproductive cycle in fertility treatment, to reduce the pain and blood loss in heavy menstrual bleeding, and to treat troublesome menopausal symptoms in hormone replacement therapy (HRT).

HORMONAL CONTROL OF THE FEMALE REPRODUCTIVE CYCLE

The ovary contains, matures, and releases the female oocytes, and is the body's main source of oestrogen. In turn, it is regulated by the hypothalamic–pituitary axis (Fig. 5.2). The hypothalamic hormone GnRH stimulates release of two pituitary hormones, FSH and LH. Between them, FSH and LH drive the regular maturation and release of one or more oocytes from the ovary, which in most women occurs roughly once every 28–30 days and is the physiological basis of the female reproductive cycle. Puberty commences when GnRH production from the hypothalamus triggers FSH and LH release from the anterior pituitary, which in turn establishes the ovarian cycle.

The Female Reproductive Cycle

The changing hormone levels and main physiological events of the female reproductive cycle are shown in Fig. 5.16.

Conventionally, the first day of the cycle is taken as the first day of the menstrual period, and bleeding usually lasts for 3–5 days. During this time, in the ovary, one or more follicles, each containing an immature oocyte, begin to develop. This is driven by FSH from the anterior pituitary (Fig. 5.16A). The developing follicle secretes oestrogen, so as it develops and gets bigger, oestrogen levels in the blood steadily rise (Fig. 5.16B). This feeds back onto the anterior pituitary and stimulates it to produce increasing levels of FSH, which sustains and promotes the developing follicle and ensures that oestrogen levels in the first half of the cycle continue to increase. At about the midpoint of the cycle, oestrogen levels become so high that they trigger a surge of LH from the pituitary (Fig. 5.16C). This is the event that stimulates ovulation (Fig. 5.16E): the maturing follicle ruptures and releases the oocyte, which is then usually swept into the uterine (Fallopian) tubes and travels towards the uterus. The oocyte has a brief lifespan of only about 48 hours: if fertilisation does not take place in this time, it dies. Following ovulation, the follicle that released it, now called the corpus luteum, continues to function as an endocrine gland, but its main product now is progesterone (Fig. 5.16D), and oestrogen level remains much lower than that in the first half of the cycle. The combination of circulating oestrogen and progesterone suppress the anterior pituitary, so that FSH and LH levels now begin to fall. This has two main consequences. With low levels of circulating

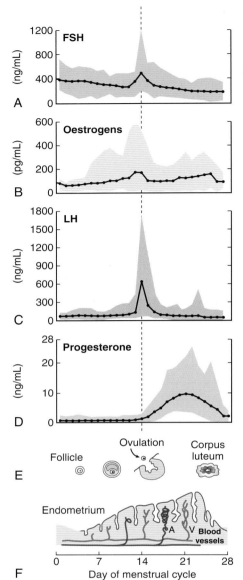

FSH from the anterior pituitary remains high in the first half of the cycle to drive follicle development in ovary but falls in the second half.

Oestrogen from the developing follicle rises steadily in the first half of the cycle and peaks mid-cycle, triggering the LH surge that causes ovulation.

The LH surge mid-cycle initiates ovulation and sustains the corpus luteum in the first part of the second half of the cycle.

Progesterone from the corpus luteum in the second half of the cycle suppresses LH and FSH release from the anterior pituitary, leading after a few days to death of the corpus luteum, falling progesterone and oestrogen levels, and initiating a new cycle.

The developing follicle produces oestrogen in the first half of the cycle. After ovulation, the corpus luteum is the source of rising progesterone and some oestrogen.

The uterine lining thickens under the influence of oestrogen in the first half of the cycle. Progesterone in the second half of the cycle further thickens and vascularises it.

Fig. 5.16 The changing plasma hormone levels and main physiological events of the female reproductive cycle. The solid curves represent mean values and the shaded area shows the maximum and minimum values, i.e. the complete range of values obtained in the experiment. (Modified from Ritter JM, Flower RJ, Henderson G, et al. (2020) Rang & Dale's pharmacology, 8th ed, Fig. 36.2. Oxford: Elsevier.)

FSH, no more follicles begin development in the ovary because there is the possibility of the current cycle ending in pregnancy. LH supports the corpus luteum. In the early stages of the second half of the cycle, while LH levels are still high, the corpus luteum maintains its output of progesterone and oestrogen, required for enriching the uterine lining with blood vessels and glands in preparation for possible implantation of a fertilised ovum (Fig. 5.16F). If there is no pregnancy, falling LH levels because of pituitary suppression by progesterone and oestrogen lead to deterioration and death of the corpus luteum. Progesterone and oestrogen levels therefore also fall, the uterine lining regresses, menstruation starts, the suppression of the anterior pituitary is released, and FSH and LH levels begin to rise again, initiating a new ovarian cycle.

HORMONAL CONTRACEPTION

Oestrogen and progesterone can be used together in a combined contraceptive preparation. Progesterone-only contraceptive preparations are also available.

The Combined Oral Contraceptive

The combination of oestrogen and progesterone in these preparations mimics conditions in the second half of the reproductive cycle: that is, after ovulation, when the corpus luteum is secreting progesterone and oestrogen into the bloodstream, inhibiting FSH and LH release from the pituitary, suppressing development of further follicles and preventing the LH rise that triggers ovulation. This is their main contraceptive action, but they cause other contributory physiological changes, including thickening

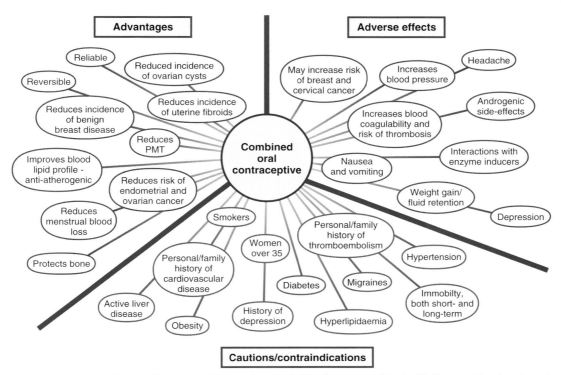

Advantages

Reliable

Reversible

Reduced incidence of ovarian cysts

Reduces incidence of benign breast disease

Reduces incidence of uterine fibroids

Reduces PMT

Improves blood lipid profile - anti-atherogenic

Reduces risk of endometrial and ovarian cancer

Reduces menstrual blood loss

Protects bone

Combined oral contraceptive

Adverse effects

May increase risk of breast and cervical cancer

Increases blood pressure

Headache

Increases blood coagulability and risk of thrombosis

Androgenic side-effects

Nausea and vomiting

Interactions with enzyme inducers

Weight gain/ fluid retention

Depression

Smokers

Personal/family history of thromboembolism

Women over 35

Hypertension

Personal/family history of cardiovascular disease

Diabetes

Migraines

Immobilty, both short- and long-term

Active liver disease

History of depression

Hyperlipidaemia

Obesity

Cautions/contraindications

Fig. 5.17   Key advantages, adverse effects, cautions, and contraindications associated with the combined oral contraceptive.

the mucus plugging the cervical canal, making it harder for sperm to journey from the vagina into the uterus. Generally, the woman takes a daily hormone-containing pill for 21 days and then has 7 pill-free days (sometimes there are seven inactive pills, so that the daily routine of pill-taking is maintained). Patches and vaginal rings that slowly release the hormones into the bloodstream are also available if the woman is unwilling or unable to take a daily pill. The most common oestrogen is **ethinyloestradiol**, either at low dose (20 µg daily) or standard strength (30–35 µg daily), combined with a progestogen. Taken according to manufacturers' instructions, the combined oral contraceptive (COC) is almost 100% effective in preventing pregnancy. Bleeding experienced during each pill-free week is usually lighter with less discomfort or pain than menstruation, and the COC may sometimes be prescribed to treat pre-menstrual tension, reduce excessive menstrual blood loss, or alleviate what can be disabling pain and cramps accompanying the monthly period. The COC reduces the incidence of uterine fibroids, ovarian cysts, and benign breast disease, and fertility usually returns within a few months of withdrawing the drug. Key advantages, disadvantages, cautions, and contraindications relating to the COC are summarised in Fig. 5.17. Note that much of this is also relevant to the use of these hormones in HRT.

Pharmacokinetics

The general pharmacokinetic profiles of the individual hormones are described above. The natural hormone, progesterone, is not used because it is rapidly and extensively metabolised by enzymes in the intestinal lining and in the liver, so its plasma levels are unpredictable and poorly sustained. Synthetic progestogens, first developed in the 1950s, are used instead: examples include **norethisterone**, **desogestrel**, and **gestodene**. An important drug interaction involves increased hormone metabolism by several enzyme inducers. Oestrogen and some progestogens are metabolised in the liver by the cytochrome P450 enzyme family, and drugs that induce cytochrome P450, including some anticonvulsants (e.g. **carbamazepine, phenytoin**), some antimicrobials (e.g. **rifampicin, antiretrovirals, griseofulvin**), and **St. John's wort** enhance hormone clearance and can reduce contraceptive effectiveness. Women should be advised to use an additional method of contraception while taking the interacting drug and for 4 weeks after stopping it.

Adverse Effects

For most women, adverse effects are relatively minor and acceptable when weighed against the prospect of an unwanted pregnancy: commonly they include nausea, mood swings, fluid retention, and a tendency to weight gain. Women prone to migraine may find that this gets worse, and they should be instructed to report any changes in headache frequency or intensity.

Increased Blood Pressure. The COC can increase blood pressure in some women. The risk increases the longer the contraceptive is used and is more likely in women with predisposing factors or pre-existing high blood pressure. The reason behind COC-induced hypertension is not clear, although there are a few possible contributing factors. For example, oestrogen activates the renin-angiotensin system, increasing sodium and water retention, although this is associated mainly with higher-dose oestrogen preparations. It also impairs the anti-thrombotic properties of blood vessel linings. Additionally, progesterone can increase the breakdown of **bradykinin** and other vasodilators. The mechanism is therefore probably multi-factorial, but although COC-induced hypertension is occasionally severe, it is mild to moderate in most women and usually returns to normal once the drug is stopped. Progesterone-only preparations are not associated with a rise in blood pressure.

Androgenic Adverse Effects. These are caused by the synthetic progestogen and can include acne and hirsutism.

Venous Thromboembolism. Both oestrogen and progesterone increase the risk of venous thromboembolism, e.g. deep venous thrombosis and pulmonary embolism. Newer (third-generation) progestogens such as **gestodene** and **desogestrel** are more potent and less androgenic than older progestogens such as **norethisterone** and **levonorgestrel** but have a higher risk of thromboembolism. The risk is highest in the first year of treatment and in women with pre-existing risk factors, e.g. smoking, overweight, and obesity, but are not as high as the increased risk associated with pregnancy. Even though progestogens are pro-thrombotic when used in combination with oestrogen, studies have shown that the progestogen-only oral contraceptive does not carry an increased risk of thromboembolism (although there is evidence that there may be a causative association between injectable progestogens and thrombosis). The reason for this is not clear.

Myocardial Infarction and Stroke. The increased incidence of venous thromboembolism is probably responsible for the slightly increased risk of angina, myocardial infarctions, and stroke seen with the COC. Women with additional cardiovascular risk factors, e.g. increased age, overweight or obesity, smokers, high blood pressure, diabetes, and a personal or family history are particularly at risk and should be carefully assessed before a decision to prescribe COC is made. It may be that a progestogen-only preparation is a better choice in these patients because it does not increase cardiovascular risk.

Neoplasia. The risks of certain cancers (e.g. breast and cervical) may be slightly increased but the risks of endometrial and ovarian cancers are slightly reduced in COC users. Changes in cancer risk are oestrogen-dependent and are not seen with progestogen-only contraceptives.

Progestogen-Only Preparations

Because oral progestogens are so rapidly metabolised and cleared from the blood, it is critical that doses are taken strictly at 24-hour intervals; if a tablet is late or missed, levels become so low that contraceptive cover is compromised. Oral progestogen contraceptives must be taken daily, with no pill-free break as with the COC. These agents may be suitable for women for whom oestrogen-containing preparations are not recommended, e.g. smokers, older women, women with hypertension, or women with cardiovascular risk factors. They are also useful in short-term cover for times when oestrogen might be contra-indicated, e.g. in breast-feeding, periods of immobility, and before and after surgery, when the risk of thrombosis is elevated.

Side-effects include breakthrough bleeding and headaches. Intra-uterine devices impregnated with a progestogen and long-acting progestogen depot injections are also available. Interaction with enzyme-inducing drugs, as described above for the COC, can also reduce contraceptive effectiveness of oral progestogen-only agents and progestogen-only implants, and a barrier method of contraception should additionally be used. **Medroxyprogesterone acetate**, a progestogen used as a depot injection for contraception, is metabolised by a different enzyme family and so is not subject to this form of interaction; no additional contraceptive precautions are needed when used with an enzyme inducer.

HORMONAL CHANGES AT MENOPAUSE

Natural menopause is caused by ovarian failure. It usually occurs between the ages of 45 and 55 years, by which time nearly all the follicles have either matured and ruptured during a reproductive cycle or have degenerated, a fate suffered by more and more follicles as they age. As follicles are lost, oestrogen levels progressively decline, because the ovarian follicles are the main source of oestrogen. Falling oestrogen levels are detected by the hypothalamus and anterior pituitary, which significantly step up GnRH and FSH/LH production in a useless attempt to restore oestrogen production. Low levels of oestrogen and high levels of FSH and LH are characteristic of the early stages of menopause. Post-menopausal women can suffer significantly because of oestrogen deficiency, and HRT is used to alleviate the condition. Removal of the ovaries and ovarian damage, e.g. by irradiation, both induce artificial menopause at any age.

Signs and Symptoms of Oestrogen Deficiency

Oestrogen protects bones, and the skeleton of post-menopausal women becomes lighter and less calcified (osteoporosis), with an increased risk of fracture. The cardioprotective effect of oestrogen is lost, and the rates of ischaemic heart disease in post-menopausal women become equivalent to age-matched men. Reproductive tissues responsive to oestrogen undergo degenerative changes: for example, vaginal dryness is common, and breasts lose their glandular structure, which is replaced with fatty tissue. Hot flushes, sudden and intense rises in body temperature accompanied by flushing and sweating, are very common and range from mild, occasional events to hourly, disabling episodes associated with significant anxiety and distress. The cause of hot flushes is not fully understood, but it is believed that abnormal blood vessel structure and responsiveness is involved. For example, the severity of hot flushes correlates with evidence for subclinical cardiovascular disease, e.g. calcification of the aorta and thickening of blood vessel walls. Another contributory factor may be abnormal hypothalamic function. The hypothalamus contains the body's temperature regulation centre, and hot flushes may be due to sudden and inappropriate hypothalamic activation of heat loss mechanisms. Other unpleasant effects of diminished oestrogen include decreased libido, changes in sleep patterns, problems with concentration, mood swings, weight gain, and depression.

Focus on: Hormone Replacement Therapy

A significant minority of women experience such severe symptoms at menopause that they seek medical advice. Hormone replacement therapy (HRT) was first offered in the 1960s, and its popularity and use has oscillated ever since, reflecting episodes of bad publicity associating it with increased risks of premature death, cardiovascular disease, and cancer. Its benefits in terms of reversing the symptoms of oestrogen deficiency and improving quality of life, including maintaining bone health, eliminating hot flushes, and preventing the emotional and cognitive effects seen in menopause, are well established and not in dispute: HRT has made an enormous difference to the lives of countless menopausal women. Current evidence suggests that although HRT is associated with increased risk of certain cancers, it does not cause premature death. The risks and benefits of HRT vary depending on the age of the woman, time since menopause, mode of administration, dosage, and treatment regime, and so should be assessed for each individual woman. The important points are summarised below.

Hormone Replacement Therapy and Cancer

In its early days, HRT was offered as oestrogen-only supplements, but within a decade it became clear that this increased the risk of endometrial cancer. Introducing a progestogen into the preparation actually reduces the risk of endometrial cancer, although it is now recognised that combined preparations increase the risk of breast cancer. In women without a uterus, consequently for whom endometrial cancer is not a concern, oestrogen-only preparations may be appropriate. The increased risk for breast cancer is generally accepted to be slight and may be less than other risk factors, e.g. obesity and high alcohol intake. The excess risk disappears within 5 years of stopping treatment. HRT also slightly increases the risk of ovarian cancer, although the excess risk disappears within 5 years of stopping treatment.

Hormone Replacement Therapy and Cardiovascular Disease

Early studies suggested that HRT increased the risk of cardiovascular disease and its consequences, including stroke and myocardial infarction. Recognition of sources of error in these studies and results of newer studies have reversed this perception, and there is increasing evidence that HRT is cardioprotective, reducing the risks of heart disease, thromboembolism, and stroke, likely more marked in younger women, those within 10 years of menopause, and those without pre-existing cardiovascular risk factors.

Hormone Replacement Therapy and Thromboembolism

HRT increases the coagulability of blood and so increases the risk of thromboembolism, especially in the first year of use and in women with pre-existing risk factors such as smoking, diabetes, and overweight/obesity. This risk may be less when oestrogen is delivered by transdermal patches rather than orally. Progesterone formulation may also be important: evidence shows that micronised progesterone carries less risk for thromboembolism than synthetic progestogens. Micronised progesterone is derived from plants but is chemically identical to the human hormone and formulated as tiny particles that are absorbed more efficiently than synthetic progestogens, improving its bioavailability.

Hormone Replacement Therapy and Bone Health

HRT consistently reduces bone loss, increases bone mineral density, and reduces the risk of fracture. This protective effect persists for a variable length of time after cessation of treatment, depending on the length of treatment: the longer the treatment time, the more extended the protection after stopping.

HORMONAL TREATMENT OF FEMALE INFERTILITY

Female infertility is sometimes due to anatomical abnormalities, e.g. inflammation, fibrosis, and obstruction somewhere in the tract by conditions including endometriosis and pelvic inflammatory disease, or by fibroids or malignancy. Infertility may also be secondary to hypothalamic, pituitary, or ovarian failure, associated for example with polycystic ovary disease or congenital failure of ovarian development, in which case the normal cyclical release of hormones essential for follicular development, ovulation, and preparation of the uterine lining is disrupted or absent. Pharmacological interventions to restore fertility include treatment with **FSH** and **oestrogen** to stimulate follicular development and ovulation. In women whose hypothalamus is failing to secrete GnRH, an infusion pump to administer **GnRH** in pulses, mimicking natural release patterns, can be used; the exogenous GnRH stimulates FSH and LH from the pituitary, initiating ovarian activity.

Clomifene

Clomifene binds to and blocks oestrogen receptors in the anterior pituitary and hypothalamus (Fig. 5.18). Unable to detect the presence of oestrogen in the blood, the hypothalamus and pituitary hugely increase GnRH, FSH, and LH output. This massively stimulates the ovaries, initiating follicular development, oestrogen secretion, and ovulation. The likelihood of multiple pregnancies is increased with clomifene treatment. It is not recommended for more than six cycles because its stimulatory action on the ovary has been associated with increased risk of ovarian cancer.

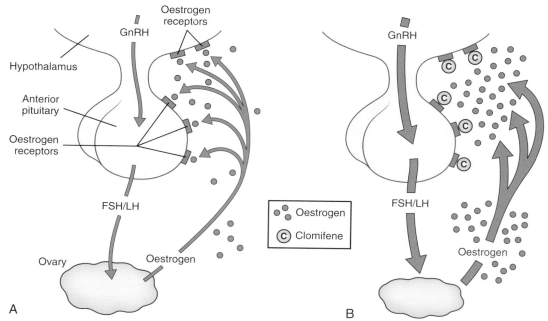

Fig. 5.18 The mechanism of action of clomifene. A. The ovary secretes oestrogen in response to follicle-stimulating hormone (FSH) and luteinising hormone (LH) from the anterior pituitary. The hypothalamus and anterior pituitary have oestrogen receptors to allow them to continually measure blood oestrogen levels and adjust their own hormone output accordingly. B. In the presence of clomifene, oestrogen receptors are blocked and the anterior pituitary and hypothalamus can no longer detect oestrogen in the blood. They therefore increase gonadotropin-releasing hormone (GnRH), FSH, and LH output, causing massive ovarian stimulation.

MALE REPRODUCTIVE FUNCTION

Unlike in females, male fertility is not cyclical, and once established at puberty can often be maintained well into old age. The principal androgen, testosterone, is used to stimulate testicular development and initiate puberty in testosterone-deficient males and to treat some hormone-responsive breast cancers in women, because testosterone has anti-oestrogenic properties in the breast.

Anti-Androgens

Examples: cyproterone acetate, flutamide, bicalutamide

Anti-androgens, drugs that block testosterone receptors, are used in testosterone-related disorders. These include prostatic hyperplasia and prostate cancer, early (precocious) puberty in young boys, and hair loss. They are used in the management of hypersexuality and compulsive sexual behaviours, which can be highly disruptive to normal life, cause significant distress and anxiety in the affected male, and contribute to unacceptable, risky, or deviant behaviours. By directly reducing testosterone action, they reduce libido and diminish sexual activity. They are also used in the treatment of a range of cancers in both men and women, although legislation varies in different countries and much work in this area is in its early stages. Some anti-androgenic agents have shown efficacy in some triple-negative breast cancers—i.e. breast cancers that do not express oestrogen, progesterone, or HER2 receptors and for which anti-oestrogen, anti-progesterone, or anti-HER2

agents are of no use. Triple-negative disease can be difficult to treat, but a subset of these cancers express androgen receptors, and initial studies suggest that they may respond to anti-androgens. Likewise, a proportion of ovarian cancers express ARs, and early clinical trials have confirmed that **enzalutamide** may be an effective treatment in some of these patients.

REFERENCES

Deacon, C.F., Lebovitz, H.E., 2015. Comparative review of dipeptidyl peptidase-4 inhibitors and sulphonylureas. Diabetes Obes. Metab 18 (4), 333–347.
Grisham, R., Giri, D., Henson, M., et al., 2019. 38 Phase II study of enzalutamide in androgen receptor positive (AR+) recurrent ovarian cancer: final results. Int. J. Gynecol. Cancer 29, A23.
Newson, L.R., 2016. Best practice for HRT: unpicking the evidence. Br. J. Gen. Pract 66 (653), 597–598.
Sola, D., Rossi, L., Schianca, G.P.C., et al., 2015. Sulfonylureas and their use in clinical practice. Arch. Med. Sci 4, 840–848.

ONLINE RESOURCES

Cagnacci, A., Venier, M., 2019. The controversial history of hormone replacement therapy. Medicina (Kaunas) 55 (9), 602. Available at: https://doi.org/10.3390/medicina55090602.
Collaborative Group on Hormonal Factors in Breast Cancer, 2019. Type and timing of menopausal hormone therapy and breast cancer risk: individual participant meta-analysis of the worldwide epidemiological evidence. Lancet 394 (10204), 1159–1168. Available at: https://doi.org/10.1016/S0140-6736(19)31709-X.
White, J.R., 2014. A brief history of the development of diabetes medications. Diabetes Spectr 27 (2), 82–86. Available at: https://doi.org/10.2337/diaspect.27.2.82.

Analgesics and Anti-Inflammatory Drugs

6

THE PHYSIOLOGY OF PAIN

From a survival point of view, pain is an important protective mechanism that informs us of disease and injury and encourages us to seek appropriate help, to avoid situations that may make the pain worse, and to protect damaged body parts while they heal. Pain is a complex phenomenon, heavily influenced by psychological, emotional, social, cultural, and cognitive factors. However, for most people it is a strongly negative experience, and the global market for drugs that relieve pain (analgesics) runs into tens of billions of pounds.

DEFINITION AND CLASSIFICATION OF PAIN

In 2020, the International Association for the Study of Pain (IASP) defined pain as 'an unpleasant sensory and emotional experience associated with or resembling that associated with actual or potential tissue damage'. Acute pain tends to start suddenly, is associated with and appropriate to a clearly defined cause, such as post-operative pain or the pain of a sprained ankle, and resolves when the injury heals. Chronic pain is pain that lasts for 3 or more months. The IASP considers chronic pain in two categories: chronic primary pain, which is pain not clearly accounted for by another disease state (for example, non-specific musculoskeletal pain), and chronic secondary pain, where the pain is directly caused

by an underlying condition (such as cancer or rheumatoid arthritis).

KEY DEFINITIONS

- Nociceptive pain:
  pain caused by stimulation of pain receptors (nociceptors) in the tissues, by physical damage, and/or by inflammatory mediators
- Neuropathic (neurogenic) pain:
  pain caused by damage to the nervous tissue
- Analgesia:
  reduction or loss of the sensation of pain. An analgesic drug reduces or abolishes pain.
- Hyperalgesia:
  abnormally increased pain response to painful stimuli
- Allodynia:
  a pain response to a stimulus that should not normally be painful, e.g. light touch

PAIN PATHWAYS AND PAIN SIGNALLING

Pain signals from injured peripheral tissues travel along a chain of sensory nerves up the spinal cord to key areas in the brain responsible for the perception, processing, and

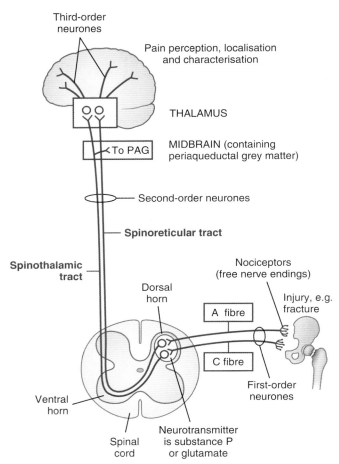

Fig. 6.1 Ascending pain pathways. First-order neurones carrying pain signals synapse in the dorsal horn of the spinal cord with second-order neurones. Second-order neurones travel via the spinothalamic and the spinoreticular tracts to the thalamus and synapse with third-order neurones. PAG, Periaqueductal grey matter.

modulation of pain (Fig. 6.1), and they activate nerve pathways that control the body's response. These nerves communicate using several neurotransmitters, including endogenous **opioids**, **noradrenaline**, gamma-amino butyric acid (**GABA**), **serotonin** (5-HT), and **substance P**. In the context of pain management, this is important because it means that there are multiple sites where a pain signal can potentially be interrupted or modified. Sensory receptors in the tissues that detect painful stimuli are called nociceptors. Nociceptors are unmyelinated free nerve endings, and the pain signals generated when they are activated are transmitted to the spinal cord by sensory nerves called first-order neurones or primary afferents. There are two main types of first-order neurones: Aδ (A-delta) and C fibres. Aδ fibres are larger than C fibres and are myelinated; hence, they have fast conduction speeds and carry the initial, sharp, 'fast' sensation of pain – for example, the acute, stabbing pain immediately following a skin cut. They respond to mechanical and thermal stimuli. C fibres are small and non-myelinated, and transmit slow, dull, burning, chronic pain – for example, the throbbing, duller, persistent pain following the acute pain of a skin cut. C fibres respond to a range of noxious stimuli including mechanical, thermal, and chemical input. Chemical stimulation of nociceptors may be due to

exposure to corrosive substances including acids or alkalis and a wide range of inflammatory mediators released following tissue damage.

The axons of the first-order neurones enter the dorsal horn of the spinal cord and synapse with the second sensory nerve of the pain pathway, called the second-order neurone. The neurotransmitter here is usually substance P or glutamate. Second-order neurones cross to the opposite side of the spinal cord and from the dorsal to the ventral horn and carry pain signals to the thalamus in one of two main pathways (tracts): the spinothalamic tract or the spinoreticular tract. In the midbrain, neurones from the spinothalamic tract project to the periaqueductal grey matter (PAG), a region important in descending inhibition. In the thalamus, the second-order neurones synapse with third-order neurones, which project to a range of brain centres involved in pain perception and processing. Some third-order neurones project to the limbic system, which determines the emotional response to pain. Others project to the somatosensory cortex, which localises the pain and interprets its intensity and characteristics. Other centres in the cerebral cortex evaluate the pain in terms of previous experience and expectations, which in turn help to determine the response to pain.

CENTRAL MODULATION OF PAIN SIGNALS

In 1965, Melzack and Wall published a seminal paper in pain theory. They suggested that pain signal transmission from one nerve in the pain pathway to the next could be suppressed by other nerves acting at these synapses, and that input from larger nerves is given priority over input from smaller nerves. The analogy that this acts like a gate, which prevents pain transmission when closed, gave rise to what is called the gate control theory. It explains why rubbing a bumped head helps the pain: the pain signals transmitted to the spinal cord along medium-sized Aδ and small C fibres are blocked out by the mechanical stimulation of rubbing the area, which transmits sensory information along much larger Aβ fibres. It is now known that there are multiple sites in the pain pathways of the central nervous system (CNS) where internal mechanisms may reduce, block, or sometimes enhance a pain signal. The capacity of the CNS to block pain sensation has an obvious protective function: pain can be an overwhelming experience that demands full attention, which may prevent an individual from escaping a dangerous situation or making other potentially critical decisions. One important pain control mechanism operates in the spinal cord: descending inhibition.

Descending Inhibition

The key brain area that controls descending inhibition is the PAG, a region in the midbrain surrounding the central aqueduct, which links the third and fourth ventricles. In the 1960s, research showed that electrical stimulation of the PAG during surgery in rats produced complete analgesia and the animals showed no signs of being in pain, and although it is now known that the PAG has a range of other functions including vocalisation and emotional responses, most investigation has focussed on its role in pain inhibition. Nerve pathways extending from the PAG travel down through the medulla, descend in the spinal cord, and synapse in the dorsal horn at the synapse between the first- and second-order neurones in the pain pathway (Fig. 6.2). These descending pathways are activated when ascending pain signals travel

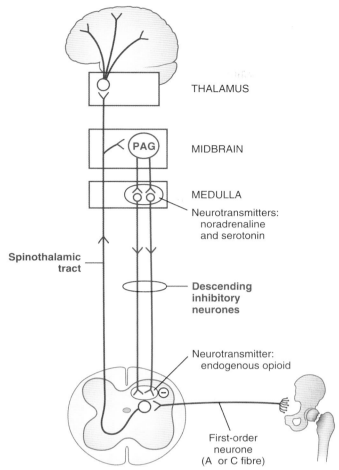

Fig. 6.2 Descending inhibition in the dorsal horn of the spinal cord. Ascending pain signals in the second-order neurones of the pain pathway travel to the periaqueductal grey matter (PAG) in the midbrain. This activates inhibitory descending nerves, which block the release of the neurotransmitter responsible for transmitting the pain signal between the first- and second-order neurones in the dorsal horn.

(Figure labels: THALAMUS; MIDBRAIN; PAG; MEDULLA; Neurotransmitters: noradrenaline and serotonin; Spinothalamic tract; Descending inhibitory neurones; Neurotransmitter: endogenous opioid; First-order neurone (A or C fibre))

up the spinothalamic tract and signal to the PAG, and they are inhibitory. When they fire, they inhibit the release of substance P or glutamate, and therefore, block transmission of pain signals between the first- and second-order pain neurones in the dorsal horn.

These inhibitory pathways use three main neurotransmitters: endogenous opioids acting on mu (μ) opioid receptors (MORs), serotonin acting on 5-HT receptors, and noradrenaline acting on α-adrenoceptors. All of these are important targets for analgesic drugs. Opioids like **morphine** are μ receptor agonists and so directly activate MORs on nerves in the pathway. Tricyclic antidepressants like **amitriptyline** block the reuptake of noradrenaline and serotonin from synapses, increasing their concentration there, prolonging their activity and the inhibition of the pain signals. The analgesic action of **gabapentin** and similar drugs is not fully understood but is thought to be partly due to enhancement of the action of serotonin in the descending pathways. Other mechanisms, including higher centres of the brain and other sensory input, may activate the PAG, meaning that the experience of pain can be significantly altered by distraction, emotional states, or prior experience.

SENSITISATION IN PAIN PATHWAYS

Sensitisation is increased sensitivity of pain nerves to sensory stimuli and occurs both in the peripheral nervous system (PNS) (peripheral sensitisation) and the CNS (central sensitisation). Peripheral sensitisation is part of the normal response to acute injury: reducing the activation threshold of nociceptors makes them more sensitive to stimuli and increases awareness of the injury and makes it harder to ignore. Peripheral sensitisation causes the increased tenderness of injured tissues; this encourages us to protect the damaged area while it heals.

In chronic pain of either nociceptive or neuropathic origin, functional and physical changes occur in pain pathways, which alter the processing and response to pain. The World Health Organisation considers chronic pain as a disease state, and effective treatment presents particular challenges. Chronic pain is associated with central sensitisation, in which pain pathways in the CNS become increasingly sensitive, leading to hyperalgesia. In addition, this dysfunctional response may also cause allodynia, the sensation of pain in response to harmless stimuli. Because central pathways are affected, the hyperalgesia can be widespread and affect body parts not involved in the principal disease process, leading to generalised pain.

OPIOIDS

KEY DEFINITIONS

- Opium:
  the juice extracted from the seed head of the opium poppy *Papaver somniferum* (in Greek: 'poppy that brings sleep')
- Opiates:
  the naturally occurring (endogenous) opioids in opium, including morphine and thebaine
- Opioid:
  any agent with opiate-like activity, including endogenous opioids, substances naturally occurring in opium, and all synthetic and semisynthetic agents, e.g. diamorphine, fentanyl

Cave paintings, clay tablets, and other artefacts from a range of ancient civilisations indicate that humankind has used opium for at least 5000 years, both for recreational and medicinal purposes. Opium contains several pharmacologically active agents including **morphine**, **thebaine**, and **papaverine**. Thebaine is too toxic to be given in its natural form but is used to synthesise certain opioid drugs including **oxycodone**, **buprenorphine**, and **naloxone**. Opioids are used in modern medicine for a range of purposes, but most significantly as analgesics: they are potent pain relievers, so effective in fact that despite their potentially lethal side-effects, they are still the first-line agents in the management of moderate to severe pain.

The active opiate content of crude opium is highly variable depending on the conditions under which the poppy was grown, leading to significant variation in the potency and activity of different opium batches. At the beginning of the 19th century, opium was widely available and sold over the counter to the general public in a range of formulations including lozenges, tablets, and tinctures (a drug dissolved in alcohol). Other than the obvious dangers of such a dangerous preparation being freely available with no restriction or regulation, the potency of these formulations could not be controlled or predicted. In 1803, **morphine** was purified from opium by a German apothecary called Friedrich Sertürner. This meant that dosages could be accurately quantified, which in theory should improve safety. Commercial morphine production began in earnest in the 1820s, and when the hypodermic needle was invented in the 1850s, the popularity of purified morphine skyrocketed. Although it provided previously unsurpassed benefits for physicians managing their patients' pain, it also led to widespread addiction in all strata of society with associated criminality and major family and societal problems. In response to the growing awareness of such negative opioid-related repercussions, in 1912, several countries including the US, Russia, and the UK signed the International Opium Convention. It was the first attempt to control the distribution, manufacture, and sale of opioids, and in modern times most global countries have regulatory legislation around their use.

Opioid Receptors

There are three main types of opioid receptors in the CNS and PNS: μ (mu), δ (delta), and ϰ (kappa), called MOR, DOR, and KOR, respectively. The brain, peripheral nerves, and some other body tissues produce a family of endogenous opioids, the **endorphins** and **enkephalins**, which act on opioid receptors and provide the body's internal pain management system. When the endogenous opioids were discovered in the 1970s, it was realised that the opium preparations that mankind had been using as analgesics for thousands of years worked by mimicking the action of the endogenous opioids and activating internal analgesia mechanisms. In terms of pain relief and most other clinically observed opioid effects, MOR is the most important opioid receptor type, and the endogenous opioids and clinically useful opioid analgesics are all agonists here. However, the KOR and DOR also play a role in analgesia, and the overall effect of an opioid, including its adverse effects, are produced by the drug interacting with all three receptor types.

MOR Distribution

MORs are found in high concentrations in pain pathways in the CNS, including in the dorsal horn of the spinal cord,

as well as brain regions involved in emotion, mood, feeding, hormonal control, respiration, and immune function. They are also found on peripheral sensory nerves, where they inhibit pain signals. Opioid action here contributes to their analgesic effect. Ongoing research is directed towards developing opioids that do not cross the blood–brain barrier and so would be free of central adverse effects like dependence and respiratory depression, but which could provide effective analgesia via this peripheral activity. MORs are also present on nerves in the gastrointestinal system, where they reduce motility and secretion. Additionally, MORs are found in non-neural tissue, including joint tissues, immune cells, and endocrine cells.

MOR Signalling

All opioid receptors are linked to inhibitory G-proteins (G_i) and inhibit adenylyl cyclase (see p. 32 and Fig. 3.7). When an opioid agonist binds to its receptor on a nerve cell membrane and activates this signalling pathway, potassium channels open, allowing potassium to enter the cell. This desensitises (hyperpolarises) the nerve and makes it less likely to fire. In addition, calcium channels are closed, preventing calcium from entering; calcium entry into nerve cells is needed for activation. By interfering with the movement of these two key ions across the nerve cell membrane, opioids prevent the nerve from releasing its transmitter, dampen neuronal transmission, and block synaptic communication (Fig. 6.3). This is reflected in the key effects of opioids including blockade of pain signals, sedation, inhibition of smooth muscle contraction, and respiratory depression.

ACTIONS OF OPIOIDS

Opioids produce a range of physiological effects via their action on opioid receptors.

Analgesia

Opioids produce effective analgesia mainly through their action on MORs in both the CNS and PNS, particularly in nociceptive pain; they are of limited use in neuropathic pain. They reduce neuronal excitability and transmitter release in pain pathways, including in the mechanism of descending

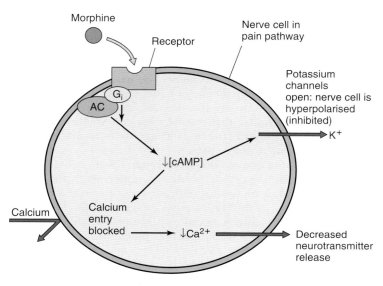

Fig. 6.3 Morphine receptor signalling and inhibition of neurotransmitter release. (Modified from Minneman KP and Wecker L (2005) Brody's human pharmacology: molecular to clinical, 4th ed. St. Louis: Mosby.)

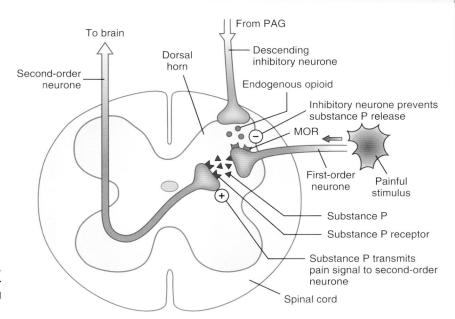

Fig. 6.4 Opioid inhibition of pain signal transmission between the first- and second-order neurone in the spinal cord. MOR, Mu opioid receptor; PAG, periaqueductal grey matter.

inhibition (Fig. 6.4). Fig. 6.4 shows the synapse in the dorsal horn between the first- and second-order pain neurones in more detail. Incoming pain signals activate this synapse; the excitatory neurotransmitter here is usually substance P or glutamate, which depolarises the second-order neurone and transmits the pain signal up the spinal cord towards the brain. The descending nerve from the PAG synapses here and releases endogenous opioid, which acts on MORs on the first-order nerve ending. This inhibits release of its excitatory transmitter and blocks transmission of the pain signal between the first- and second-order neurones. Opioid drugs mimic the action of the endogenous opioid transmitter by binding directly to the MORs.

Opioids usually induce a profound sense of well-being, relaxation, and deep contentment, and produce a sensation of dissociation from pain; this euphoric effect is often beneficial in pain relief.

Sedation

Opioids sedate and may induce sleep by inhibiting central pathways responsible for arousal and wakefulness. This may worsen their respiratory depressant effect but can be clinically useful because it may relieve distress and anxiety. Alternatively, sedation may be unwanted: for example, it may limit activities of daily living for people using opioids to manage chronic pain.

Respiratory Depression

Neurones in the respiratory centre in the brainstem are normally very sensitive to even slight increases in carbon dioxide levels and respond by increasing respiratory rate and depth of breathing. Opioids depress this response, allow carbon dioxide levels to rise, and produce hypoventilation, hypercarbia (high blood carbon dioxide levels), apnoea, reduced respiratory rate, and potentially respiratory arrest. Opioid-induced respiratory depression is more marked and therefore most dangerous when brain activity levels are suppressed, e.g. in sleep, in anaesthesia, or in the presence of other central depressants like **alcohol** or **benzodiazepines**.

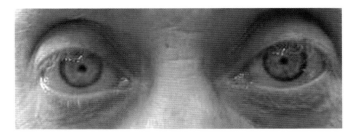

Fig. 6.5 Opioid-induced miosis. (From Stern TA, Fava M, Wilens TE, et al. (2018) Massachusetts General Hospital. Tratado de psiquiatría clínica, 2nd ed. Madrid: Elsevier Spain.)

Habitual opioid use leads to a developing tolerance, but respiratory arrest is still the most common cause of death in opioid overdose.

Miosis

Opioids act directly on the oculomotor nerve (cranial nerve III), which controls the muscle of the iris of the eye and therefore pupil diameter. They constrict the circular muscle in the iris and reduce the size of the pupils (miosis). In overdose, pupil size may be pinpoint (Fig. 6.5).

Nausea and Vomiting

Opioids directly stimulate MORs in the chemosensitive trigger zone (CTZ), located in the medulla of the brain. The CTZ has an important protective function: it contains specialised receptors that detect potentially toxic substances in the cerebrospinal fluid, and because it lies outside the blood–brain barrier, blood-borne toxins as well. Stimulation of the CTZ triggers the vomiting centre in the brain and elicits the vomiting reflex. Opioids also reduce GI motility, which contributes to nausea and vomiting. Up to 40% of individuals experience nausea following opioid administration, and a significant number actively vomit. Pre-treatment or concurrent treatment with an anti-emetic, e.g. **cyclizine** or **ondansetron**, can prevent this.

Gastrointestinal Effects

The walls of the GI tract contain extensive networks of nerves (the enteric nervous system) which regulate its function. Enteric nerves release a range of neurotransmitters, including endogenous opioids, which act on MORs in GI smooth muscle to reduce motility and secretions and increase sphincter tone. Administered opioids also act on these MORs and therefore slow gastric emptying, which can significantly delay the delivery of swallowed medication into the duodenum and delay absorption. Constipation is a common and very troublesome adverse effect of opioids. However, due to their ability to put GI smooth muscle into stasis, opioids have been used for thousands of years to treat diarrhoea. **Loperamide** is a MOR agonist used by mouth for this purpose. It is poorly absorbed, so its action is largely restricted to the GI tract, and it does not cross the blood–brain barrier in high enough concentrations to produce central effects. Other GI consequences of opioid use include bloating, abdominal distension and discomfort, and sometimes gastro-oesophageal reflux. Tolerance tends not to develop to GI side-effects, which persist during treatment, a particular challenge when opioids are used to manage chronic pain. In addition to non-specific management (e.g. high-fibre diets, good fluid intake, and laxatives), opioid-induced constipation can be treated with **methylnaltrexone bromide**, an opioid receptor antagonist that does not cross the blood–brain barrier; it therefore blocks peripheral receptors, including those in the GI tract, without interfering with the central analgesic action.

Cough Suppression

Opioids suppress cough, i.e. they have an antitussive action, but the mechanism by which they do this is not completely clear. They inhibit central neurones involved in cough pathways, but there is probably also a peripheral component: for example, they may decrease the sensitivity of sensory nerves in the airways and reduce their response to irritants. For example, nebulised **diamorphine** is used to relieve persistent cough in bronchial carcinoma. The antitussive action of opioids does not correlate with their analgesic effect, so that even weak opioid analgesics like **codeine** effectively suppress cough.

Immunosuppression

The interaction between opioids and immunity is complex and our understanding is quite incomplete. There is substantial evidence that opioids, especially in long-term use, are immunosuppressant, and may increase the risk of infection. Opioids act on MORs on the cell membrane of a range of important immune cells, including T-cells, B-cells, and macrophages, and suppress their activity. Immune cells themselves release opioids, leading to some researchers speculating that activation of the body's immune system may also switch on an analgesic effect, which may offer another possible target in designing new analgesic drugs. Opioids have no anti-inflammatory effect; in fact, **morphine** triggers histamine release from mast cells, which can cause itch and sufficient vasodilation to cause a drop in blood pressure.

Tolerance

Tolerance (and dependence) to opioids develops because continual exposure to the drug changes the response of the receptors and reduces drug action. This means that the drug dose must be increased to maintain its effect. Tolerance develops very slowly to GI effects and to miosis, whereas it develops quickly to opioid-induced respiratory depression, euphoria, emesis, and analgesia, especially if the drug is used intravenously. This means that habitual opioid users may require 50 times the standard dose to achieve a desired euphoric effect without obvious respiratory depression, but still experience significant constipation and pupillary constriction. Several mechanisms by which tolerance develops have been identified. One way involves the uncoupling of the receptor from its signalling pathways, like cutting through the wire of a doorbell; the drug binds to its receptor but cannot produce an effect inside the cell because the receptor is no longer connected to its transduction pathways. Other tolerance mechanisms include increased activation of excitatory nerve pathways to oppose the inhibitory action of the opioids. There is a degree of cross-tolerance between clinically used opioids, and switching between different agents when tolerance becomes a problem with one can help to maintain their usefulness.

Addiction and Dependence

Opioids are strongly associated with the development of addiction, the inability to stop using a substance. Historically, opioid addiction has fuelled major social and economic issues, and a current global opioid addiction epidemic is causing significant health and social problems. Pleasurable and addictive behaviours are self-reinforcing because they activate reward centres of the brain, particularly in an interconnected circuit called the mesocorticolimbic pathway, which connects several brain areas involved in motivation, reinforcement, and reward (p. 40). A range of pleasurable activities can stimulate these reward pathways, including sexual behaviour, eating enjoyable foods, and taking any of a wide range of recreational and lifestyle drugs including **alcohol** and **nicotine**. This creates self-reinforcing loops that motivate an individual to repeat the pleasurable behaviour. The key transmitter in these pathways is **dopamine**, sometimes called the 'pleasure hormone' because of its role in reward pathways and in the development of dependence and addiction. Opioids markedly increase dopamine release in these pathways and thus reinforce the desire to persist with opioid consumption. Regular use of opioids over even a few weeks causes adaptive changes in these dopamine pathways, which become dependent upon the new, higher levels of dopamine and do not function adequately without them. If dopamine levels begin to fall because opioid levels fall, the individual experiences a range of well-defined and highly unpleasant withdrawal symptoms, which motivates them to take more opioids and restore dopamine levels. Opioid withdrawal causes sweating, tremor, anxiety, anorexia, insomnia, diarrhoea, and goosebumps, caused by contraction of the piloerector muscles controlling the tiny hairs of the skin: this is the origin of the phrase 'going cold turkey' to indicate someone undergoing withdrawal.

THE MAIN OPIOIDS

Morphine is the gold-standard analgesic to which new analgesic drugs are compared during clinical trials, but a range of synthetic and semi-synthetic agents have been developed to improve efficacy and reduce adverse effects. Synthetic drugs, e.g. **fentanyl** and **pethidine**, may have significantly different chemical structures than morphine, accounting for clinically different adverse effects and routes of metabolism (Fig. 6.6).

Uses of Opioids

Opioids are extensively used as analgesics in both acute and chronic pain, usually for moderate to severe pain of nociceptive origin. Other uses include:

- relief of persistent cough, e.g. in bronchial carcinoma

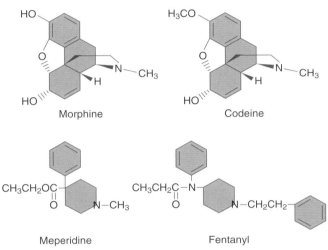

Fig. 6.6 The chemical structures of synthetic drugs with opioid activity, e.g. fentanyl and pethidine, are different from naturally occurring opioids, e.g. morphine and codeine. (From Hemmings H and Egan T (2019) Pharmacology and physiology for anesthesia, 2nd ed, Fig. 17.1. Philadelphia: Elsevier.)

- relief of dyspnoea, e.g. in heart failure and pulmonary oedema
- pre-medication, to relieve anxiety, sedate, and provide analgesia
- treatment of diarrhoea

Morphine

Crude opium usually contains between 9% and 15% morphine, and global supplies of the drug still rely on extracting it from the poppy seed head because all attempts to synthesise it have failed.

Pharmacokinetics

Morphine is usually given orally, intravenously, rectally, or intrathecally. Absorption from intramuscular sites can be slow and unpredictable, and so this is usually not the route of choice. It has a half-life of 4–6 h and is available in modified release preparations to extend its duration of action. Morphine is subject to significant first-pass metabolism, so care is needed in patients with liver impairment in whom the drug effect can be significantly enhanced. The metabolism of the main opioids, showing morphine as the main agent, is shown in Fig. 6.7. Opioid metabolism produces several metabolites, including **codeine** and active metabolites such as normorphine, dihydrocodeine, and morphine-6-glucuronide, which contribute significantly to morphine's clinical effects.

Diamorphine (Heroin)

This semi-synthetic derivative of morphine was first synthesised in 1874. It is more potent and more lipid-soluble than morphine and is not licensed for medical use in many countries because of its significant abuse potential. Reflecting the lack of legislation at the time around drug regulation and marketing, it was advertised initially by the drug company Bayer under the trade name **Heroin** as a treatment for

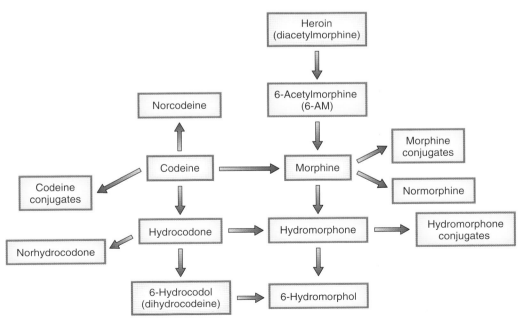

Fig. 6.7 **Metabolism of the main opioids.** (From Dasgupta A and Sepulveda JL (2013) Accurate results in the clinical laboratory, Fig. 15.1. San Diego: Elsevier.)

a range of conditions including respiratory and cardiovascular disorders (Fig. 6.8) and was available for public purchase. It was also recommended as a safer, non-addictive alternative to morphine even though it is neither.

Pharmacokinetics

Diamorphine is a pro-drug and metabolised to **morphine** in the liver (Fig. 6.7). Given orally, it is subject to very high first-pass hepatic metabolism and almost completely converted to morphine; it is therefore not given by mouth. Given by injection, its increased lipid solubility means it rapidly crosses the blood–brain barrier, where it is converted to morphine in brain tissues. Because it has no intrinsic action of its own, but its increased solubility enhances its entry into the CNS, diamorphine is sometimes referred to as a morphine delivery agent. This rapid uptake by the CNS gives heroin a faster and more potent onset of action, one reason for its widespread illicit use. It can also be given intranasally, subcutaneously, and by inhalation. Recreational users may smoke or inhale ('snort') it.

Codeine

Codeine is used to relieve mild to moderate pain, as a cough suppressant, and to treat diarrhoea.

Pharmacokinetics

Codeine is given orally and is well absorbed from the GI tract. It is a pro-drug and relies upon metabolism by the hepatic CYP2D6 enzyme to convert it to **morphine** for its activity. Only around 10% undergoes conversion to morphine, the reason why it is a less potent analgesic, although it is an effective cough suppressant and causes significant constipation. It is generally well tolerated, although genetic variations in CYP2D6 activity affects its metabolism to morphine. In rapid and ultra-rapid metabolisers, rapid conversion of codeine to morphine can worsen opioid adverse effects such as respiratory depression, whereas in poor metabolisers, the therapeutic effects of the drug can be delayed and reduced (Fig. 6.9; see also Pharmacogenomics, p. 3).

Fentanyl

Fentanyl is a synthetic opioid structurally similar to **pethidine** (Fig. 6.6), with potent MOR agonist activity. It was first produced in 1960 by Janssen and is currently in widespread use globally to manage severe pain in various clinical settings including cancer and acute post-surgical pain. It is around 100 times more potent as an analgesic than morphine. Although it produces the typical range of opioid-induced adverse effects including respiratory depression and constipation, it is

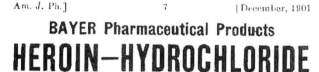

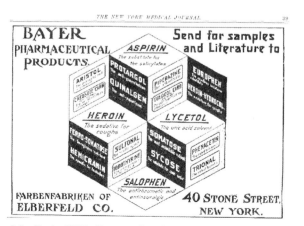

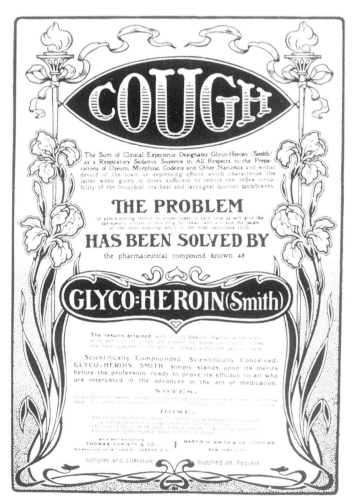

Fig. 6.8   Early 1900s Bayer advertisement for heroin. (From Koob GF, Arends MA, and le Moal M (2015) Drugs, addiction, and the brain, Fig. 5.3. San Diego: Academic Press.)

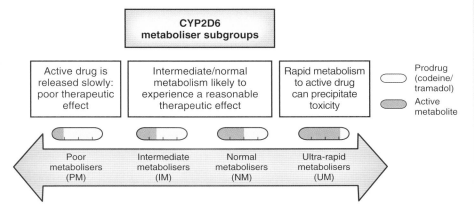

Fig. 6.9 The impact of metabolism on activation of the pro-drugs codeine and tramadol. Poor metabolisers activate the drugs slowly, and analgesia may be slow or incomplete. Fast metabolisers activate the drugs quickly, which can cause toxicity. (Modified from Magarbeh L, Gorbovskaya I, le Foll B, et al. (2021) Reviewing pharmacogenetics to advance precision medicine for opioids. *Biomedicine & Pharmacotherapy.* 142: 112060.)

less likely to cause histamine release, hypotension, and itch than morphine, which has contributed to its rising popularity. Other drugs in the fentanyl group include **sufentanil**, **alfentanil**, and **remifentanil**.

Pharmacokinetics

Fentanyl has a rapid onset of action, acting within 5 minutes, although this depends on the route of administration – it is faster with intravenous and intranasal administration but slower with transdermal patches. It has a shorter duration of action (30–40 minutes) than morphine, although this is extended with transdermal or buccal preparations because the drug is absorbed slowly. Fentanyl is metabolised in the liver by cytochrome P450 enzymes, and so other agents that inhibit cytochrome P450, including **verapamil**, some **antifungal agents**, and **erythromycin**, can reduce fentanyl metabolism and increase plasma levels sufficiently to depress respiration.

Pethidine

Pethidine (also called **meperidine**) was discovered in 1939 by researchers screening a range of compounds for antimuscarinic activity. By chance, it was noticed that it also produced opioid-like activity in the test animals, and it was rapidly developed as an analgesic. It acts on both MORs and KORs, although its molecular structure is different from morphine (Fig. 6.6), and as a result, its pharmacological effects are not always the same as the naturally derived opioids. It is 10 times less potent as an analgesic than morphine and causes respiratory depression, constipation, and histamine release, but is much less likely to cause nausea and vomiting and is less sedative. Because it has antimuscarinic activity, it also causes typical antimuscarinic adverse effects including dry mouth, blurred vision, and bradycardia.

Pharmacokinetics

Pethidine is only moderately well absorbed orally and is usually given parenterally, with a half-life of 2–3 h. It undergoes significant first-pass metabolism in the liver, and care is needed in patients with impaired liver function, in whom the half-life can be significantly extended. One of its metabolites, **norpethidine**, has some analgesic activity but can cause significant CNS excitation, including hallucinations and seizures, if the drug accumulates (for instance, in overdose or in renal impairment).

Methadone

Methadone is a synthetic opioid with a long (24 h) half-life because the drug leaves the bloodstream and accumulates in the tissues where it is slowly released. It binds to MORs and produces a similar range of pharmacological activity to morphine, including effective analgesia, euphoria, cough suppression, constipation, and respiratory depression. Because of its sustained action, it is mainly used in opioid withdrawal programmes and in maintenance treatment in opioid-dependent people.

Pharmacokinetics

Methadone is well absorbed orally and is also available for injection; its onset of action is usually between 30 and 60 minutes and its duration of action 4–6 h. It is heavily plasma protein-bound, which in addition to high levels of tissue binding contributes to its long half-life. It is metabolised in the liver and eliminated by the kidney.

Tramadol

Tramadol is an interesting opioid analgesic because its action is attributable to at least two different mechanisms acting synergistically. This synthetic drug is structurally related to **morphine** and is a weak agonist at MORs with much lower affinity than morphine. In addition to its opioid activity, it also acts as a serotonin and noradrenaline reuptake inhibitor (**SNRI**). It blocks the reuptake of serotonin and noradrenaline in serotonergic and noradrenergic nerve pathways, including descending inhibitory pathways (Fig. 6.2) involved in pain modulation. This increases the level of these transmitters, and therefore enhances the activity of the inhibitory neurones in blocking transmission of pain signals from the first-order to the second-order neurones. SNRIs are used to treat depression and anxiety (p. 58), both associated with chronically painful conditions, and this action of tramadol may contribute to its analgesic effect in these disorders. It is useful in a wide range of situations, including neuropathic pain, post-operative pain, osteoarthritis, and rheumatoid arthritis.

Pharmacokinetics

Because it increases serotonin levels, tramadol may cause serotonin syndrome. It may also reduce the anti-emetic action of **ondansetron**, an anti-emetic commonly used to counteract opioid-induced nausea and vomiting. Ondansetron blocks 5HT$_3$ receptors, opposing the raised serotonin levels caused by tramadol. There is evidence that higher doses of tramadol are needed to control pain in the presence of ondansetron, and that the anti-emetic action of ondansetron is reduced in the presence of tramadol.

Tramadol is a pro-drug and genetic variations in the enzyme that activates it, CYP2D6, can reduce or increase the rate at which the active agent is released, which in turn can affect its analgesic action (Fig. 6.9).

OPIOID REVERSAL AGENTS

MOR antagonists used to reverse opioid overdose include **naloxone** and **naltrexone**. **Naloxone** is a fast-acting antagonist at all opioid receptor subtypes with a half-life of 1–2 h depending on the route of administration (Fig. 6.10). It is usually given intravenously, sometimes by infusion, or intramuscularly: it is not active when given orally. Intranasal preparations are available in some countries, including the UK, the US, and Europe. Non-injectable preparations can have significant advantage for first-responders in emergency situations, including family and friends of users who may not be appropriately trained to give injections, and avoid the risk of needlestick injuries in all settings. Naloxone is generally safe to use, although it produces withdrawal symptoms, including restlessness, nausea, and vomiting. If given to reverse opioids given for pain, it reverses analgesia and

has been associated with cardiovascular events including arrhythmias and hypertension in susceptible people, thought to be secondary to sympathetic activation following the sudden return of pain. **Naltrexone** is used orally to prevent relapse in former users of opioids. Recently, very low doses of naltrexone have been shown to improve certain symptoms in multiple sclerosis, including cognitive function and mental health. Although the mechanism of action in this regard is unclear, it may be that low-grade blockade of opioid receptors may upregulate endorphin production.

NEW DIRECTIONS

There would be huge clinical value in new opioid drugs with equivalent analgesic potency to current agents, but with fewer adverse effects. One promising direction of research is based on the observation that adjusting the precise molecular shape of the drug can determine the signalling pathway activated in the cell when it binds to the opioid receptor. The pharmacological effects of opioids binding to the MOR are due to activation of signalling pathways within the cell, and recently it has become clear that different drug effects are caused by different signalling pathways. The analgesic effect of opioids in pain pathways is due to G_i-protein activation (see p. 32), but respiratory depression and constipation seem to be the result of the MOR activating a different pathway in the nerve, called the β-arrestin pathway. Standard MOR agonists, e.g. **morphine**, activate both pathways, but it was realised that if an opioid drug could be designed to activate G-protein signalling but not the β-arrestin signalling pathway, it could produce an effective analgesic without these additional adverse effects. Research in this area has produced a group of opioids called biased ligands, because they select one signalling pathway over another, and which may represent one of the most significant advances in analgesia development for some time. The first drug in this group to reach clinical practice, **oliceridine** (TRV130), was approved by the FDA in 2020, and other agents are currently in development. Oliceridine is a MOR agonist that preferentially activates G_i-protein signalling over β-arrestin signalling, and so gives analgesia with fewer adverse effects, particularly respiratory depression. Its mechanism of action is shown in Fig. 6.11.

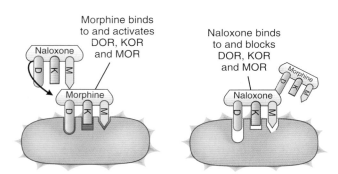

Fig. 6.10   The mechanism of action of naloxone. Naloxone binds to all types of opioid receptor (mu, kappa, and delta) with an imperfect fit, so it acts as a competitive antagonist to morphine. (Modified from Tyerman J, Cobbett S, Harding MM, et al. (2023) Medical-surgical nursing in Canada, 5th ed, Fig. 10.9. Toronto: Elsevier.)

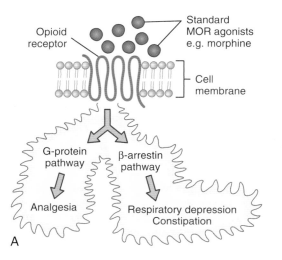

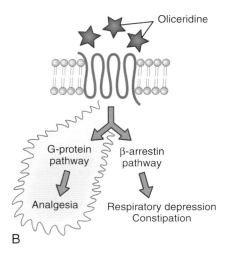

Fig. 6.11   Mechanism of action of oliceridine. A. Standard mu opioid receptor agonists (e.g. morphine) activate G_i-protein and β-arrestin pathways in the cell, resulting in adverse effects as well as analgesia. B. Oliceridine selectively activates the G_i-protein pathway, resulting in analgesia with minimal respiratory depression or constipation.

INFLAMMATION AND ANTI-INFLAMMATORY DRUGS

Inflammation is the response of tissue to injury and the inflammatory response is a complex and important protective mechanism that limits damage, prevents, or limits infection and promotes healing. It involves a complex interplay between the damaged tissue cells, local nerves, and blood vessels and defensive and immune cells recruited to the area. All these cells and tissues synthesise and release a range of mediators and cytokines that regulate inflammation and any associated immune response. Many of the anti-inflammatory drugs in common use work by blocking the production or the activity of one or more groups of these important pro-inflammatory chemicals.

Pathophysiology of the Inflammatory Response

The four main signs of the inflammatory response are redness (erythema), swelling, heat, and pain at the site. Depending on the site and severity of the injury, there may also be reduced or loss of function of the affected part. Tissue damage with or without microbe entry triggers a response in defensive sentinel cells in the tissue, like macrophages and mast cells, whose role is to initiate and regulate the tissue response to injury. Non-specific antimicrobial defence mechanisms including the complement cascade are activated. Blood vessels supplying the area dilate to increase blood flow. This causes localised redness and warmth, and the increased blood flow improves oxygen and nutrient supply to the damaged tissues, as well as bringing in additional leukocytes for defence and repair. In addition, blood vessel walls become more permeable because the endothelial cells that line them pull apart from each other, opening gaps between them and allowing increasing amounts of fluid to escape from the bloodstream into the tissues. This increased permeability also allows leukocytes to adhere to the blood vessel wall and to migrate out of the blood more easily into the tissues. Here they combat infection and begin to clear away dead and dying body cells in preparation for regeneration and repair. A wide range of leukocytes, including neutrophils, eosinophils, macrophages, and lymphocytes are involved in inflammation and immunity, and their recruitment and activation by inflammatory mediators promotes the development of the inflammatory response. Fig. 6.12 shows an overview of a typical inflammatory response.

Table 6.1 and Fig. 6.13 show some of the most important inflammatory mediators and their roles in the inflammatory response. Leukocytes migrating into the area produce a range of cytokines including **interleukins** and **tumour necrosis factor** (TNF). Damaged cells produce **prostaglandins** (PGs) and **leukotrienes**, and damaged blood vessel endothelium releases **nitric oxide**. Mast cells release **histamine** and injured sensory nerves release **substance P**. Plasma-derived proteins include **bradykinin** and **complement proteins**, and platelets release **serotonin** and **platelet activating factor** (PAF).

Inflammatory Mediators and Pain

Tissue swelling compresses and stimulates sensory nerves, contributing to the pain of inflammation, but inflammatory pain is also generated because mediators like **bradykinin** directly activate nociceptors. Prostaglandins are sensitising agents that act directly on peripheral nociceptors to increase their sensitivity to other agents such as bradykinin. There is also strong evidence that they are released in pain pathways in the CNS and enhance transmission of pain signals.

Anti-inflammatory drugs relieve pain mainly through suppressing inflammation in the injured tissue. There is strong evidence that anti-inflammatory drugs increase healing times in a range of situations including post-operatively and following bone fracture; this emphasises the important role of the inflammatory response in tissue healing and repair.

GLUCOCORTICOIDS

The adrenal cortex produces a range of steroid hormones, including mineralocorticoids, some sex hormones, and glucocorticoids. The main glucocorticoid in humans is **cortisol**, which is usually referred to as **hydrocortisone** when used therapeutically. In addition, a range of synthetic and semi-synthetic agents is available. Glucocorticoids have multiple, wide-ranging effects on immunity, inflammation, and energy metabolism, and so great care is needed when using them.

Glucocorticoids and the Stress Response

Glucocorticoids are sometimes called the stress hormones because they are essential to the body's response to stress and are essential to life: removal or failure of the adrenal glands causes a rapid decline in health and inevitable death unless steroid replacement therapy is initiated. Physiological stressors are defined as any stimulus that disrupts homeostasis, and the body is constantly exposed to such stressors, most of them mundane and everyday (the fall in blood sugar when the last meal was some time ago, fatigue, running for a bus, worry over a forthcoming exam or starting a new job). More significant stressors include infection, injury, surgery, chronic illness, pain, and psychological and emotional stress. In health, the adrenal cortex secretes cortisol in a clear diurnal pattern reflecting the sleep-wake cycle (Fig. 6.14). Assuming a normal day–night sleep cycle, cortisol levels are lowest in the late evening and into the night, rising towards morning, and then falling over the course of the day. Additionally, there are likely to be multiple smaller surges over the course of the day, caused by whatever stressors are experienced. Chronic stress in whatever form causes sustained and prolonged cortisol secretion, which is associated with a range of negative consequences described below.

Control of Cortisol Secretion

Cortisol secretion by the adrenal cortex is regulated by the anterior pituitary and the hypothalamus in the functional relationship called the hypothalamic–pituitary–adrenal (HPA) axis. This is described in more detail in Chapter 5 and shown in Fig. 5.2. Physiological stress triggers release of corticotropin-releasing hormone (CRH) from the anterior pituitary. CRH travels the short distance in the portal blood vessels linking the hypothalamus to the anterior pituitary and stimulates release of adrenocorticotrophic hormone (ACTH) into the bloodstream. ACTH in turn stimulates the adrenal cortex to release cortisol.

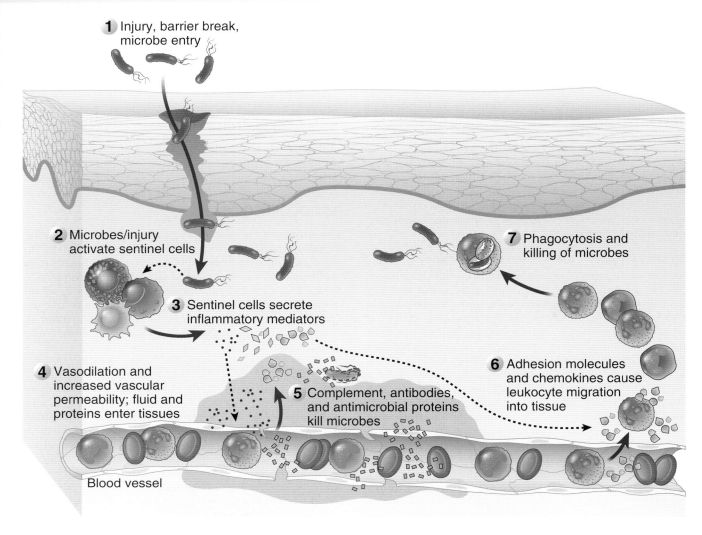

1 Injury, barrier break, microbe entry

2 Microbes/injury activate sentinel cells

3 Sentinel cells secrete inflammatory mediators

4 Vasodilation and increased vascular permeability; fluid and proteins enter tissues

5 Complement, antibodies, and antimicrobial proteins kill microbes

6 Adhesion molecules and chemokines cause leukocyte migration into tissue

7 Phagocytosis and killing of microbes

Blood vessel

Fig. 6.12 The acute inflammatory response. Stages 1–7 are described in the text. (From Abbas AK, Lichtman AH, and Pillai S (2021) Cellular and molecular immunology SAE, 10th ed, Fig. 4.14. New Delhi: Elsevier India.)

Physiological Effects of Cortisol

To help manage the physiological demands of stress, cortisol has profound effects on the major energy metabolism pathways – the use of glucose, protein, and lipids. In general, cortisol mobilises the body's stored energy resources and limits their non-essential use to keep their blood levels high so that they are available for essential tissues. This produces hyperglycaemia, hyperlipidaemia, and increased circulating amino acid levels. Cortisol also has profound anti-inflammatory and immunosuppressant properties, achieved through a range of mechanisms. The main physiological actions of cortisol are summarised in Table 6.2. The widespread activity of this family of hormones in so many areas of body metabolism and function means that the potential for adverse effects when using them therapeutically is very high.

Mechanism of Action of Glucocorticoids

Steroid hormones are synthesised from cholesterol, and so are highly fat-soluble. They cross the cell membrane and enter the cytoplasm, where they bind to a specific steroid-binding protein. This complex then enters the nucleus where it binds to its target gene. It has been estimated that glucocorticoids regulate one-fifth of the cell's genome, emphasising the widespread range of effects produced by these hormones. Depending on the steroid hormone and the target cell, this binding may either activate the gene and initiate synthesis of the protein for which the gene codes, or block gene activation and inhibit protein synthesis (Fig. 6.15). This usually means that it can take hours or even longer for prescribed steroid drugs to take effect because of the time required for levels of the target protein to either rise or fall. It also means that their duration of action is often much longer than the plasma half-life might suggest: the steroid activates or deactivates the gene, but the biological consequence of that is the result of stimulation or inhibition of protein synthesis, ongoing processes sustained over extended periods. For example, the plasma half-life of **cortisol** is only 1–2 h, but its duration of action is up to 12 h. In terms of their anti-inflammatory action, glucocorticoids bind to genes that produce pro-inflammatory proteins and switch them off. For example, they inhibit the production of cyclo-oxygenase (COX), the enzyme that produces

Table 6.1   The Actions of Key Inflammatory Mediators

Mediator	Main source	Main inflammatory action
Bradykinin	From the precursor kininogen circulating in the plasma	• Vasodilation and increases vascular permeability • Activates nociceptors • Contracts smooth muscle, e.g. in the gastrointestinal tract
Histamine	Mast cells (co-released with heparin)	• Vasodilation and increases vascular permeability • Causes itch • Contracts smooth muscle, e.g. in the respiratory system • Important mediator in allergic inflammation
Prostaglandins (PGs): PGE_2 is the main pro-inflammatory PG	Injured tissues	• PGE_2 causes vasodilation and increases vascular permeability • Promotes the action of bradykinin on nociceptors
Leukotrienes	Leukocytes Injured tissues	• Attracts and activates leukocytes • Vasodilation • Bronchoconstriction
Substance P	Injured sensory nerves	• Releases histamine from mast cells • Vasodilation • Irritates mucous membranes and triggers secretion of mucus • Transmits pain signals in the central nervous system
Interleukins: IL-1 is the main pro-inflammatory interleukin	Leukocytes	• Activate and promote leukocyte action in inflammation • Trigger the release of a wide range of other inflammatory agents
Complement	Plasma	• Activates white blood cells and increases phagocytosis • Stimulates clotting
Serotonin (5-HT)	Platelets	• Vasodilation and increased vascular permeability • Stimulates nociceptors • Bronchoconstriction and stimulation of gastrointestinal smooth muscle
Platelet activating factor (PAF)	Platelets	• Promotes clotting • Vasodilation and increased vascular permeability • Attracts white blood cells • Increases the sensitivity of nociceptors to painful stimuli • Promotes PG formation
Nitric oxide (NO)	Blood vessel endothelium	• Vasodilation • Has direct antimicrobial activity against a range of pathogens
Tumour necrosis factor (TNF)	Leukocytes	• Activates complement • Increases clotting • Promotes fever

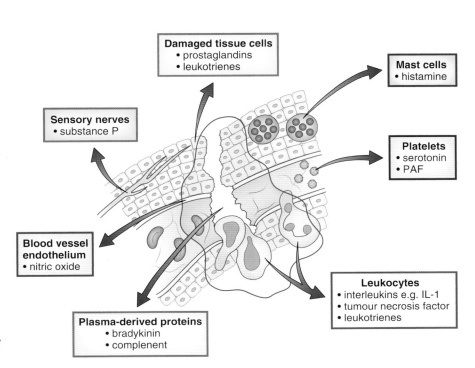

Fig. 6.13 Mediators of the inflammatory response and their source cells.

pro-inflammatory Prostaglandins. Additionally, they bind to genes that produce proteins that suppress or reverse inflammation, switching them on: for example, they increase production of **interleukin 1**, an anti-inflammatory cytokine released from white blood cells. They therefore have sweeping anti-inflammatory and immunosuppressant properties, blocking multiple aspects of the inflammatory and immune responses.

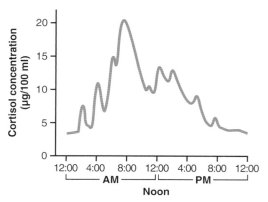

Fig. 6.14   Typical pattern of cortisol secretion over a 24-h period. (From Hall JE and Hall ME (2021) Guyton and Hall textbook of medical physiology, 14th ed, Fig. 78.9. Philadelphia: Elsevier.)

GLUCOCORTICOIDS IN THERAPEUTICS

Glucocorticoids are used in a wide range of acute and chronic inflammatory and immune conditions to suppress inflammation and modulate immune responses. They are essential therapy in adrenal insufficiency or failure or following adrenalectomy and are used for their immunosuppressant action in malignancies of lymphoid tissue and leukaemia. Because of their wide-ranging adverse effects, they are used at the lowest effective concentration and for as short a time as possible. Potency varies significantly between different preparations, and low to moderate potency agents are used wherever possible; high-potency glucocorticoids are only used if necessary and with great care. Box 6.1 lists doses of some commonly used glucocorticoids required to give an anti-inflammatory effect equal to 5 mg of **prednisolone**.

Routes of Glucocorticoid Administration

Because these agents are highly fat-soluble, they are well absorbed orally and from sites of injection. Most glucocorticoids are available in a range of formulations for oral, topical, inhalational, or parenteral administration. To minimise adverse effects, topical or local administration is preferred to systemic wherever possible, allowing a high drug concentration to be achieved locally. For example, steroids are given by inhaler in maintenance therapy of asthma, and only used orally or intravenously in exacerbations. Steroids are efficiently absorbed across the skin, especially if it is thin

Table 6.2   The Main Physiological Actions of Cortisol

	Mechanism	Result
Glucose metabolism	• Stimulates gluconeogenesis (glucose production from non-carbohydrate molecules, e.g. amino acids) • Reduces glucose uptake by body cells • Increases insulin resistance	• Hyperglycaemia
Protein metabolism	• Breakdown of protein stores (mainly muscle) • Inhibits protein synthesis by most tissues	• Elevates blood amino acid levels • Muscle wasting
Fat metabolism	• Breaks down triglycerides from fat stores to release free fatty acids • Redistributes fat stores	• Hyperlipidaemia • Shifts body cell metabolism from glucose as the main energy source to fats
Immune and inflammatory responses	• Inhibits recruitment and activity of a wide range of immune and inflammatory cells • Widespread blockade of pro-inflammatory mediator production • Atrophy of lymphoid tissue • Reduces vascular permeability • Inhibits fibroblast activity	• Effective immunosuppression • Marked anti-inflammatory activity • Leukopenia (reduced blood white cell count) • Increased risk of infection • Protects blood volume and supports blood pressure • Reduces collagen production and impair wound repair
Musculoskeletal system	• Inhibits osteoblast (bone-building cells) activity • Stimulates osteoclast (bone-absorbing cells) activity • Inhibits chondrocytes (cartilage-forming cells)	• Reduces bone density and loss of bone mass • Reduces bone growth in children
Central nervous system	• Steroid receptors found throughout the central nervous system • Steroids regulate several brain functions including the sleep-wake cycle, hunger, learning, and memory	• Stimulates appetite • Increases alertness • May induce euphoria • May induce psychiatric conditions, e.g. psychosis, depression, or anxiety • Reduces cognitive function
Sodium and water retention (mineralocorticoid activity)	• Many glucocorticoids also have mineralocorticoid (p.177) activity	• Na+ and water retention in the renal tubule • Increased K+ excretion • Increased body water • Increased blood pressure

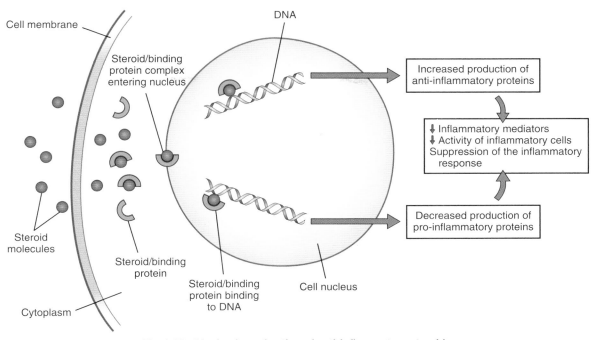

Fig. 6.15 Mechanism of action of anti-inflammatory steroids.

Box 6.1 Equivalent Anti-Inflammatory Doses of a Range of Glucocorticoids Compared with 5 mg of Prednisolone

The significant differences indicate the potency range of these drugs, with hydrocortisone being the least potent and betamethasone the most potent.

Hydrocortisone	20 mg
Deflazacort	6 mg
Prednisolone	5 mg
Triamcinolone	4 mg
Dexamethasone	750 µg
Betamethasone	750 µg

(e.g. in children or the elderly) or broken, which must always be borne in mind with topical use. A person applying a topical steroid should wear gloves to protect themselves and take care when applying to avoid adjacent healthy skin, because glucocorticoids cause skin atrophy.

ADVERSE EFFECTS OF GLUCOCORTICOIDS

Glucocorticoids are usually well tolerated when used in low doses in short courses. The risk of adverse effects increases with prolonged treatment, higher doses, systemic use, and increased potency. Although these agents are widely used in chronic conditions, they may be supplemented with other immunomodulatory drugs, for example, **methotrexate** in rheumatoid disorders, to reduce steroid doses and minimise the long-term impact of their unwanted effects. It must of course be noted that such supplemental drugs also cause adverse effects.

Cushing's Syndrome

In 1912, Harvey Cushing described the signs and symptoms of excessive glucocorticoid production by the adrenal gland, and the syndrome produced by prolonged glucocorticoid excess was named after him. Iatrogenic Cushing's syndrome, caused by administered glucocorticoids, is relatively common because of the widespread use of these agents in medicine, and it consists of a wide constellation of signs and symptoms listed below and shown in Fig. 6.16.

- Hyperglycaemia, which may precipitate diabetes mellitus
- Breakdown of muscle, particularly limb muscles, causing wasting and weakness
- Mobilisation of fats from adipose tissue: hyperlipidaemia; redistribution of adipose tissue, giving abdominal obesity, moon face, buffalo hump, and sometimes exophthalmos as adipose tissue is deposited behind the eyeballs
- Mineralocorticoid activity: fluid retention, hypertension, raised intracranial pressure
- Immunosuppression, poor inflammatory response, and increased risk of infection; acne
- Poor tissue repair; delayed healing; peptic ulceration
- Abnormal connective tissue formation: cataracts; easy bruising because blood vessel walls are fragile; striae as connective tissue in the skin becomes weakened; skin atrophy and thinning; alopecia
- Loss of bone mass: osteoporosis; increased risk of fracture; loss of height because of vertebral compression; vertebral deformity
- Psychological effects including euphoria, psychosis, depression, anxiety
- Increased appetite: weight gain, obesity, anti-emetic
- Menstrual disturbances and hirsutism in women
- Growth retardation in children

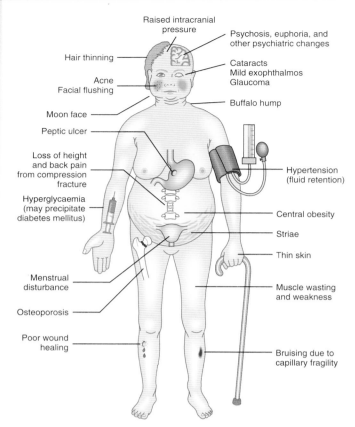

Fig. 6.16   The main features of Cushing's syndrome. (Modified from Innes JA (2016) Davidson's essentials of medicine, 2nd ed, Fig. 10.6. Edinburgh: Elsevier.)

Suppression of Endogenous Glucocorticoid Secretion

Systemically administered glucocorticoid drugs maintain artificially high plasma levels, which feed back on the hypothalamus and anterior pituitary to suppress release of CRH and ACTH respectively. This removes the internal hormonal stimulus for adrenal production of endogenous cortisol. The adrenal cortex therefore halts cortisol secretion, and adrenal atrophy occurs. At the end of a course of glucocorticoids, it is important to step down treatment over time rather than withdrawing suddenly. Stepping down slowly reduces blood steroid levels slowly, giving the HPA axis time to detect the change and respond to it. The hypothalamus and pituitary gland resume production of CRH and ACTH, respectively, which stimulates the adrenal gland to resume natural cortisol secretion. Abruptly discontinuing steroid administration after an extended course of treatment may lead to life-threatening adrenal crisis. Depending on the length of treatment, the dose given, and the potency of the steroid used, it can take the adrenal glands up to eight weeks to return to full function, although in some individuals adrenal suppression may persist for much longer.

Adrenal suppression in people taking steroid treatment means that the normal increased production of glucocorticoids in response to stress does not occur. Steroid doses need to be increased in illness, infection, trauma, and prior to surgery and other stressful situations, and individuals should always carry a steroid card to alert medical teams to this in the event of accident or illness.

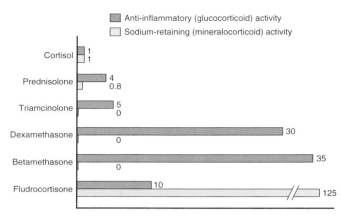

Fig. 6.17   The relative glucocorticoid and mineralocorticoid activity of some steroid drugs.

GLUCOCORTICOID DRUGS

Examples: betamethasone, dexamethasone, hydrocortisone, prednisolone, triamcinolone

The choice of drug is made based on several considerations, including its mineralocorticoid (sodium- and water-retaining) activity. A glucocorticoid with significant mineralocorticoid activity is inappropriate in conditions where fluid retention could be damaging, e.g. in raised intracranial or intraocular pressure, where increased fluid load would worsen the condition. On the other hand, when adrenal failure requires replacement therapy, mineralocorticoid activity is useful because it is part and parcel of the normal physiological function of the missing hormones. Fig. 6.17 illustrates the relative glucocorticoid and mineralocorticoid potencies of a few steroids, including the mineralocorticoid **fludrocortisone**. For comparative purposes, cortisol is assigned the value of 1 for both glucocorticoid and mineralocorticoid activity and the other agents are evaluated in comparison to this: for example, **betamethasone** is on average 35 times as potent a glucocorticoid as **cortisol** but possesses almost none of its mineralocorticoid action. Potency, half-lives, and duration of action of some of the main glucocorticoids are given in Table 6.3.

NON-STEROIDAL ANTI-INFLAMMATORY DRUGS

Non-steroidal anti-inflammatory drugs (NSAIDs) are the mainstay in the management of a wide range of acute and chronic inflammatory conditions. The history of the original NSAID, aspirin, dates back to ancient Egypt and Sumeria, whose physicians were using willow extracts as early as 3000 BC to treat painful or inflammatory conditions. In 400 BC in ancient Greece, Hippocrates is known to have prescribed a willow bark extract to women in labour, although whether it helped is not recorded. The Reverend Edward Stone, an English clergyman, submitted a report to the Royal Society in 1763 containing data and observations from five years of his experiments examining the effects on willow bark extract in the treatment of fevers.

In 1828, **salicin**, the active ingredient in willow, was isolated and named by the German chemist Joseph Buchner. Although salicin is an effective anti-inflammatory, it is an irritant when taken orally, ulcerating the membranes of the

Table 6.3   Potency, Plasma Half-Life, and Duration of Action of Some Typical Glucocorticoids

Duration of action	Drug	Plasma half-life (h)	Duration of action (h)	Additional comments
Short-acting	Hydrocortisone	2–4	8–12	Used in replacement therapy and short-term management of inflammatory conditions
Intermediate acting	Deflazacort	1–2	12–36	Pro-drug derived from prednisolone; activated in the liver
	Prednisolone		12–36	**Prednisone** is a pro-drug, activated to prednisolone in the liver
	Triamcinolone	2–5	12–36	Synthetic derivative of cortisol
Long-acting	Betamethasone	35–55	36–72	Betamethasone (and beclomethasone) esters very effective in low doses as topical/inhaled preparations
	Dexamethasone	2–4	36–72	Effective anti-emetic activity

mouth, throat, and oesophagus, and causing significant nausea, vomiting, and gastric pain. In 1897, Felix Hoffmann, a German chemist working for Bayer, showed that adding an acetyl group to the salicin molecule significantly reduced its irritant properties, and Bayer went on to manufacture and market the new drug, acetylsalicylic acid, under the trade name **Aspirin**.

Aspirin rapidly became the most popular painkiller worldwide, but its mechanism of action was not explained until the 1970s when Professor John Vane, working at the University of London, showed that aspirin inhibits an enzyme called cyclo-oxygenase (COX). COX produces prostaglandins, a family of inflammatory mediators generated in large quantities in injured tissues, and which promote all aspects of the inflammatory response. Inhibiting this enzyme blocked PG production and suppressed inflammation. Vane was a co-winner of the Nobel Prize in 1982 for this work.

Aspirin's popularity as an anti-inflammatory analgesic was tempered by the fact that its adverse effects can be severe and potentially fatal, which drove research to find safer alternatives including **ibuprofen** and **naproxen**. In addition, new uses for this old drug were being explored: several large studies in the 1990s and 2000s demonstrated clear benefit of aspirin use in cardiovascular disease and cancers.

THE BIOLOGY OF PROSTAGLANDINS

PGs were discovered by the Swedish physiologist Ulf von Euler in 1935. He called them prostaglandins because he found them in semen and assumed the prostate gland was the source. We now know that they derive from arachidonic acid, an important constituent of cell membranes, and so all body tissues can produce them.

Biosynthesis of Prostaglandins

Fig. 6.18 shows the pathway by which PGs are produced. It names two important enzymes involved: phospholipase A_2 and COX.

Phospholipase A_2 releases arachidonic acid from the cell membrane into the cell cytoplasm. **Glucocorticoids** inhibit this step, one of the many anti-inflammatory actions of these steroids. Arachidonic acid is the precursor for several inflammatory mediators, the most important being the PGs

and the leukotrienes (see p. 167 and Fig. 8.12). COX converts arachidonic acid into unstable intermediates, PGG_2 and PGH_2, which are then converted into the five main PGs – PGD_2, PGE_2, $PGF_2\alpha$, PGI_2 (prostacyclin), and thromboxane (TX) A_2 – by specific synthases. COX is inhibited by NSAIDs and also by **paracetamol,** which is interesting because paracetamol is not classed as an NSAID due to its lack of anti-inflammatory activity.

Function of Prostaglandins

PGs are important drivers of the inflammatory response and mediate pain and fever, but in healthy tissues they have a wide range of roles, sometimes called housekeeping functions, essential to the normal functions of the cell. They include cell growth and division, thermoregulation, blood clotting and cardiovascular function, appetite and feeding behaviours, protection of the gastric lining, and smooth muscle contraction, and are involved in the physiology of pain. Many of the most significant adverse effects of NSAIDs arise because they block production of housekeeping PGs in healthy tissues, as well as inflammatory PGs in injured tissues.

COX-1 and COX-2. COX is present in two main isoforms: COX-1 and COX-2. Both produce PGs from arachidonic acid, but they are expressed in different concentrations and in different tissues, depending on the stimulus. COX-1 is continually produced in small quantities by most healthy body tissues and is mainly but not exclusively involved in producing the 'housekeeping' PGs. It is sometimes referred to as the 'constitutive' isoform because its continual production suggests it performs necessary, constitutional functions. COX-2, on the other hand, is generated in very large quantities following tissue damage and is responsible for the high levels of the pro-inflammatory prostaglandins produced following injury. It is sometimes referred to as the 'inducible' isoform because its levels can be rapidly induced by tissue injury. It is also involved in the pathogenesis of cancer, promoting cell division and metastasis. However, it is not the case that COX-1 is solely responsible for the effects of PGs in healthy tissues and COX-2 is only produced in injured or diseased tissues. COX-2 is important in healthy cardiovascular function: it regulates blood flow in key organs including the heart and the kidneys and has vasodilator and

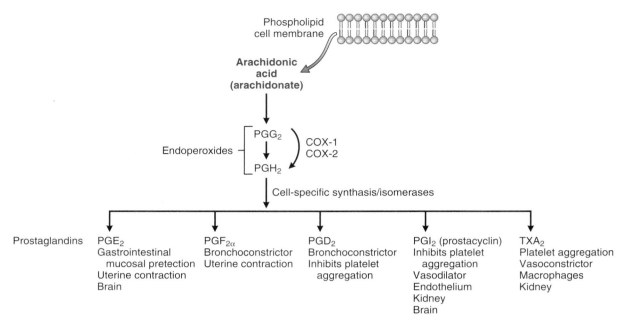

Fig. 6.18   The biosynthesis of prostaglandins and leukotrienes from arachidonic acid. (Modified from Waller DG, Sampson A, and Hitchings A (2022) Medical pharmacology and therapeutics, 6th ed, Fig. 29.1. Oxford: Elsevier.)

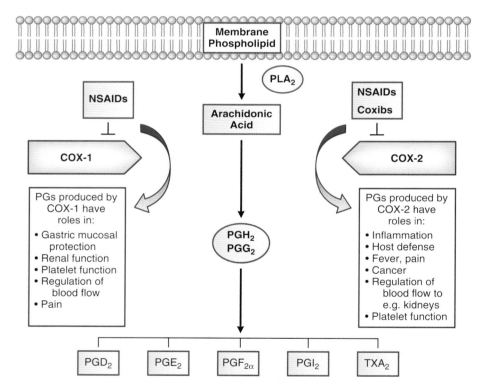

Fig. 6.19   The two main isoforms of COX. (Modified from Bonavida B and Johnson DE (2019) Targeting cell survival pathways to enhance response to chemotherapy Vol 3, Fig. 6.2. San Diego: Academic Press.)

antithrombotic activity. Fig. 6.19 and Table 6.4 summarise the main roles of COX-1 and COX-2 in PG production in healthy and injured/diseased tissues. Traditional NSAIDs including **ibuprofen** and **aspirin** block both COX-1 and COX-2, although not necessarily with equal affinity. Selective COX-2 inhibitors such as **rofecoxib** will be discussed in more detail.

The therapeutic (i.e. anti-inflammatory) effects of NSAIDs are attributable to blockade of the action of COX-2 released by injured tissues, which in turn blocks the production of pro-inflammatory PGs. However, NSAIDs also block COX-1 and COX-2 in healthy tissues, accounting for most of their adverse effects.

Prostaglandins in Inflammation and Pain

In damaged tissues, phospholipase A_2 and COX-2 levels rise rapidly and PG production increases sharply. The main agent produced in inflammation is PGE_2, which causes vasodilation, increases vascular permeability, and sensitises pain receptors. NSAIDs are effective anti-inflammatory agents,

Table 6.4 COX-1 and COX-2 Activity in Healthy and Injured/Diseased Tissues

	In healthy tissues ('housekeeping' functions)	In injury or disease
COX-1	Aggregates platelets (produces platelet TXA_2) Protects gastric mucosa (produces PGE_2) Regulates blood flow	Pain signalling May contribute to chronic inflammation Increases blood pressure
COX-2	Protects blood flow, e.g. in kidneys and heart (prostacyclin) Protects gastric mucosa (mainly PGE_2) Inhibits platelet aggregation (prostacyclin) Uterine contraction in labour ($PGF_{2\alpha}$)	Produces pro-inflammatory prostaglandins (mainly PGE_2) Produces fever (PGE_2) Promotes tumour growth and metastasis May contribute to the pathology of Alzheimer's disease

and their analgesic activity is most effective in pain of inflammatory origin.

Prostaglandins in Fever

The temperature control centre of the brain lies in the hypothalamus, which contains a network of heat-sensitive neurones that maintain core body temperature at around 37°C (98.6°F). In response to a range of inflammatory or infective substances circulating in the bloodstream, the hypothalamus can adjust this internal thermostat to increase body temperature. Substances that cause fever are called pyrogens. As with other aspects of the inflammatory response, fever is protective because increased body temperature usually inhibits microbial growth and enhances the activity of defence cells including phagocytes. Most pyrogens are derived from microbes and include some bacterial toxins and **lipopolysaccharide** (LPS) from bacterial cell walls. In addition, some products of damaged tissues, and some inflammatory mediators, such as **interleukin-6**, act as endogenous pyrogens. Pyrogens increase PGE_2 synthesis by COX-2 in the hypothalamus and this is the key event that sets the hypothalamic thermostat to the higher level and causes fever. NSAIDs reduce fever because by blocking this pyrogen-induced rise in PGE_2, the hypothalamic thermostat remains at normal core temperature level.

PGE_2 and the Stomach Lining

This important housekeeping function is performed by PGE_2 secreted in the stomach mainly but not exclusively by the action of COX-1: COX-2 is also thought to contribute. PGE_2 stimulates gastric mucus production, increases blood flow through the mucosa, stimulates bicarbonate production, and reduces gastric acid production. All these measures protect the integrity of the gastric mucosa and enhance its ability to regenerate damaged cells.

Gastrointestinal Adverse Effects of NSAIDs. By reducing PGE_2 production, NSAIDs block its protective actions, explaining their profoundly irritant effect on the gastric mucosa. Agents with a high affinity for COX-1, like **aspirin, naproxen,** and **ibuprofen**, are most likely to cause gastrointestinal irritation. Because NSAIDs are acidic drugs, they remain un-ionised in the acidic stomach fluids and are taken up and concentrated in the gastric mucosal cells, promoting their irritant effect. Enteric-coated and parenteral formulations reduce but do not eliminate gastric irritation, because circulating drug is taken up from the bloodstream into the gastric mucosal cells. GI side-effects include nausea, vomiting, abdominal pain, dyspepsia, gastric ulceration, gastric bleeding, and perforation. Pre-existing inflammatory GI disease (e.g.

TXA_2 - pro-clotting	PGI_2 - anticlotting
Vasoconstriction	Vasodilation
Platelet aggregation	Inhibition of platelet aggregation

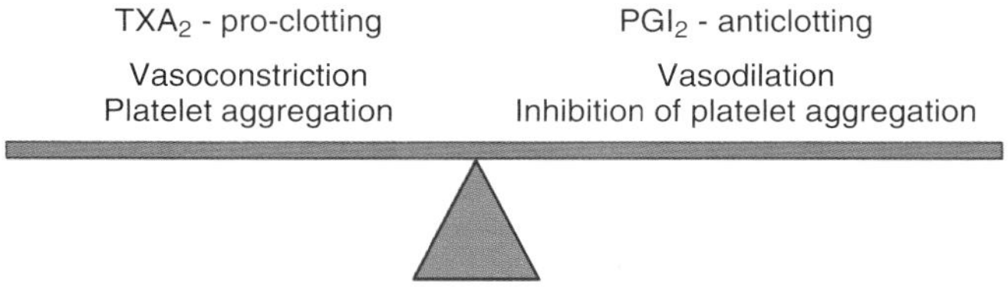

Fig. 6.20 Opposing actions of thromboxane A2 and prostacyclin in clotting.

inflammatory bowel disease) increases the risk. Rectal administration causes local irritation and bleeding. Chronic low-grade gastrointestinal bleeding may cause anaemia.

NSAIDs can be given in combination with **misoprostol**, a synthetic analogue of PGE_2, which inhibits gastric acid secretion, increases gastric mucus and bicarbonate production, and promotes healing of the stomach mucosa. Another useful combination is with a proton-pump inhibitor such as **omeprazole**. These gastroprotective agents reduce the incidence and severity of gastrointestinal side-effects. It is also recommended to take NSAIDs with food.

PGI_2, TXA_2, and Blood Clotting

This important housekeeping function mainly involves two PGs: PGI_2 (prostacyclin) and TXA_2 (Fig. 6.20). PGI_2 is produced in the healthy endothelium lining blood vessels by the actions of both COX-1 and COX-2. It causes vasodilation and inhibits platelets, and therefore has an anticoagulant effect, maintaining the fluidity of blood. TXA_2 is produced by COX-1 in platelets, and it activates platelets and causes vasoconstriction, both of which predispose to clotting. In the healthy, uninjured vascular bed, the balance between these two agents is important in keeping the blood flowing but ensuring that rapid clotting can take place if necessary. **Aspirin** is over 130 times more selective for platelet COX-1 than for COX-2 and accumulates rapidly in platelets at even low doses. This explains why low-dose aspirin is such an effective antithrombotic agent and why much higher doses are needed to block PG production in inflammation, which is mediated by COX-2. In addition, aspirin irreversibly blocks platelet COX-1, and so its antiplatelet action is much more prolonged than its effect in other tissues, strongly tipping the balance towards inhibition of clotting.

Regulation of Cardiovascular Function, Including Renal Blood Flow

Prostacyclin is an important regulator of blood flow; this important housekeeping function protects blood flow to, among other organs, the kidney and heart. Its potent vasodilator and antithrombotic actions have led to its use in the treatment of pulmonary hypertension and to prevent platelet aggregation during haemodialysis. COX-2 appears to be particularly important for producing vascular prostacyclin, and NSAIDs that are more selective for COX-2 inhibition than COX-1, like **diclofenac**, and COX-2 selective agents, such as **celecoxib,** are more strongly associated with adverse cardiovascular events than those that block both forms equally.

In the kidney, prostacyclin controls the diameter of renal blood vessels and is responsible for renal autoregulation, the ability of renal blood vessels to control local blood flow and pressure to protect them from changes in systemic pressure. Systemic blood pressure in healthy people fluctuates significantly across a wide range; for example, in sleep, it can fall to very low levels but rise temporarily into the hypertensive range during heavy exercise. It is important that the renal vasculature is protected from circulating vasoconstrictors and rising systemic blood pressure because not only would this damage the delicate renal glomeruli, but also rising pressure here would increase glomerular filtration rate and increase sodium and water loss. This could be undesirable: for example, blood pressure rises in exercise, which would then lead to excessive salt and water loss at a time when the body needs to preserve both. In the face of fluctuating systemic pressures, renal blood vessels adjust their diameter to compensate and to maintain glomerular filtration pressures at the appropriate values to control the body's salt and water balance. Prostacyclin-mediated vasodilation keeps pressure low in the renal vasculature even when systemic blood pressure is high and is therefore a key player in renal autoregulation.

Renal and Cardiovascular Adverse Effects of NSAIDs. NSAIDs block the synthesis of renoprotective prostacyclin and are therefore highly renotoxic. They increase sodium and water retention, increase blood pressure, and can trigger acute kidney injury, especially in older people whose renal function may already be in decline. Because they increase blood pressure, NSAIDs reduce the effect of antihypertensive medication, including **diuretics** and **angiotensin-converting enzyme (ACE) inhibitors**.

Apart from aspirin, all NSAIDs increase the risk of cardiovascular events, including myocardial infarction, both in people with cardiovascular risk factors (e.g. ischaemic heart disease) and without. Extended use and higher doses increase risk. It has been suggested that because of the widespread use of NSAIDs in the general population, a significant proportion of myocardial infarctions and other cardiovascular adverse effects may be attributable to NSAID use. This is thought to be due to NSAID-mediated blockade of COX-1 and COX-2 activity, reducing prostacyclin levels in blood vessels.

Prostaglandins in Tumour Growth and Development

COX-2 levels are significantly increased in a range of cancers, including breast, lung, and prostate tumours, and produce elevated levels of PGE_2, which promotes tumour cell division and contributes to tumour growth and metastatic potential. NSAIDs are sometimes used as adjuncts to chemotherapy in the treatment of some cancers and there is research interest in developing specific PGE_2-receptor

antagonists, which could be used to suppress tumour growth. There is also evidence that NSAIDs reduce the risk of developing certain cancers, including prostate, breast, and colorectal malignancies.

Prostaglandins in the Nervous System

PGs produced in the CNS have been associated with a range of neurological disorders, including Alzheimer's disease, multiple sclerosis, and sleep disorders. They do not directly stimulate pain receptors in the tissues, but they sensitise them to the action of mediators that do, including bradykinin, and release of PGs in the brain facilitates pain signalling.

NON-SELECTIVE COX-1 AND COX-2 INHIBITORS

Examples: aspirin, diclofenac, ibuprofen, naproxen

Most NSAIDs block both COX-1 and COX-2, although not necessarily with equal affinity. Fig. 6.21 shows the relative selectivity of a range of NSAIDs for the two isoforms. NSAIDs are used as analgesics, anti-inflammatories, and antipyretics in a wide range of acute and chronic conditions, including rheumatic and musculoskeletal disorders, colds and other viral infections, headache, and dysmenorrhoea. They are most effective in mild to moderate pain but are also used in combination with **opioids** in the management of moderate to severe pain, as in cancer. In this situation, they reduce inflammation in the tissues affected by the growth and expansion of a solid tumour and can reduce the dose of opioids required in pain management. There are about 50 NSAIDs available worldwide, and the annual value of the global market runs into tens of billions of pounds sterling.

Adverse Effects of NSAIDs

Adverse effects of this group of drugs tend to be broadly similar, because they all inhibit COX and prevent PG production. The mechanisms underpinning their gastrointestinal and cardiovascular side-effects are discussed above.

NSAIDs are the most common cause of drug allergy and may affect up to 1 in 50 people. It is much more common in certain groups, including people with asthma, nasal polyps, or a history of allergy. Allergy can manifest as skin rashes, rhinitis, and/or asthma. Around 15% of people with asthma experience worsening of their asthma if exposed to NSAIDs. This is because by inhibiting the conversion of arachidonic acid to PGs, more arachidonic acid is available for conversion to leukotrienes via the action of lipoxygenase (Fig. 8.12). The cysteinyl leukotrienes are bronchoconstrictors and exacerbate symptoms in some people with asthma.

NSAIDs should be used with care or completely avoided in some groups of people. They are contraindicated in people with a history of NSAID allergy. They are best avoided in people with active or previous GI bleeding, but if there is no effective alternative (e.g. in severe rheumatic disorders), then they are used with cytoprotective treatments like **misoprostol**, **proton-pump inhibitors**, or **antacids**. They should be used carefully, if at all, in individuals with a range of cardiovascular diseases including heart failure and hypertension, with asthma, or with bleeding disorders. The incidence and severity of side-effects increase with age, but in all ages they should be used at the lowest possible dose for the shortest possible time. **Paracetamol** is usually the preferred alternative analgesic, especially in older people.

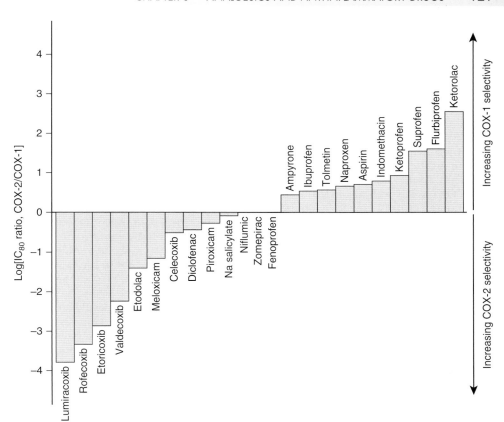

Fig. 6.21 The relative selectivity of a range of non-steroidal anti-inflammatory drugs for COX-1 and COX-2. (From Thompson SA, Courtney PM, and Fillingham YA (2023) Complications in orthopaedics: adult reconstruction, Fig. 3.4. New Delhi: Elsevier.)

Aspirin

Aspirin is currently used in medical practice mainly as an antithrombotic agent, and its prior use as an anti-inflammatory has largely fallen out of favour because of adverse effects. Aspirin is highly selective for platelet COX-1 and accumulates selectively in platelets. At much lower doses (75 mg/day) than are needed for effective anti-inflammatory action, it gives prolonged inhibition of platelet activity by irreversibly blocking platelet COX-1, permanently preventing it from producing the pro-clotting PG TXA_2. This means the effects of aspirin last for the lifespan of the platelet (about 10 days).

Pharmacokinetics

Aspirin (acetylsalicylic acid) is a pro-drug and is rapidly broken down in the plasma and the liver to release the active agent, salicylic acid. Oral doses are rapidly and completely absorbed. Because it is an acidic drug, it is not ionised in the stomach and so there is some gastric absorption; however, most is absorbed in the small intestine. The plasma half-life of acetylsalicylic acid is less than 20 minutes, and the half-life of salicylic acid is 3–4 h. Salicylic acid is metabolised in the liver, and the main metabolic pathway involved is saturated at higher doses. This means that the drug can accumulate and the half-life of the drug increases. This can happen at the upper end of the therapeutic dose range, and so clearance times in overdose or in liver impairment can be significantly extended. Metabolites are mainly excreted in the urine, although this is strongly influenced by urinary pH. Normal urine is acidic, which increases the reabsorption of salicylic acid from the filtrate back into the bloodstream (see also p. 19). Increasing urinary pH (i.e. making it more alkaline, for example, by administration of bicarbonate) increases urinary excretion and is a key element in the treatment of aspirin overdose.

Adverse Effects

Aspirin can cause any or all of the NSAID adverse effects described above. Because of its antiplatelet action, it can increase bleeding times and the risk of haemorrhage; the risk of major haemorrhage increases with age. Additionally, it can cause a condition called Reye's syndrome in children. This is characterised by encephalopathy and fatty liver failure and is fatal in a high proportion of cases. It was most commonly seen in children recovering from a viral illness and who were treated with aspirin, an observation that led to the recommendation that it should not be used in children under the age of 12. Implementation of this recommendation led to an immediate and dramatic fall in the incidence of Reye's syndrome, which is now rarely seen.

Salicylism. Aspirin toxicity (salicylism) is characterised by headache, nausea, and vomiting. There is also hyperventilation, because aspirin directly stimulates the respiratory centre; this increases carbon dioxide loss and causes respiratory alkalosis. Hyperventilation and vomiting lead to dehydration. Aspirin is neurotoxic and causes a range of neurological signs and symptoms including tinnitus, nausea, vomiting, seizures, and cardiorespiratory depression.

Diclofenac

Diclofenac was developed in the mid-1960s as the product of rational drug design, based on the structures of pre-existing NSAIDs. It reversibly inhibits both COX-1 and COX-2 and is available in oral and parenteral formulations, including rectal preparations and topical gel. Its plasma half-life is around 2 h, but its duration of action is usually between 8 and 12 h. It has been associated with higher cardiovascular risks than other NSAIDs, probably due to a relative selectivity for COX-2 inhibition over COX-1, thus reducing prostacyclin levels in the cardiovascular system.

Ibuprofen

Ibuprofen, synthesised by Boots in the 1960s, is now globally the most common NSAID. It is a propionic acid derivative, not a salicylate, and reversibly inhibits both COX-1 and COX-2. It is well absorbed orally, has a plasma half-life of about 2 h, is over 99% bound to plasma proteins, and almost completely metabolised in the liver to inactive products.

Naproxen

Naproxen reversibly inhibits both COX-1 and COX-2 and, like ibuprofen, is a propionic acid derivative. Its plasma half-life is between 12 and 15 h, and so can be given only twice a day.

Piroxicam

Piroxicam is well absorbed following oral administration, is mainly metabolised in the liver, and has a long plasma half-life (more than 30 h), which means it needs only once daily administration. It is associated with more significant GI toxicity and serious skin reactions than other NSAIDs and is not normally a first-choice NSAID when initiating anti-inflammatory treatment.

Coxibs

The coxibs are COX-2 selective inhibitors and were developed in the 1990s, when it was believed that COX-1 and COX-2 had clearly separated roles in prostaglandin production. COX-1 was clearly associated with housekeeping functions including protection of the stomach lining. The researchers who initially identified COX-2 could only induce their experimental tissues to produce it by exposing the tissue to pro-inflammatory stimuli, and so it was initially thought that COX-2 was only expressed following tissue damage and that it was exclusively responsible for the production of inflammatory PGs. Several drugs, including **celecoxib**, **etoricoxib**, and **rofecoxib**, were developed to selectively inhibit COX-2 and released onto the global market. These agents cause less GI irritation and bleeding than non-selective NSAIDs and so are better tolerated in longer-term use. However, they should still be used with care in those with GI disorders because they can exacerbate inflammatory bowel disease and increase the risk of bleeding from GI ulcers. They are unlikely to worsen asthma but should be avoided in people with a history of allergy to NSAIDs. As with the non-selective agents, they increase the risk of cardiovascular events and impair kidney function, probably because they block COX-2-mediated prostacyclin production in blood vessels. Roche withdrew **rofecoxib** in 2004 because clear evidence was emerging linking the drug to increased risk of heart attacks and strokes. **Celecoxib** has a plasma half-life of 8–12 h and is given orally. It is well absorbed and metabolised in the liver. **Etoricoxib** has a longer half-life of around 20 h and is given once daily.

PARACETAMOL

Paracetamol is an effective antipyretic and is analgesic in mild to moderate pain. The mechanism of action of paracetamol is not fully understood and although it reversibly inhibits COX, it seems likely that other mechanisms contribute to its pharmacological activity. It does not block COX in peripheral tissues, so it has no anti-inflammatory action, does not irritate the stomach, and has no effect on platelets. It inhibits COX-1 in the CNS, which may explain its antipyretic action. When paracetamol is used in combination with an NSAID like **ibuprofen**, the analgesic effect is better than either drug used alone, suggesting that paracetamol has an additional pain-relieving action that does not involve COX inhibition. Paracetamol is metabolised in the liver and some of its metabolites may contribute to its analgesic action by increasing activity in pain modulation pathways in the brain, and it is possible that further research in this area will produce new analgesic drugs.

Pharmacokinetics

Paracetamol is well absorbed when given orally or rectally. Its plasma half-life is 2–3 h and it is metabolised in the liver; some of its metabolites may be responsible for at least some of the analgesic action of the drug. It is generally well tolerated and is often the preferred analgesic in children, older people, and individuals unable to tolerate NSAIDs. Overdose, however, can lead to serious liver injury and fatal liver failure. Paracetamol is metabolised in the liver to more than one product. Around 10% is metabolised to n-acetyl-p-benzoquinone imine (NAPQI), which is highly hepatotoxic: it binds irreversibly to liver proteins, causing cellular necrosis. At therapeutic levels of paracetamol, and with normal liver function, the liver rapidly and efficiently converts NAPQI to non-toxic compounds; this reaction requires glutathione. Liver stores of glutathione are limited, however, and at higher paracetamol doses, the levels of NAPQI exceed available levels of glutathione, allowing NAPQI levels to rise and cause liver injury (Fig. 6.22). The standard treatment for paracetamol overdose is **n-acetylcysteine (NAC)**, given orally or intravenously. NAC increases glutathione levels and increases the liver's ability to clear NAPQI. It provides complete protection from liver injury if given within 8 h of paracetamol ingestion.

ANTIHISTAMINES

Histamine is an important inflammatory mediator, synthesised from the amino acid histidine by the enzyme histidine decarboxylase and broken down via two main metabolic pathways catalysed by diamine oxidase (also called histaminase) and histamine N-methyl transferase respectively (Fig. 6.23).

Histamine is implicated in a range of inflammatory and allergic disorders including atopic dermatitis and allergic rhinitis (hay fever).

HISTAMINE

Most body tissues synthesise histamine, which has several actions in regulating inflammatory and immune functions. It acts via four types of histamine receptor: the H_1, H_2, H_3, and H_4 receptors. The location and distribution of these receptors varies, which determines the effect of histamine on a specific tissue. The main actions of histamine are as an inflammatory mediator, a regulator of gastric acid secretion, and a neurotransmitter in the brain.

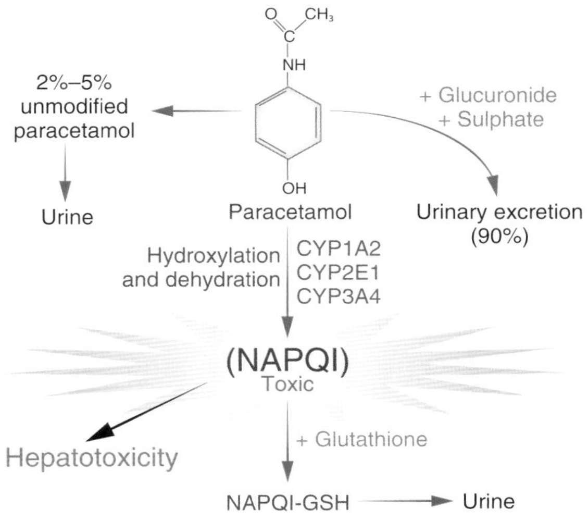

Fig. 6.22 Metabolism of paracetamol and the hepatotoxic metabolite NAPQI. (Modified from Ha CE and Bhagavan NV (2023) Essentials of medical biochemistry, 3rd ed, Fig. 35.9. San Diego: Academic Press.)

Histamine and Inflammation

Tissues exposed to the external environment – the skin, GI tract, and respiratory passageways – have large populations of mast cells and therefore high histamine levels. The strategic placement ensures that any antigen exposure or injury to these external-facing tissues is met with a rapid and protective inflammatory response, and it explains why allergy usually involves respiratory, cutaneous, and/or GI symptoms. Histamine is stored in mast cells with other pro-inflammatory substances and released into the local environment when the mast cell is activated. Basophils are another important source of histamine. Acting on H_1 receptors in the smooth muscle of blood vessels and airways and on secretory epithelia, histamine causes vasodilation, increased vascular permeability and swelling, pain and itch, bronchoconstriction, and increased secretions. Drugs that block the effects of histamine at H_1 receptors, e.g. **chlorphenamine** and **fexofenadine**, are called **antihistamines** and are commonly used to treat allergic inflammation. H_4 receptors were only discovered in 2001 and are found mainly on inflammatory and immune cells including lymphocytes and eosinophils, the latter of which is strongly associated with allergy. There is increasing evidence that much of histamine's pro-inflammatory actions are mediated by acting on H_4 receptors, and so they are the subject of current research in the hope that H_4 antagonists may offer a new group of anti-inflammatory and immunomodulatory drugs.

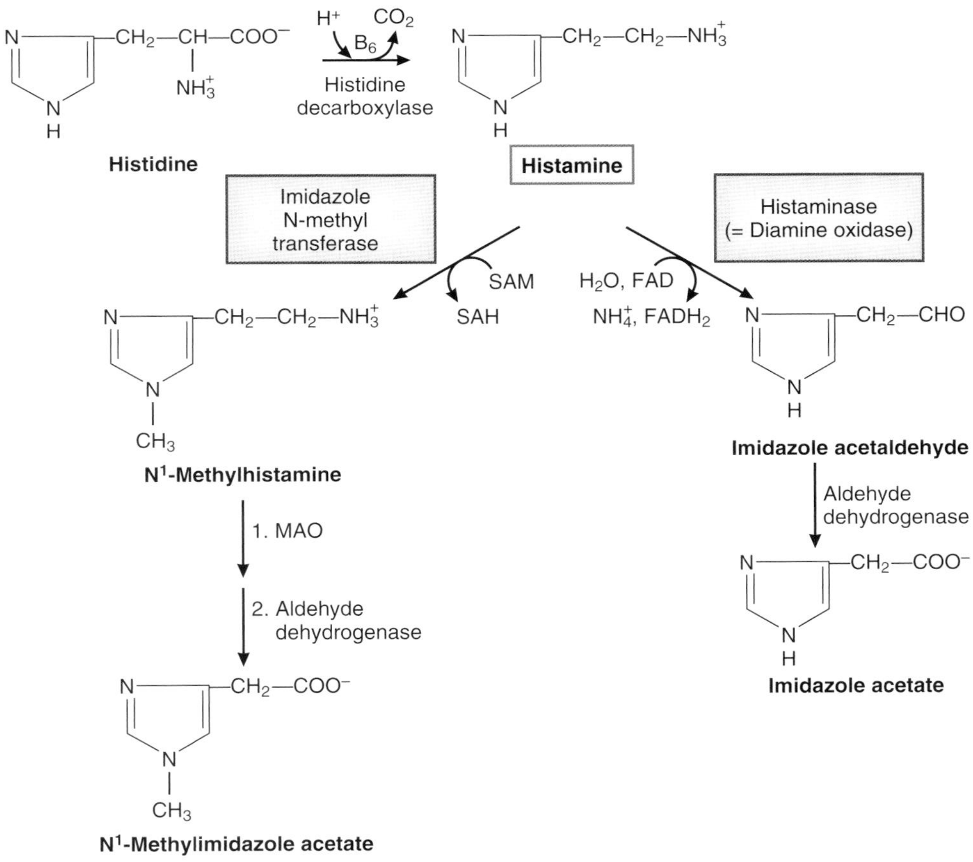

Fig. 6.23 Synthesis and breakdown of histamine. (Modified from Meisenberg G and Simmons WH (2012) Principles of medical biochemistry, 3rd ed, Fig. 16.23. Philadelphia: Saunders.)

Histamine in Allergy

In allergy (immediate or type I hypersensitivity), exposure to a usually harmless antigen stimulates an excessive and inappropriate immune response. Signs and symptoms depend on the site of exposure to antigen and on the degree of the immune response. Local responses, e.g. following an insect bite, include redness, swelling, itch, and pain at the site. Inhaled allergens, e.g. in hay fever, cause swelling and increased nasal secretions, sometimes also involving the eyes and ears. This causes runny nose, nasal congestion, sneezing, and red, itchy eyes characteristic of the disorder. If the bronchial tree is involved, there is bronchoconstriction and increased secretions, causing wheeze and cough, as in asthma. Ingested substances in food allergy cause abdominal cramping, nausea, vomiting, and diarrhoea. In the most severe form, anaphylaxis, widespread release of histamine gives blood levels high enough to cause systemic and life-threatening bronchoconstriction and upper airway swelling. In addition, systemic vasodilation and loss of blood volume because of histamine-induced increased vascular permeability reduces blood pressure and leads to profound shock, and there is usually a widespread skin rash, urticaria, or other skin symptoms.

Histamine and Gastric Acid Secretion

Histamine release from histaminocytes in the stomach triggers gastric acid release from parietal cells. Parietal cells possess H_2 receptors, and drugs used to block this action of histamine and to treat conditions associated with excess stomach acid are called H_2 receptor antagonists. They include **cimetidine** and **famotidine** (see also Ch. 10).

Histamine as a Neurotransmitter

Histamine is a neurotransmitter in the brain, acting on H_1, H_2, and H_3 receptors. It is released in vomiting pathways linking the inner ear and the brain, triggering nausea and vomiting induced by motion sickness and vertigo (see Fig. 10.13). It is also released by a collection of nerves running from the hypothalamus to the cortex and the reticular activating system, which are involved in regulation of the sleep-wake cycle. These nerves are active during waking hours and the histamine they release maintains alertness, and at night their activity stops to allow sleep. Antihistamines that cross the blood–brain barrier are commonly used as anti-emetics (e.g. **cinnarizine** and **cyclizine**) and/or sedatives (e.g. **promethazine**).

ANTIHISTAMINES

Antihistamines antagonise the action of histamine at H_1 receptors and are widely used as anti-inflammatories, especially in allergic inflammation, as anti-emetics, and as sedatives. Research in the first decades of the twentieth century demonstrated and explained the role of histamine in allergy and anaphylaxis, and the first antihistamines were introduced in the 1930s. Most antihistamines are available as oral preparations, and some are available for topical application to the skin, eye, or ear. They are not useful in the emergency treatment of anaphylaxis, because histamine is not the only mediator involved.

First-Generation Antihistamines

Examples: chlorphenamine, cyclizine, cyproheptadine, diphenhydramine, promethazine

Diphenhydramine and **chlorphenamine**, which are still widely used today, became available in the 1930s. These and other older drugs are sometimes referred to as first-generation or sedating antihistamines because they cross the blood–brain barrier and sedate, impair memory and cognitive function, and can decrease sleep quality. **Promethazine** is particularly sedative. Additionally, they are associated with a range of adverse effects because they block other receptor types including muscarinic receptors and so can have significant antimuscarinic adverse effects, including urinary retention, dry mouth, constipation, and tachycardia. First-generation antihistamines can interfere with cardiac conductivity and cause arrhythmias, including QT prolongation and torsades de pointes, and can cause hypotension. In general, these agents are best avoided in older people because newer drugs are considered to be safer and superior choices. Most have fairly long half-lives: the half-life of chlorphenamine can vary between 12 and 40 h depending on the individual's ability to metabolise it. **Cyclizine** is used as an anti-emetic.

Second- and Third-Generation Antihistamines

Examples: cetirizine, fexofenadine, loratadine

Newer drugs, the so-called second- and third-generation antihistamines, were developed to reduce adverse effects associated with older agents. In most circumstances, and particularly in older people, they are preferred to the first-generation agents in the treatment of allergic and inflammatory conditions because they have fewer side-effects and are considered safer. Their ability to cross the blood–brain barrier is much more limited than the first-generation agents, although some cause some sedation: **loratadine** and **fexofenadine** are two of the least sedating agents but may still impair co-ordination, judgement, and reaction speed in some individuals. **Fexofenadine** is a third-generation agent: it is the active metabolite of an earlier second-generation drug, **terfenadine**, which was withdrawn from the market because of cardiotoxicity. As a group, they generally have a faster onset of action than the first-generation drugs. Most have a duration of action of between 3 and 6 h and are deactivated in the liver. **Loratadine** is an exception; it is converted to an active metabolite that has a plasma half-life of around 20 h, and this drug can be given only once daily.

REFERENCES

Bannister, K., Dickenson, A.H., 2017. The plasticity of descending controls in pain: translational probing. J. Physiol. 595 (13), 4159–4166.
Melzack, R., Wall, P.D., 1965. Pain mechanisms: a new theory. Science 150 (3699), 971–979.
Praveen Rao, P.N., Knaus, E., 2008. Evolution of nonsteroidal anti-inflammatory drugs (NSAIDs): cyclooxygenase (COX) inhibition and beyond. J. Pharm. Pharm. Sci. 11 (2), 81s–110s.
Steed, C., 2016. The anatomy and physiology of pain. Surgery 34 (2), 55–59.
Trang, T., Al-Hasani, R., Salvemini, D., et al., 2015. Pain and poppies: the good, the bad and the ugly of opioid analgesics. J. Neurosci. 35 (41), 13879–13888.
Valentino, R.J., Volkow, N.D., 2018. Untangling the complexity of opioid receptor function. Neuropsychopharmacology 43, 2514–2520.

RESOURCES

Church, M.K., Church, D.S., 2013. Pharmacology of antihistamines. Indian J. Dermatol. 58 (3), 219–224.

Emanuel, M.B., 1999. Histamine and the antiallergic antihistamines: a history of their discoveries. Clin. Exp. Allergy 29 (S3), 1–11.

Laight, D., 2018. Accounting for cardiovascular risk when prescribing NSAIDs. Prescriber, pp. 15–20.

Thangam, E.B., Jemima, E.A., Singh, H., et al., 2018. The role of histamine and histamine receptors in mast-cell mediated allergy and inflammation: the hunt for new therapeutic targets. Front. Immunol. 9, 1873.

7 Drugs and Cardiovascular Function

FOCUS ON

INTRODUCTION

Worldwide, cardiovascular disease, including coronary heart disease and stroke, is the most common non-communicable disease. The morbidity, mortality, and economic cost imposed on healthcare systems by this disease burden is enormous. In this chapter, the main groups of drugs used to treat some important cardiovascular disorders are described and related in the Focus sections to their use in specific conditions. Although the material here is divided for convenience into drugs acting on the heart and drugs acting on blood vessels, cardiovascular physiology is an integrated balance of both cardiac and blood vessel activity, and many drugs discussed below affect the function of both.

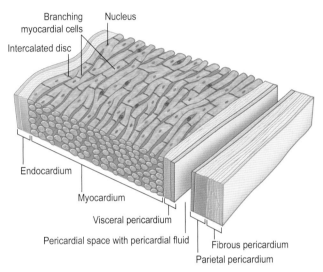

Fig. 7.1 The layers of the heart wall. (Modified from Waugh A and Grant A (2020) Ross & Wilson anatomy and physiology in health and illness, 14th ed, Fig 5.9A. Oxford: Elsevier.)

THE MYOCARDIUM

The layers of the heart wall are shown in Fig. 7.1. The heart chambers, and the valves that control flow through the heart and into the aorta and pulmonary arteries, are lined with a single-cell thick endothelium. This provides a smooth, glossy surface to facilitate low-friction, non-turbulent blood flow. The outer layer, the pericardium, is a protective double membrane enclosing the pericardial sac, which contains pericardial fluid to lubricate the beating of the heart. The middle layer, the myocardium or heart muscle, is the thickest layer and is composed of branched cardiac myocytes which are structurally and functionally different from smooth and skeletal muscle cells.

Blood Supply to the Myocardium

The myocardium receives about 5% of the cardiac output via the coronary arteries, which open from the aorta just above the aortic valve where the aorta arises from the left ventricle. The oxygen needs of the myocardium are high: at resting heart rates, myocardial oxygen consumption is 8 mL of oxygen per minute per 100 g of tissue. This rises to 70 mL of oxygen per minute per 100 g during strenuous exercise. For comparison, the brain consumes 3 mL of oxygen per minute per 100 g tissue, and contracting skeletal muscle uses 50 mL of oxygen per minute per 100 g of tissue.

CONTRACTILITY OF THE MYOCARDIUM

As with other muscle types, the myocardium needs calcium (Ca^{2+}) for contraction. Fig. 7.2 shows the mechanism by which stimulation of the cardiac myocyte, e.g. by sympathetic nerve activity or by sympathomimetic drugs, increases Ca^{2+} levels in the cell. Sympathetic nerves release noradrenaline at the axon terminal, which binds to postsynaptic β_1-adrenoceptors and activates a pathway that generates cyclic AMP (cAMP). cAMP opens Ca^{2+} channels in the myocyte membrane, allowing Ca^{2+} to enter the cell from the extracellular fluid. This triggers release of much larger quantities of Ca^{2+} from the sarcoplasmic reticulum, the organelle that

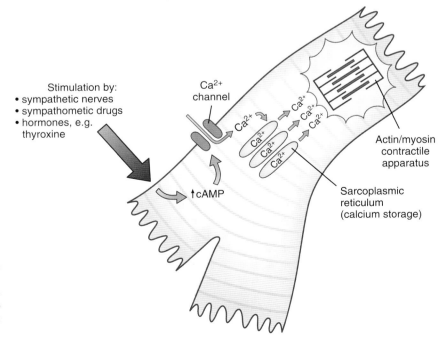

Fig. 7.2 The importance of calcium in initiating cardiac myocyte contraction. Sympathetic stimulation increases cyclic AMP levels in the cell, which opens calcium channels in the cell membrane. Rising calcium levels trigger release of more calcium from intracellular stores and activate actin and myosin.

stores the cell's Ca^{2+}. Intracellular Ca^{2+} levels rise rapidly, which activates the actin–myosin proteins that generate contraction. Certain drugs, e.g. **digoxin**, increase Ca^{2+} levels and cell contraction by mechanisms other than cAMP stimulation (see Fig. 7.8). Drugs that increase Ca^{2+} levels in the myocyte increase the contractility of the heart, and drugs that reduce them reduce cardiac contractility.

The Relationship Between Cardiac Output, Preload, and Afterload

KEY DEFINITIONS

- Cardiac output (CO):
  the volume of blood one ventricle ejects in 1 minute
- Stroke volume (SV):
  the amount of blood ejected by the ventricle in a single contraction
- Preload:
  the degree of stretch in the ventricular wall just before it contracts
- Afterload:
  the resistance against which the ventricle must push to eject blood into the circulation
- End-diastolic volume:
  the volume of blood in the ventricle immediately before it contracts

Cardiac output is calculated by the following equation:

$$CO = HR \times SV$$

where HR is heart rate and SV is stroke volume. Factors, including drugs, that increase or decrease either Heart rate or SV consequently affect cardiac output, although when functioning normally, the cardiovascular system (CVS) makes appropriate adjustments to maintain cardiac output if one parameter changes. For example, in a warm environment, peripheral blood vessels dilate to increase heat loss through the skin, which reduces systemic blood pressure (BP). To maintain blood flow to the tissues, sympathetic stimulation increases heart rate to compensate and maintain cardiac output. Cardiac output is an important determinant of BP. Falling cardiac output tends to reduce BP, and rising cardiac output tends to increase it.

Preload is the degree of stretch in the ventricular wall just before it contracts and is mainly determined by the volume of blood in the ventricle, called the end-diastolic volume (EDV, Fig. 7.3). The higher the EDV, the more stretched the ventricular wall and the higher the preload. The EDV in turn is determined by the venous return. The more blood returning to the ventricle through the venous system, the fuller the ventricle is and the more work it must do to eject it. In the healthy ventricle, increasing EDV actually increases the force of contraction because the increased blood volume stretches the myocardium, and as with other muscle tissue, a degree of stretch increases the force of muscular contraction. This ensures that the myocardium adjusts its contractility to match the amount of work it must do to eject the blood from the heart chambers. Drugs that reduce preload, e.g. **β-blockers**, reduce cardiac workload but can reduce cardiac output.

Afterload is the pressure against which the ventricle must push to eject blood into the arterial system (Fig. 7.3). This increases when arterial BP is high, either because of high circulating blood volume or because there is increased vasoconstriction in the peripheral arterial networks. Drugs that reduce afterload, e.g. **vasodilators**, reduce cardiac workload and increase cardiac output.

THE CARDIAC CONDUCTING SYSTEM

The heart possesses the property of autorhythmicity, meaning that it generates its own action potentials and is not dependent on external signals to trigger contractions. The main pacemaker is the sinoatrial (SA) node, located in the upper wall of the right atrium. Heart rhythms originating here are called sinus rhythms. The SA node is a group of electrically active but unstable cells, which depolarise spontaneously and regularly, generating the impulses that spread through the heart muscle along a network of specialised conducting fibres to trigger each heartbeat (Fig. 7.4). Depolarisation is highly dependent on the opening of Ca^{2+} channels in the SA nodal cells, allowing Ca^{2+} from the extracellular fluid to enter and intracellular Ca^{2+} levels to rise. This explains why **Ca^{2+}-channel blockers** reduce HR when in sinus rhythm. The intrinsic discharge rate of the SA node is around 120 bpm, but the resting heart rate is usually much slower than this because the vagus nerve (cranial nerve X), a parasympathetic nerve, exerts a continuous inhibitory influence. This is called vagal tone, and this action explains why some drugs that block the action of the parasympathetic nervous system, including drugs with antimuscarinic side-effects, increase heart rate. Increased sympathetic activity and the action of a range of

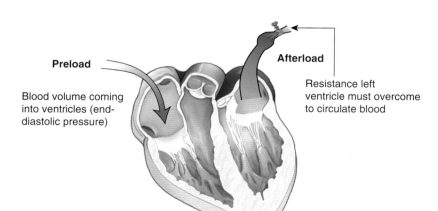

Preload

Blood volume coming into ventricles (end-diastolic pressure)

Afterload

Resistance left ventricle must overcome to circulate blood

Fig. 7.3 Preload and afterload. (Modified from Irwin S and Tecklin SJ (2005) Cardiopulmonary physical therapy: a guide to practice, 4th ed. St. Louis: Mosby.)

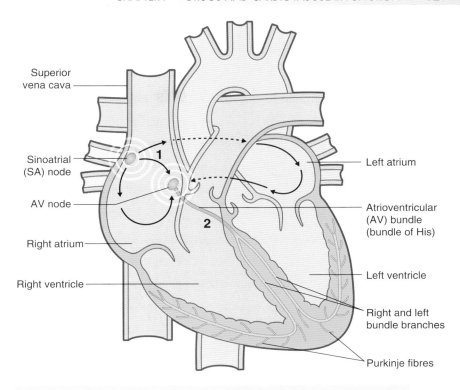

Fig. 7.4   The conducting system of the heart.
(Modified from Waugh A and Grant A (2020) Ross & Wilson anatomy and physiology in health and illness, 14th ed, Fig 5.9A. Oxford: Elsevier.)

1. Electrical impulses spread from the SA node through the atria to the AV node
2. The AV node forwards electrical impulses to the ventricles

hormones, e.g. **thyroxine** and **adrenaline**, increase the rate of SA nodal firing and increase heart rate.

Travelling along a specialised network of conducting fibres within the myocardium, each impulse from the SA node spreads through the atria and via the atrioventricular (AV) node and bundle branches to the Purkinje fibres in the ventricles. This produces co-ordinated and synchronous contraction, starting in the atria and spreading to the ventricles. Impulse conduction slows as it travels through the AV node, to allow the atria to finish emptying into the ventricles before ventricular contraction begins.

Secondary Pacemakers

The SA node is the primary pacemaker in the heart because it spontaneously discharges faster than any other area of the conduction system. However, if the SA node fails or if the conduction pathway carrying its impulses to the AV node are blocked or damaged, the AV node can take its place, discharging much more slowly (40–60 times per minute). This gives the heart a backup pacemaker, which preserves life, although an heart rate so slow greatly limits exercise tolerance. Like the SA node, the AV node is supplied by the vagus nerve (parasympathetic input), which slows conduction between atria and ventricles; sympathetic stimulation increases the rate and frequency of AV conduction. As with the SA node, AV node depolarisation requires increased Ca^{2+} levels in its cells. This is achieved by the opening of Ca^{2+} channels in the nodal cell plasma membranes, allowing Ca^{2+} to enter from the extracellular fluid, and so **Ca^{2+}-channel blockers**, which prevent Ca^{2+} entry, effectively delay AV conduction speeds.

Sometimes, an area of tissue somewhere in the heart may develop abnormal pacemaker activity and, by generating its own action potentials, it can disrupt normal conduction pathways and interfere with normal cardiac contraction. The abnormal tissue is called an ectopic focus, and ectopic beats are a common cause of arrhythmia.

AUTONOMIC CONTROL OF THE CARDIOVASCULAR SYSTEM

The autonomic nervous system (ANS) regulates physiological processes not under conscious control and is described on p. 45. Autonomic input to the heart and blood vessels is a very important contributor to cardiovascular function, and several important drugs exert their clinical effect either by enhancing or inhibiting it. Fig. 7.5 (see also Figs. 4.4A and B) summarises the autonomic nerve supply to the heart and blood vessels, identifying the receptor subtypes present at each site and the neurotransmitters released at each synapse. Both sympathetic and parasympathetic pathways from the central nervous system (CNS) to the heart and blood vessels contain two nerves, which synapse at a ganglion. The neurotransmitter released at both sympathetic and parasympathetic ganglia is acetylcholine (ACh) acting on nicotinic receptors on the post-synaptic neurone. Post-synaptic neurones in the sympathetic pathways release noradrenaline at their target organs, but the receptor subtypes differ between the heart and blood vessels: the heart has β1-adrenergic receptors, and blood vessels have mainly α1 adrenergic receptors, although some also have $β_2$-receptors. Post-synaptic

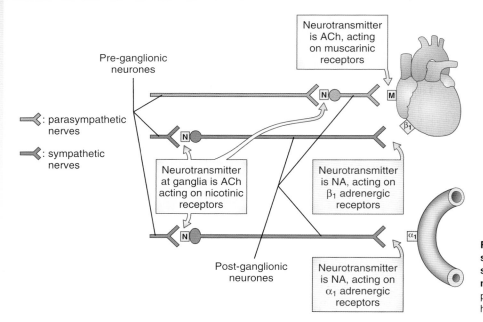

Pre-ganglionic neurones

Neurotransmitter is ACh, acting on muscarinic receptors

: parasympathetic nerves

: sympathetic nerves

Neurotransmitter at ganglia is ACh acting on nicotinic receptors

Neurotransmitter is NA, acting on β_1 adrenergic receptors

Post-ganglionic neurones

Neurotransmitter is NA, acting on α_1 adrenergic receptors

β_1

α_1

Fig. 7.5   Summary of the autonomic nerve supply to the heart and blood vessels, showing receptor types and neurotransmitters. Sympathetic supply in red, parasympathetic supply in blue. Most blood vessels have no parasympathetic blood supply.

parasympathetic neurones release ACh at the target tissue, which acts on muscarinic receptors.

Most blood vessels have only sympathetic supply, which usually causes vasoconstriction (e.g. in the gastrointestinal tract and the skin). In some blood vessel beds, however, for example the coronary arteries, sympathetic activity causes vasodilation to supply the myocardium in times of stress.

SYMPATHETIC ACTIVITY AND CARDIOVASCULAR SYSTEM FUNCTION

Sympathetic activity increases in times of stress (flight or fight). Increased activity in sympathetic nerve fibres supplying the SA node increases the heart rate (positive chronotropy), and nerve fibres supplying the myocardium increase the strength of contraction (positive inotropy) via release of noradrenaline acting on β_1-receptors. Sympathetic stimulation of blood vessels via their α_1 receptors usually causes vasoconstriction. Sympathetic activity stimulates the renin–angiotensin–aldosterone system (RAAS, see Fig. 7.13), causing general vasoconstriction and water and sodium retention. This in turn increases circulating blood volume and increases BP.

The hormone **adrenaline**, which is closely related to noradrenaline (see Fig. 4.12), is released from the adrenal cortex and has exactly the same activity on adrenergic receptors as noradrenaline. Drugs that stimulate adrenergic receptors are called sympathomimetics.

PARASYMPATHETIC ACTIVITY AND CARDIOVASCULAR SYSTEM FUNCTION

Parasympathetic activity predominates over sympathetic activity when at rest (rest and digest). Increased activity in parasympathetic nerve fibres supplying the SA node slows the heart rate (negative chronotropy) and, in parasympathetic nerve fibres supplying the myocardium reduce the strength of contraction (negative inotropy), via release of ACh acting on muscarinic receptors. Most blood vessels have no parasympathetic blood supply, but those that do,

including salivary and digestive glands, dilate in response to parasympathetic stimulation.

DRUGS AND THE HEART

KEY DEFINITIONS

- Positive/negative inotrope:
  a drug that increases/decreases the strength of cardiac contractions
- Positive/negative chronotrope:
  a drug that increases/decreases heart rate

DRUGS THAT AFFECT CARDIAC CONTRACTILITY

Drugs with positive inotropic and/or positive chronotropic effects can improve heart function in a range of conditions including heart failure, shock, and some cardiomyopathies. Drugs that reduce cardiac contractility are used to reduce the workload and oxygen consumption of the heart in conditions such as angina.

Drugs with positive chronotropic and/or inotropic activity may act by increasing Ca^{2+} levels in the myocyte by one of a few mechanisms. Conversely, drugs with negative inotropic and/or chronotropic activity are often associated with reduced intracellular Ca^{2+}.

SYMPATHETIC AGONISTS

Examples: adrenaline, dobutamine

Sympathomimetics that stimulate cardiac β_1-receptors have positive inotropic and chronotropic effects. β_1-receptors in the cardiac myocyte membrane are linked to biochemical pathways in the cell that generate cAMP, which activates a range of processes that facilitate contraction, including opening Ca^{2+} channels in the cell membrane. The Ca^{2+} that enters the cell stimulates further Ca^{2+} release from the sarcoplasmic reticulum, activating the intracellular contractile mechanism (Fig. 7.6). Sympathomimetics also cause vasoconstriction, partly by a direct action on α_1 receptors on blood vessels, but also via the vasoconstrictor action of angiotensin II, released by activation of the RAAS (see Fig. 7.13). This increases BP, which is further enhanced by RAAS-induced fluid retention and increased circulating blood volume.

Adrenaline acts at both α- and β-receptors and so affects the heart and blood vessels, and is used in acute cardiac emergencies including cardiac arrest, as well as in anaphylaxis. **Dobutamine** is more active on β-receptors than α-receptors, so it has more effect on the heart than the vasculature and is used to support heart function in a range of situations including cardiogenic shock.

β_2-agonists, used as bronchodilators in asthma and other obstructive airways disorders, are discussed on p. 164.

Pharmacokinetics

Sympathomimetics should either be avoided completely or used very carefully with other drugs that increase sympathetic neurotransmitter levels, including **amitriptyline** and **doxepin**, because their common action of increasing sympathetic activity increases preload and afterload, placing additional strain on the heart. **Adrenaline** is used by injection or by infusion. When given intravenously, it is rapidly removed from the bloodstream and taken up into sympathetic nerves, so it has a rapid onset of action but its duration of action is short. It is mainly metabolised in the liver and its breakdown products are excreted in the urine. It is a powerful vasoconstrictor because it also activates α_1 receptors in blood vessels, which helps to slow its absorption and extend its duration of action when given intramuscularly. **Dobutamine** has a very short half-life of around 2 minutes and is given by intravenous infusion.

Adverse Effects

Sympathomimetics increase the risk of cardiac arrhythmias and can cause tachycardia and hypertension. They increase the workload and the oxygen requirements of the heart and can precipitate angina in people with pre-existing cardiac ischaemia. Other adverse effects related to their sympathetic action include palpitations, cold fingers and toes (Raynaud's phenomenon), hyperglycaemia, and tremor.

SYMPATHETIC ANTAGONISTS

A wide range of drugs is available to block sympathetic effects at both α- and β-receptors.

α-Adrenergic Antagonists (α-Blockers)

Prazosin and **doxazocin** (see below) are selective α_1-blockers, and effectively block sympathetic-mediated vasoconstriction, causing widespread vasodilation and a rapid fall in BP. Some adrenoreceptor antagonists, e.g. **labetalol** and **carvedilol** (see below), block both α- and β-receptors.

β-Adrenergic Receptor Antagonists (β-Blockers)

β-blockers reduce heart rate, cardiac contractility, and cause vasodilation by reducing the influence of the sympathetic nervous system on the heart and blood vessels. They also inhibit sympathetic activation of the RAAS. They are used in hypertension, angina, and some arrhythmias. The family of β-blockers includes agents that non-selectively block two or more β-receptor subtypes, e.g. **propranolol**, which blocks β_1-, β_2-, and β_3-receptors, as well as drugs with a degree of selectivity for particular subtypes, e.g. **atenolol,** which is relatively selective for β_1-receptors. It is important when choosing a β-blocker for use in cardiac conditions to be aware that non-selective agents block both β_1- and β_2-receptors, widening the potential range of adverse effects. Agents that selectively block β_1-receptors are referred to as cardioselective. Some β-blockers, e.g. **labetalol** and **carvedilol,** also block α_1-receptors on blood vessels and so can cause vasodilation, which may be beneficial, for example in hypertension. It is important to note that although subtype-selective agents are preferentially active on one subtype, they also affect other subtypes, usually in a dose-dependent manner; for example, cardioselective agents such as **atenolol** may also cause bronchoconstriction by blocking β_2-receptors in the airways, especially at higher doses (Fig. 7.7).

β-Blockers and Blood Glucose Control. β-blockers can interfere with regulation of blood glucose levels. Sympathetic stimulation increases blood glucose, because in a fight-or-flight situation, key body tissues such as the heart and skeletal muscle need a good energy supply. Sympathetic stimulation of β_2-receptors in the pancreas inhibits

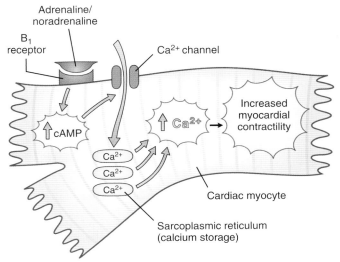

Fig. 7.6 The action of β_1-agonists on cardiac myocytes. The β-receptor is linked to pathways that increase cyclic AMP levels, which in turn increases intracellular calcium levels and activates actin and myosin contractile filaments.

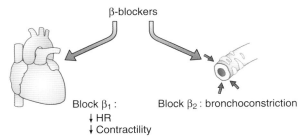

Fig. 7.7 The effects of β-receptor blockade on the heart and airways.

insulin release, which allows blood glucose levels to rise. β-receptor blockade can therefore cause hypoglycaemic episodes and particular care must be taken in diabetes. In addition, β-blockers can mask the signs of an impending hypoglycaemic episode, which can be troublesome for some diabetics. Falling blood glucose levels reflexively activate the sympathetic nervous system, producing a range of symptoms including increased heart rate, tremor, irritability, and sweating, signalling potential hypoglycaemia. This early warning system is blunted or absent in the presence of β-blockers.

Hypoglycaemia secondary to β-blockers can be treated with **glucagon** (p. 85). β-blockers can also cause hyperglycaemia, mainly in type 2 diabetes, probably because they block insulin release from the pancreas.

β-Blockers and Bronchoconstriction. Non-selective β-blockers block not only cardiac β_1-receptors, but also the β_2-receptors found in the airways, which cause bronchodilation. Blockade here can cause significant airflow restriction in susceptible people, including asthmatics (Fig. 7.7).

β-Blockers and the Renin–Angiotensin–Aldosterone System. The sympathetic nervous system activates the RAAS (see Fig. 7.13), causing systemic vasoconstriction and increasing renin release and sodium and water retention. This increases circulating blood volume and increases BP. β-blockers blunt the effects of the RAAS, an important contribution to their overall antihypertensive effect.

Pharmacokinetics

Some β-blockers, including **propranolol**, **pindolol,** and **labetalol,** are more fat-soluble than water-soluble, and so enter liver cells and are metabolised. Others, like **atenolol** and **sotalol**, are more water-soluble, and so are less well metabolised in the liver and depend upon renal function to clear them from the bloodstream. The half-lives of β-blockers is generally short, between 2 and 12 hours, and there are sustained-release preparations available to extend the duration of action of each dose.

Adverse Effects

Many of the main adverse effects of β-blockers relate to reduced sympathetic nervous system activity. There may be hypotension and bradycardia. β-blocker-induced bradycardia can be treated with **glucagon**, which increases Ca^{2+} levels in cardiac myocytes by increasing cAMP levels and has positive inotropic and chronotropic effects. β-blockers depress myocardial contractility and so should be used very carefully in heart failure. They interfere with cardiac conduction and can cause arrhythmias and should be used cautiously if at all in heart block. They can cause cold hands and feet because they block β_2-receptors on blood vessels, which normally mediate vasodilation and maintain blood flow. This may be less common when cardioselective β_1-antagonists are used than with non-selective agents. They interfere with lipid and glucose metabolism and can cause weight gain and fatigue. The more lipid-soluble drugs, e.g. **propranolol** and **metoprolol**, cross the blood–brain barrier and cause CNS side-effects, including vivid dreams, nightmares, and other sleep disturbances. This is less common with the more water-soluble agents like **atenolol**.

Non-selective β-blockers

Examples: propranolol, sotalol, pindolol, oxprenolol

Some non-selective β-blockers, including **pindolol** and **oxprenolol**, weakly stimulate β-receptors when they bind; this gives them a degree of sympathomimetic activity. Although the ability of a β-blocker to mildly stimulate β-receptors may seem counterproductive, it does mean that the side-effects of these drugs can be attenuated; bradycardia and cold extremities, for example, can be less marked. **Propranolol** has an additional action in the heart: it has an anaesthetic-like action on the sinoatrial node, which may be important when used to treat cardiac arrhythmias.

Cardioselective β-Blockers

Examples: atenolol, bisoprolol, metoprolol

Cardioselective (β_1-selective) agents may cause fewer β_2-blockade related side-effects, including cold extremities. However, they are more likely to prevent the hypoglycaemia-induced tachycardia that warns many people with diabetes, particularly type 1, of falling blood glucose levels.

CALCIUM CHANNEL ANTAGONISTS

Also called Ca^{2+}-channel blockers, these drugs block Ca^{2+} channels in cardiac myocytes and in smooth muscle cells, which prevents the rise in intracellular Ca^{2+} essential for contraction (Fig. 7.2). Ca^{2+}-channel blockers fall into two main groups, according to their relative selectivity for cardiac muscle or for vascular smooth muscle. Agents acting preferentially on vascular smooth muscle are the **dihydropyridines** and include **nifedipine, felodipine,** and **amlodipine**, used in hypertension and angina. By relaxing vascular smooth muscle, these drugs cause systemic vasodilation, reducing BP, cardiac workload, and cardiac output consumption. They dilate the coronary arteries, improving blood flow to the heart.

Cardioselective Ca^{2+}-channel blockers include **verapamil** and **diltiazem**, used to treat cardiac arrhythmias, angina, and hypertension. They slow the heart rate, slow the speed of impulse transmission through the heart's conducting system, and cause vasodilation. cardiac output falls because of the fall in heart rate and reduced cardiac contractility, and because of this and the vasodilator effect of these drugs, BP falls.

Pharmacokinetics

Amlodipine has a long half-life of 30–50 hours because it is slowly absorbed and poorly metabolised. **Felodipine** has a half-life of 11–16 hours because it is heavily plasma protein-bound. Most drugs in this group, however, have relatively short half-lives (**nifedipine,** 2 hours; **verapamil,** 4 hours), and sustained-release preparations are available to maintain therapeutic plasma levels. Most are extensively metabolised in the liver, and enzyme inducers such as **rifampicin** and **St. John's wort** can increase their metabolism and reduce their effectiveness. On the other hand, enzyme inhibitors like **ketoconazole** and grapefruit juice can reduce metabolism of the Ca^{2+} antagonist and elevate blood concentrations to potentially toxic levels. The Ca^{2+}-channel blockers themselves interfere with the metabolism of a large number of other drugs.

Adverse Effects

Most Ca^{2+}-channel blockers, except **amlodipine**, reduce cardiac contractility and can precipitate or worsen heart failure. **Verapamil** is the most likely to do this. There may be bradycardia and poor exercise tolerance because the heart cannot respond adequately to the demands of exercise. Relaxation of GI smooth muscle causes gastric acid reflux and constipation. Vasodilation causes headache, facial flushing, and pooling of blood, especially in leg veins. This in turn causes oedema of the feet and ankles.

DIGOXIN

Cardiac glycosides, including **digoxin** and **digitoxin**, are a group of plant-derived organic compounds related to steroids. Digoxin, the main agent in clinical use, was originally extracted from the purple foxglove (*Digitalis purpurea*) and is still extracted from plants of the foxglove family because this is cheaper than manufacturing it. It is used mainly in heart failure and in some atrial arrhythmias. The doctor credited with first demonstrating its clinical effectiveness in heart failure was William Withering, who in 1795 published an account of his use of foxglove extracts in a range of patients, including those with dropsy (oedema), a common consequence of heart failure.

Digoxin blocks the Na$^+$/K$^+$ pump in the cell membrane. This pump maintains the ionic gradient across the membrane so that it remains electrically excitable. It continually pumps potassium ions into the cell in exchange for Na$^+$ ions. By blocking the Na$^+$/K$^+$ pump, digoxin increases Na$^+$ levels in the cell (Fig. 7.8). This excess Na$^+$ is pumped out of the cell using a pump which exports Na$^+$ and imports Ca^{2+}. This therefore increases intracellular Ca^{2+} levels, which increases myocyte contractility and the strength of cardiac contraction. Digoxin improves ventricular contractility and improves heart function in heart failure.

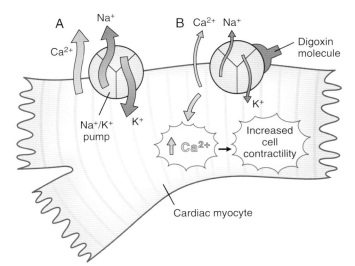

Fig. 7.8 The mechanism of action of digoxin.

Digoxin stimulates the vagal nerve, increasing parasympathetic activity in the heart: this action slows electrical discharge from the SA node and reduces the speed of impulse transmission through the AV node. This slows the heart down, so that although digoxin has a positive inotropic effect, it is a negative chronotrope. This reduces the heart's workload and oxygen consumption, useful in the failing heart and when treating arrhythmias featuring tachycardia, such as atrial fibrillation.

Pharmacokinetics

Digoxin is given orally and is generally well absorbed. Some antibiotics, including **erythromycin** and **gentamicin,** destroy microbes in the GI tract that normally deactivate oral digoxin and can significantly increase absorption and blood levels. Digoxin is very water-soluble, and so is poorly metabolised in the liver and has a long half-life of about 36 hours. Clearance therefore depends on renal elimination, and care must be taken in people with reduced kidney function. It has a narrow therapeutic index, and even small increases in plasma levels can precipitate toxicity.

Adverse Effects

Digoxin toxicity is potentially life-threatening and can develop even when plasma levels are within the therapeutic range. Although digoxin is used to treat certain atrial arrhythmias, it can cause a range of abnormal rhythms, including ventricular ectopic beats, because by interfering with the Na$^+$/K$^+$ pump, it increases the excitability of the myocyte membrane. It may slow down AV nodal conduction enough to cause heart block, and cause bradycardia because of its inhibition of the SA node. One important interaction is with **diuretics**, which may cause excessive K$^+$ excretion and hypokalaemia and are often co-prescribed with digoxin in heart failure. Hypokalaemia increases the risk of digoxin-induced arrhythmias, so it is important to ensure K$^+$ levels remain within the normal range, giving K$^+$ supplements if necessary. Digoxin also has a range of non-cardiac side-effects, including nausea and vomiting, mainly due to stimulation of the chemosensitive trigger zone. Other neurological effects include dizziness, fatigue, and a yellowing of vision, the latter because of inhibition of the Na$^+$/K$^+$ pump in the light-sensitive cones of the retina.

PHOSPHODIESTERASE INHIBITORS

Examples: enoximone, milrinone

Phosphodiesterase (PDE) is the enzyme that breaks down cAMP (see Fig. 3.7). When its action is inhibited, cAMP levels in the cardiac myocyte rise, Ca^{2+} levels increase, and contractility improves, without increasing heart rate. PDE inhibitors improve heart function in heart failure but can trigger potentially life-threatening ventricular arrhythmias, seen in more than 1 in 10 patients. They are given by infusion. **Milrinone** has a plasma half-life of 2 hours and depends on good kidney function for clearance because it is not metabolised in the liver. **Enoximone** has a longer half-life of 8 hours and undergoes hepatic metabolism, so should be used carefully in people with liver impairment. Both agents cause vasodilation and possibly hypotension.

Focus on: Drug Treatment of Heart Failure

Heart failure is a syndrome that occurs when the heart becomes unable to meet the needs of the body. This may be due to a disorder or disease of the heart itself that impairs its pumping efficiency or due to a non-cardiac condition that places additional demands on it, e.g. thyrotoxicosis or lung fibrosis. Heart failure usually involves the ventricles, and more commonly the left because its workload is greater. The main causes of heart failure are listed in Box 7.1.

Pathophysiology of Heart Failure

When a ventricle begins to fail, forward movement of blood becomes sluggish, reducing blood flow through body tissues and creating back pressure in the failing chamber and the blood vessels feeding blood into it. Left ventricular failure reduces output of blood via the aorta to body organs, leading to systemic hypoxia. As blood accumulates in the left ventricle, pressure rises, eventually backing up through the left atrium and into the pulmonary veins. This increases pressure in the pulmonary circulation, with pulmonary congestion and oedema. Right ventricular failure reduces blood flow into the pulmonary circulation, and as blood backs up through the right atrium, it causes congestion in the venous circulation.

Once the heart begins to fail, it usually initiates a self-perpetuating circle of events that accelerates progressive deterioration of its function. The failing heart pumps out less blood with each contraction, leading to a reduced cardiac output, falling BP, and diminished perfusion of vital organs including the kidneys. This stimulates compensatory mechanisms via the sympathetic nervous system in an attempt to restore cardiac output, summarised in Fig. 7.9. Reduced renal blood flow activates the RAAS (Fig. 7.13), leading ultimately to the release of angiotensin II, which causes widespread vasoconstriction and stimulates water and Na⁺ retention. Both mechanisms help to support BP, but at the expense of increasing preload and afterload, imposing higher demands on the already failing heart. Sympathetic stimulation releases **adrenaline** and increases activity in sympathetic nerve supply to the heart, causing tachycardia and increasing the force of contraction. This measure increases the performance of the heart in the early stages of failure, but these additional demands increase its oxygen requirements and accelerate its deterioration.

Box 7.1 The Main Causes of Heart Failure

Myocardial infarction, usually due to coronary artery atherosclerosis
Hypertension
Valvular disease, including stenosis
Cardiac myopathy
Restrictive pericarditis
Arrhythmias
Non-cardiac disease, e.g. hyperthyroidism, chronic anaemia, pulmonary embolism, pregnancy

Drug treatment of heart failure aims to interrupt and delay the progress of the vicious cycle of deteriorating cardiac function. This includes reducing the workload of the heart by blocking excessive sympathetic nervous system activity, reducing preload and afterload, improving coronary artery blood flow to increase oxygen and glucose supply, and supporting cardiac function with drugs that improve contractility without increasing oxygen demands. The main drug groups used in the treatment of heart failure are summarised in Fig. 7.10.

Angiotensin-Converting Enzyme Inhibitors

Angiotensin-converting enzyme inhibitors (ACEIs) are key drugs in heart failure because they:
- reduce circulating blood volume, reducing preload
- cause vasodilation, reducing venous return and reducing afterload
- reduce sympathetic nervous system activity.

Their pharmacology is described below. For people who cannot tolerate ACEIs, angiotensin-receptor antagonists (ARAs) can be used; they have a similar range of effects and their pharmacology is also described below.

Diuretics

Diuretics, e.g. **bendrofluazide**, **furosemide**, and **spironolactone**, are widely used in heart failure because they promote water and electrolyte loss in the urine, reducing oedema, pulmonary congestion, and circulating

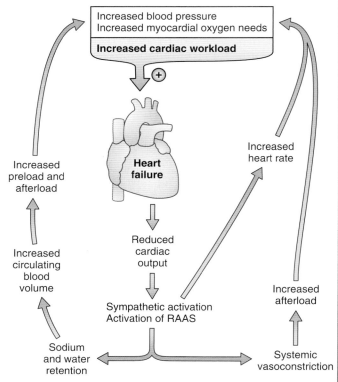

Fig. 7.9 The cycle of deterioration in heart failure. RAAS, Renin-angiotensin-aldosterone system.

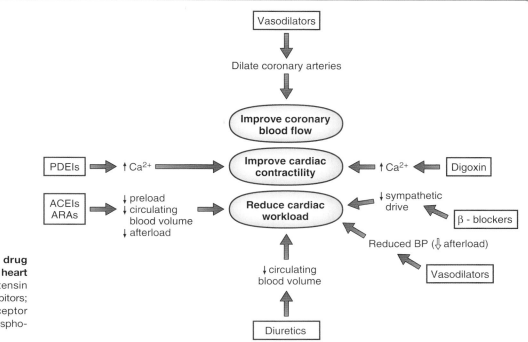

Fig. 7.10 The main drug treatment options in heart failure. ACEIs, Angiotensin converting enzyme inhibitors; ARAs, angiotensin receptor antagonists; PDEIs, phosphodiesterase 5 inhibitors.

blood volume. By reducing the volume load of the heart, the efficiency of heart contraction can be improved. Care must be taken not to over-reduce circulating blood volume, because this reduces cardiac output, causes hypotension, and may trigger kidney injury if renal blood flow falls too low. The pharmacology of diuretics is discussed in Chapter 10.

Vasodilators

Vasodilators are useful in heart failure because they:
- dilate coronary arteries, improving blood supply to the myocardium
- dilate the systemic veins, reducing venous return and preload
- dilate the arterial system, reducing afterload.
  The pharmacology of the main vasodilators is described below.

Digoxin

Digoxin is useful in heart failure because it slows the heart down, reducing its workload and its oxygen needs. Slowing the heart rate gives the heart chambers time to fill adequately and so improves contraction efficiency. It is particularly useful when heart failure is complicated by atrial arrhythmia, because of its anti-arrhythmic activity.

β-Blockers

These drugs block the sympathetic input to the heart, slow the heart rate, reduce contractility, and reduce oxygen requirements. They must be used carefully, because they depress myocardial function and may worsen heart failure; however, in low doses they improve symptoms and reduce mortality.

CARDIAC ARRHYTHMIAS

A cardiac arrhythmia is a disturbance of rate or rhythm. Some arrhythmias are very common and do not interfere significantly with the efficiency of the heart's pumping action. At the other end of the spectrum, some arrhythmias are immediately life-terminating. Arrhythmias are described according to their anatomical origin: ventricular arrhythmias arise from the ventricles, and supraventricular arrhythmias arise either from the atria or the AV node.

THE CARDIAC ACTION POTENTIAL

Initiation and spread of action potentials through the healthy heart are described above (Fig. 7.4). Normal heart rhythm generated by SA nodal activity is called sinus rhythm. In a similar way to nerve and muscle tissues elsewhere, electrical activity of the pacemaker cells, conducting tissue, and the myocytes is generated by the movement of electrically charged ions, specifically Na^+, K^+, and Ca^{2+}, across the cell membrane, which in turn is controlled by the opening and closing of ion channels.

Ion Movements and the Cardiac Action Potential

At rest, the distribution of ions across the myocyte membrane is not equal. Na^+ ions are concentrated outside the cell and K^+ ions are concentrated inside, and this unequal distribution is maintained by the continuous operation of the Na^+/K^+ pump. This unequal distribution means that the interior of the cell is more electrically negative than the outside, and the resting membrane potential sits at between -70 mV and -80 mV (Phase 4, Fig. 7.11).

When the myocyte is stimulated, Na^+ channels in its plasma membrane open, and Na^+ floods into the cell down its concentration gradient. The inside of the cell is now more electrically positive than the outside, and the membrane potential is now +20 mV. This is called phase 0 and represents depolarisation, which triggers contraction. The myocyte is now electrically unexcitable, and unlike skeletal muscle, it is important that it remains electrically unexcitable for a period of time so that the action potential travelling along conduction pathways cannot travel backwards (retrograde conduction), which would generate arrhythmias and interfere with the synchronised pumping action of the heart. Phase 0 is therefore followed by a brief period of repolarisation (phase 1) and an extended plateau phase (phase 2) of sustained depolarisation, during which the myocyte remains unexcitable (refractory). The plateau phase persists for about 0.2 seconds and is caused by opening of Ca^{2+} channels, allowing entry of Ca^{2+} ions, keeping the inside of the cell electrically positive. The Ca^{2+} channels then close and K^+ channels open, allowing K^+ ions to rush out of the cell down their concentration gradient, which repolarises it and returns the membrane potential to its resting value (phase 3). The interior of the cell is now left with high levels of Na^+ and less K^+ but the Na^+/K^+ pump, which is in continuous operation, rapidly restores this to its original state by pumping out Na^+ and importing K^+. Drugs that block Na^+ channels, e.g. **lidocaine**, and K^+ channels, e.g. **amiodarone**, disrupt and delay these electrical changes, and are useful anti-arrhythmic agents.

In the SA and AV nodes, although the key elements of depolarisation, plateau, and repolarisation are present, the action potential is a different shape (see Fig. 7.13B) and the ion that causes depolarisation is Ca^{2+}. **Ca^{2+}-channel blockers**

therefore reduce the speed of action potential conduction through the AV node and reduce the firing rate of the SA node.

Understanding the physiology of the cardiac action potential explains the mechanism of action of the main anti-arrhythmic drugs, especially as the classification of anti-arrhythmic agents relates to their physiological effects on the movement of specific ions during different phases (Fig. 7.11).

THE AETIOLOGY OF CARDIAC ARRHYTHMIAS

The two main mechanisms responsible for arrhythmias are the establishment of re-entrant circuits and the appearance of ectopic foci within the myocardium.

Re-Entrant Rhythms

These are common causes of arrhythmias and arise when an action potential is allowed to establish a self-perpetuating circuit. In the healthy heart, the impulses travel together throughout each section of tissue and cannot spread backwards or to adjacent areas because of the long refractory period following the wavefront. Impulses that do meet along adjacent pathways extinguish each other (Fig. 7.12A). Re-entrant circuits develop when two parts of the myocardium are conducting at different speeds, one slower than the other. As the slower impulse travels down its pathway, it can then excite adjacent areas of the myocardium that have conducted at normal speed and have repolarised and become excitable again (Fig. 7.12B). This sends impulses backwards up the normally conducting tissue, establishing a self-perpetuating re-entrant circuit (Fig. 7.12C). Re-entrant rhythms are common causes of tachyarrhythmias, i.e. arrhythmias associated with fast heart rates, including atrial fibrillation and flutter and ventricular tachycardia following myocardial infarction.

Ectopic Arrhythmias

If an area of heart muscle acquires increased automaticity, it can begin to generate action potentials independently of normal sinus rhythm, interfering with normal conduction pathways and co-ordinated myocardial contraction (Fig. 7.12D).

ANTI-ARRHYTHMIC DRUGS

Because they interfere with electrical activity in the heart, anti-arrhythmic drugs may themselves generate arrhythmias. By slowing the generation and transmission of impulses in normal pathways, they may allow an ectopic focus to become dominant, or may allow a re-entrant circuit to become established (Fig. 7.12). The risks of anti-arrhythmic drug-induced arrhythmias is increased in people with pre-existing heart disease, e.g. ischaemic heart disease. In addition, people with increased sympathetic drive are at higher risk because sympathomimetics are themselves arrhythmogenic; for example, sympathetic drive to the heart is increased in heart failure in an attempt to maintain cardiac output. Some anti-arrhythmic drugs, e.g. **sotalol**, **disopyramide,** and **digoxin**, are particularly associated with the production of arrhythmias.

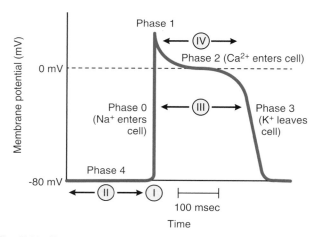

Fig. 7.11 Representative action potential from a ventricular myocyte, showing the four phases and relating them to the pharmacological action of the four classes (I–IV) of anti-arrhythmic drugs. (Modified from Brown MJ, Sharma P, Mir FA, et al. (2019) Clinical pharmacology, 12th ed, Fig. 25.1. Edinburgh: Elsevier.)

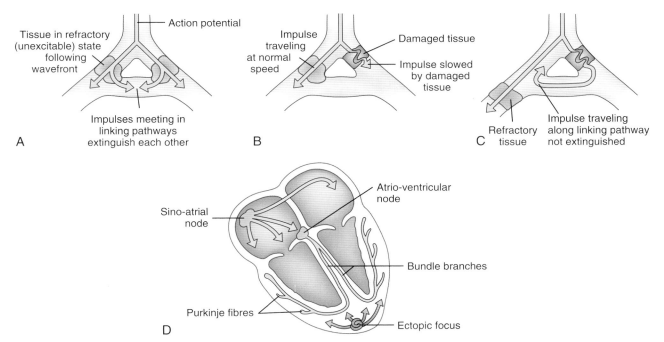

Fig. 7.12   **The genesis of cardiac arrhythmias.** A. Normal conduction pathways. B–C. Re-entrant rhythms. D. Ectopic focus.

Focus on: The Vaughan Williams Classification of Anti-Arrhythmic Drugs

The standard classification of anti-arrhythmic drugs was drawn up by Miles Vaughan Williams in 1970. The four classes reflect the main electrophysiological targets of each group of drugs, but newer drugs do not always fall tidily into this classification system, and some drugs have activity in more than one class.

Class I

These agents all block Na^+ channels and block the influx of Na^+ that depolarises the cell (phase 0), similar to the mechanism of action of local anaesthetics (p. 69). They all therefore slow the rate of depolarisation. There are three subgroups, classified according to the drug binds to and dissociates from the channel, which in turn determines the duration of the channel block.

Class Ia: **quinidine, procainamide, disopyramide**
Class Ib: **lidocaine**
Class Ic: **flecainide, propafenone**

   Fig. 7.13A shows a typical action potential from a ventricular cell treated with a class Ic agent, showing the shallower slope of depolarisation caused by the reduced rate of Na^+ entry into the cell. Class Ia and Ic agents are used in both supraventricular and ventricular arrhythmias, and class Ib drugs are only effective in ventricular arrhythmias.

Class II

Examples: propranolol, atenolol, metoprolol

   Class II agents are the β-blockers, which inhibit the effect of the sympathetic nervous system on the heart. **Adrenaline** and other sympathomimetics can cause arrhythmias by stimulating both SA and AV nodal discharge, by initiating ectopic beats and by increasing the excitability of the myocardium, and a range of arrhythmias are at least partly due to excessive sympathetic stimulation, including atrial fibrillation and post-MI. β-blockers delay AV nodal conduction and control ventricular tachycardias originating from the atria and suppress discharge from ectopic foci. Fig. 7.13B shows the effect of β-blockade on an action potential in an AV nodal cell: the action potential is both delayed and prolonged. Class II agents are used in both supraventricular and ventricular arrhythmias.

Class III

Examples: amiodarone, sotalol

   These agents are K^+-channel blockers, and so they inhibit phase 3 of the action potential and slow repolarisation of the cardiac cells. In so doing, they delay the restoration of the ion balance across the myocyte membrane and extend its refractory period. Fig. 7.13C shows the effect of a class III agent on the action potential in a ventricular myocyte. They are used in both supraventricular and ventricular arrhythmias.

Class IV

Examples: verapamil, diltiazem

   Class IV agents are the Ca^{2+}-channel blockers. They have particular activity on the Ca^{2+} channels that open to depolarise cells in the SA and AV nodes, and so reduce the rate of SA nodal firing and slow impulse transmission through the AV node. For this reason, they are most useful in treating arrhythmias originating in these parts of the heart and are not effective in ventricular arrhythmias. Fig. 7.13D shows the effect of Ca^{2+}-channel blockers on an action potential in an AV nodal cell: depolarisation is slow because depolarisation in AV and SA nodal cells is due to Ca^{2+} influx, not Na^+ influx, and repolarisation is delayed.

Continued

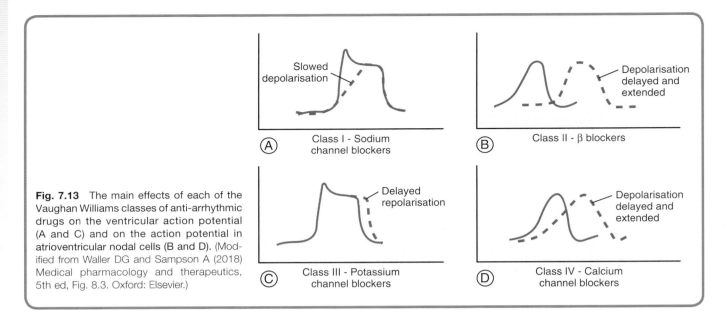

Fig. 7.13 The main effects of each of the Vaughan Williams classes of anti-arrhythmic drugs on the ventricular action potential (A and C) and on the action potential in atrioventricular nodal cells (B and D). (Modified from Waller DG and Sampson A (2018) *Medical pharmacology and therapeutics*, 5th ed, Fig. 8.3. Oxford: Elsevier.)

CLASS I AGENTS

Although all class I agents block Na^+ channels and so slow depolarisation in heart cells, this class is subdivided because some have additional channel-blocking activity, and some have more extended block than others.

Disopyramide (Ia)

Disopyramide blocks K^+ channels (class III activity) as well as Na^+ channels, so it not only delays depolarisation, it slows repolarisation too and extends the action potential and the refractory period. Along with **quinidine**, another class Ia drug, it is falling out of use because of its serious side-effects.

Pharmacokinetics

Disopyramide is given orally and has a half-life of about 6 hours. It is partly metabolised in the liver, producing a metabolite with marked antimuscarinic activity.

Adverse Effects

Antimuscarinic side-effects (reduced saliva production, bradycardia, constipation, blurred vision) can be very troublesome. Disopyramide has a significant negative inotropic action: it can cause or worsen heart failure and produce problematic hypotension. It is strongly arrhythmogenic.

Lidocaine (Ib)

Lidocaine blocks Na^+ channels in a use-dependent manner (see also Local anaesthetics, p. 69). This means that it is most effective in electrically excitable cells when they are most active and their Na^+ channels are open for most of the time. Lidocaine therefore blocks rapidly discharging, arrhythmogenic heart cells preferentially to normal tissue.

Pharmacokinetics

Lidocaine is given intravenously because if given orally, it is almost completely cleared by the liver in first-pass metabolism. It is extensively metabolised in the liver, and some of its metabolites are active. IV administration allows drug delivery to be rapidly titrated against its clinical effects. Its plasma half-life is around 2 hours, but this can be longer in liver or renal failure.

Adverse Effects

Lidocaine depresses nerve activity in the CNS and at high doses may cause drowsiness, confusion, and convulsions.

Flecainide (Ic)

Flecainide is given orally or intravenously. Although it is used in both ventricular and supraventricular arrhythmias, it is particularly effective in converting atrial fibrillation to sinus rhythm.

Pharmacokinetics

Flecainide is slowly but completely absorbed following oral administration. Its plasma half-life is around 12 hours, and there are extended-release preparations, so its action is long-lasting.

Adverse Effects

Flecainide is contra-indicated in people who have had a myocardial infarction or have heart failure, in whom the drug significantly increases the risk of fatal ventricular arrhythmias. Common side-effects include oedema, dyspnoea, and dizziness.

CLASS II AGENTS

The general pharmacology of β-blockers is described on p. 47. A number of β-blockers, including **propranolol** and **atenolol**, are used to treat arrhythmias.

CLASS III AGENTS

Sotalol

Sotalol is a β-blocker with additional class III activity: that is, it blocks K^+ channels which open to allow the cardiac myocyte to repolarise in phase 3 of the action potential. It has significant arrhythmogenic action of its own, and so is usually only used in certain serious arrhythmias, e.g. ventricular tachycardia.

Amiodarone

Amiodarone is widely used in a range of arrhythmias. Although its main action is by blocking K^+ channels and so is categorised as a class III drug, it has activity in all four classifications. It blocks Na^+ channels (class I), has β-blocker activity (class II), and blocks Ca^{2+} channels (class IV). It can be given orally or intravenously.

Pharmacodynamics
Amiodarone is highly lipid-soluble and is extensively taken up from the blood and stored in many body tissues. Its half-life is very long, between 7 and 8 weeks. Because its half-life is so long, treatment is usually initiated with a large loading dose to bring plasma levels up quickly. It is metabolised in the liver.

Adverse Effects
The incidence of side-effects with amiodarone is very high: up to 15% of patients report side-effects in the first year of treatment, rising to 50% with longer-term use. Skin reactions and nausea are common. Amiodarone contains about 37% iodine by weight, and so can interfere with thyroid function, causing either hyperthyroid or hypothyroid states. Assessing thyroid function before beginning treatment is essential. Cardiac side-effects include arrhythmias and bradycardia. In 10% of patients, corneal deposits of the drug cause visual symptoms including halos and photophobia. There may be irreversible pulmonary toxicity, which carries a mortality rate of up to 10%. Neurotoxic side-effects include peripheral neuropathy and altered taste and smell. Hepatic function should be monitored because amiodarone can cause liver impairment.

Dronedarone

Like **amiodarone**, dronedarone has activity in all four Vaughan Williams classes. It may be preferred to amiodarone because it is better tolerated and patients may be more likely to comply with treatment.

Pharmacokinetics
Dronedarone was designed to be much less fat-soluble than amiodarone in the expectation that its distribution throughout body tissues would be less extensive and it contains no iodine, so it has no thyroid toxicity. It has a much shorter half-life than amiodarone and is less arrhythmogenic.

Adverse Effects
Dronedarone shares many of amiodarone's side-effects including pulmonary toxicity and liver toxicity. It should not be used in heart failure because it increases mortality, and it can cause heart failure in people with no prior history. GI symptoms, e.g. vomiting, diarrhoea, nausea, and taste disturbances, are common.

CLASS IV DRUGS

The general pharmacology of Ca^{2+}-channel blockers is described on p. 132.

ANTI-ARRHYTHMIC DRUGS NOT COVERED IN THE VAUGHAN WILLIAMS SYSTEM
Adenosine
Adenosine is a small but important molecular mediator widespread in body fluids and has a range of biological effects. It forms the core of ATP, the cell's energy storage molecule. Adenosine is pro-inflammatory and **theophylline**, an adenosine-receptor antagonist, is used in asthma (see p. 165). In the heart, adenosine inhibits transmission in both the SA and AV nodes and is used to terminate supraventricular tachycardia.

Pharmacokinetics
Adenosine has a very short plasma half-life (less than 10 seconds) and its duration of action is less than a minute, so is given by rapid bolus injection.

Adverse Effects
These are common but short-lived because adenosine is so rapidly cleared from the bloodstream. There may be bradycardia and AV block. Adenosine is a vasodilator, so facial flushing and headache may occur. It should not be used in asthma because it can cause bronchospasm.

Digoxin
The pharmacology of digoxin is described above. It blocks AV nodal conduction and so is used to reduce transmission of impulses to the ventricles in atrial tachycardias, including atrial fibrillation and atrial flutter. Because it increases Ca^{2+} levels in myocardial cells, it increases excitability and can cause arrhythmias.

DRUGS AND BLOOD VESSELS

The health of blood vessels has an important impact on cardiovascular function. The ability of the arterial system to adjust vessel diameter is a major determinant of afterload, and so contributes significantly to the workload of the heart. Damage to blood vessel walls, for example by atheroma, can reduce blood flow to the organs they supply and is an important cause of stroke, ischaemic heart disease (IHD), and peripheral vascular disease. The ability of the vascular system to respond appropriately to neural and hormonal control mechanisms is a key element in maintaining BP within normal parameters and in adjusting blood flow to meet changing tissue needs, e.g. in exercising muscle.

BLOOD VESSEL ANATOMY AND BLOOD VESSEL DIAMETER

Arteries and veins have the same three layers of tissue: an outer protective layer (the tunica externa) and an inner lining, the endothelium or tunica intima, which is continuous with the endocardium lining the heart and is smooth to optimise non-turbulent blood flow (Fig. 7.14). The middle layer, the tunica media, varies considerably in composition depending on the vessel. In large arteries, it contains a great deal of elastic tissue to absorb the pressure wave from the heart and propel the blood forward by elastic recoil. The large arteries divide into extensive networks of small arterioles whose middle layers are very rich in smooth muscle. Contraction and relaxation of this smooth muscle constricts and dilates the vessels, adjusting flow and pressure. Because they contain so much smooth muscle and are so numerous, the muscular arterioles are the most important blood vessel in the control of systemic BP, and for this reason they are sometimes called resistance vessels. Their diameter is controlled by the autonomic nervous system, although unlike most body tissues, most blood vessels do not have both sympathetic and parasympathetic supply: most arteriolar beds have only sympathetic nerve fibres, and sympathetic stimulation usually causes vasoconstriction.

The Biological Activity of the Endothelium

The endothelium is a single-cell layer of flattened cells lining blood vessels. It is actively involved in regulation of clotting, recruitment of white blood cells in tissue injury and inflammation, and the control of blood vessel diameter. It produces several agents that relax or contract the smooth muscle in the blood vessel wall, causing vasodilation or vasoconstriction, as well as regulating the coagulability of the blood and the 'stickiness' of the endothelium, which increases in inflammation to allow white blood cells to adhere and migrate through into the tissues. Some of the most important are listed in Table 7.1, and many are important targets for drug action. Nitric oxide (**NO**) is an important vasodilator, and the nitrate vasodilators, e.g. **glyceryl trinitrate (GTN)**, increase NO levels in blood vessel walls, relax vascular smooth muscle, increase blood flow, and reduce pressure. NO has antiplatelet activity and inhibits blood clotting; there is also evidence that it reduces inflammation and the development of atherosclerotic changes in the vascular wall. Atherosclerosis is an important contributor to blood vessel disease and is discussed on p. 147. Some prostaglandins, notably prostaglandin I$_2$ (**prostacyclin**), are vasodilators and antithrombogenic. Important vasoconstrictors derived from the endothelium include **endothelin** and **angiotensin II** (see below), and key drugs used in a range of cardiovascular conditions act by antagonising their action or preventing their synthesis: for example, **bosentan** is an endothelin-receptor antagonist, and **losartan** is an angiotensin receptor antagonist.

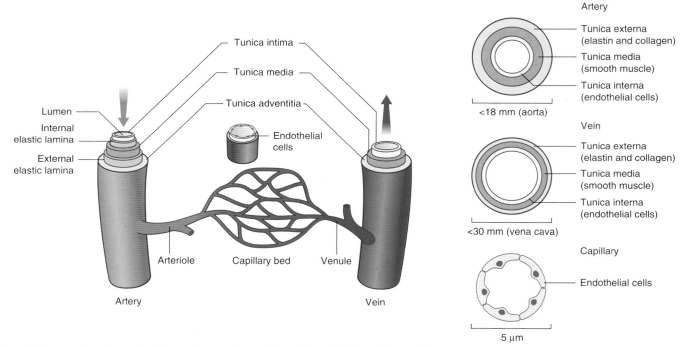

Fig. 7.14 The structure of arteries, veins, and capillaries. (From Naish J and Court DS (2019) Medical sciences, 3rd ed, Fig. 11.29. Edinburgh: Elsevier.)

Table 7.1 Endothelium-Derived Mediators

Mediator	Function	Relevant Drugs
Nitric oxide	Vasodilator; anticlotting; anti-inflammatory	Nitrate vasodilators increase nitric oxide levels
Prostacyclin	Vasodilator and anticlotting prostaglandin	Non-steroidal anti-inflammatory drugs reduce production (Fig. 6.18)
Endothelin	Vasoconstrictor	Bosantan blocks endothelin receptors
Angiotensin II	Produced by the enzyme angiotensin-converting enzyme acting on angiotensin I in pulmonary endothelium; vasoconstrictor	Angiotensin-converting enzyme inhibitors inhibit production; angiotensin-receptor antagonists block its action

CONTROL OF SYSTEMIC BLOOD PRESSURE

BP is determined by two main factors: cardiac output and total peripheral resistance (TPR), according to the following equation:

$$BP = CO \times TPR$$

Cardiac output, the volume of blood ejected from each ventricle per minute, is discussed above. TPR is determined by the degree of constriction in the arterial bed, especially the resistance arterioles. The greater the degree of constriction in arterioles, the higher the resistance to blood flow and the higher the BP. Vasodilation, on the other hand, opens up the vascular bed and BP falls. Moment-to-moment control of BP is controlled mainly by the ANS regulating heart rate, cardiac contractility, and peripheral resistance.

Total blood volume is an additional factor influencing BP. It is usually maintained within a narrow range, and in health varies little. Excess fluid is excreted, mainly by the kidney, and if the body water content falls, homeostatic mechanisms conserve fluid, for example by reducing urine volume, until intake can replace it. This is a slower, more sustained mechanism in BP regulation because changes in total body water usually take longer to become significant. The RAAS is fundamental to this process.

The Renin–Angiotensin–Aldosterone System

The RAAS operates closely with the sympathetic nervous system to regulate fluid balance, peripheral resistance, and BP. The outcomes of RAAS activity include increased Na^+ and water retention by the kidney, increased circulating blood volume, a generalised vasoconstriction, and a rise in BP.

The sequence of events involved in activation of the RAAS are shown in Fig. 7.15. The first step is release of the enzyme renin into the bloodstream from the kidney, which is triggered by three main factors:

- reduced blood flow through the renal blood vessels
- increased Na^+ levels in body fluids

- sympathetic stimulation of the kidney, which is triggered by central mechanisms detecting any fall in systemic BP. **β-blockers** inhibit this loop and help to reduce BP by blocking this sympathetically mediated activation of the RAAS.

In the bloodstream, renin converts an inactive protein called angiotensinogen to angiotensin I. Angiotensin I itself has little biological activity, but when it passes through the pulmonary capillaries in the lungs, it is converted to angiotensin II. The enzyme that catalyses this conversion is called angiotensin-converting enzyme (ACE), an important drug target in the treatment of hypertension and some kidney disorders by the group of drugs called **ACEIs**. Angiotensin II is a powerful vasoconstrictor and increases peripheral resistance. It also stimulates release of the mineralocorticoid steroid hormone **aldosterone** from the adrenal cortex. Aldosterone stimulates Na^+ and water reabsorption and promotes K^+ excretion in the renal tubules, increasing Na^+ and water load, blood volume, and BP. Certain diuretics, e.g. **spironolactone**, are aldosterone antagonists, used to increase Na^+ and water excretion in hypertension, heart failure, and other conditions associated with oedema (see also Chapter 9).

VASODILATORS

> **KEY DEFINITIONS**
>
> Vasodilator:
>   an agent that relaxes smooth muscle in arteries and veins
> Venodilator:
>   an agent whose vasodilator action is more pronounced in veins than arteries

Vasodilators relax vascular smooth muscle, increasing blood flow through the vessel. They are used to reduce BP in hypertension and to reduce afterload in heart failure. Dilation of systemic vessels improves blood supply to tissues,

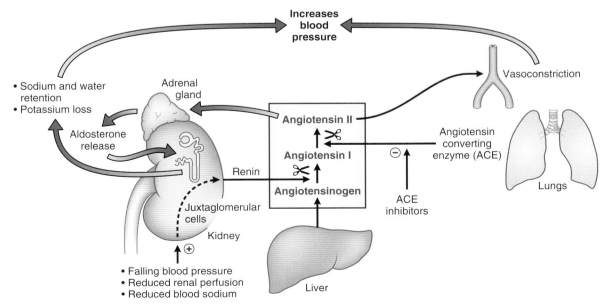

Fig. 7.15   The renin–angiotensin–aldosterone system. (Adapted from Raven JPH, Raven P, Chew SL (2023) The endocrine system, 3rd ed, Fig. 6.10. Oxford; Elsevier.)

including the heart in angina and systemic vessels in peripheral vascular disease and Raynaud's disease. Most vasodilators act on both arteries and veins, and so reduce pressure throughout the vascular system. Exceptions include the **nitrate vasodilators**, which act preferentially on veins, and **hydralazine**, which dilates arteries. Venodilators like nitrates are useful mainly in heart failure, because by opening venous capacity, more blood remains in the venous system and less is returned to the heart, reducing preload and relieving cardiac effort. Arterial dilators are more useful in hypertension, although they reduce BP, which can trigger reflexive sympathetic tachycardia.

VASODILATORS AND THE SYMPATHETIC NERVOUS SYSTEM

Sympathetic nerves supplying blood vessels release noradrenaline, which acts on α_1-receptors and usually causes vasoconstriction; α_1-receptors are the most common adrenergic receptor in blood vessels. α_1-receptor blockade therefore causes vasodilation. Some blood vessel beds also have β_2-receptors, which cause vasodilation. β-blockers can cause vascular side-effects by blocking these receptors: for example, **propranolol** causes cold hands and feet, because it blocks the vasodilator action of the sympathetic nervous system on β_2-receptors in these vascular beds and reduces blood flow.

α_1-Blockers

Examples: prazosin, doxazocin

α_1-receptor blockade causes vasodilation in arteries and veins, which decreases afterload, preload, and BP, and these drugs are used in hypertension. They are also used to treat urinary retention associated with benign prostatic hyperplasia because they relax the smooth muscle of the bladder neck and improve urine flow. **Prazosin** has also been used to improve sleep patterns in post-traumatic stress disorder. Its half-life is only 3 hours, whereas **doxazocin's** half-life is about 12 hours. Hypotension, especially early in treatment and in older people, is common.

NITRATES

Examples: Glyceryl trinitrate, isosorbide dinitrate

Nitrates have been used as vasodilators since the 1850s to treat hypertension and angina. Nitroglycerine, the original nitrate, is highly unstable (it is a key component of explosives), and early workers studying this new class of compound included Alfred Nobel, who gave his name to the most famous prize in science, and whose first invention was a detonator to control nitroglycerine explosions. Early work to produce a stable and convenient form of nitroglycerine included incorporating it into chocolate, which was nibbled at the onset of anginal pain. Nitrates increase levels of nitric oxide in smooth muscle in blood vessel walls, producing vasodilation, reducing BP, and increasing blood flow. Nitric oxide is the main endogenously produced vasodilator, and so has a key role in the control of systemic vascular resistance. It lowers free Ca^{2+} levels inside the muscle cell by increasing Ca^{2+} uptake into the storage membranes inside the cell and by blocking Ca^{2+} uptake by the cell from extracellular fluids. This reduces the amount of Ca^{2+} available to activate the actin–myosin contractile proteins and relaxes the muscle. Nitrate vasodilators cause venous dilation, which reduces venous return and preload, and arterial

dilation, which reduces afterload, relieving the workload of the heart. They dilate coronary arteries, improving blood and oxygen supply to the heart, and improve blood flow, particularly to the ischaemic areas of the myocardium.

Glyceryl Trinitrate

GTN is an important drug in the treatment of angina. Given as a sublingual spray or a tablet tucked under the tongue, it relieves anginal pain within minutes. Tablets lose their pharmacological activity within 8 weeks of opening their container because GTN is volatile and evaporates with time, but the spray formulation is stable for up to three years. It may also be given by infusion or via a skin patch.

Pharmacokinetics

GTN cannot be given orally because it is completely eliminated from the bloodstream by first-pass metabolism in the liver. Its plasma half-life is between 1 and 4 minutes, and it is effective over a period of half an hour or so. Tolerance to the vasodilator effect of the drug develops with extended administration, i.e. with infusion or with patches, and withdrawal of the drug is needed for it to regain its effectiveness. The cause of the tolerance is not understood, but it limits sustained use of nitrate vasodilators especially in chronic angina. The usual management strategy is to build in a nitrate-free period every 24 hours, usually overnight, to restore the drug's effectiveness.

Adverse Effects

Because it is such a powerful vasodilator, GTN dilates meningeal blood vessels and causes headaches, which can be severe. Other side-effects due to excessive vasodilation include facial flushing and hypotension.

Isosorbide Dinitrate

This nitrate vasodilator can be taken orally, and in addition is available in slow-release form to prolong therapeutic plasma levels. Tolerance to its vasodilator effects develops quickly, and it is usually taken in the morning, so that its levels are low overnight and the tolerance is reversed.

Ca^{2+}-CHANNEL ANTAGONISTS

Smooth muscle needs an increase in intracellular Ca^{2+} levels to activate contraction. This rise is triggered by Ca^{2+} influx through Ca^{2+} channels in the smooth muscle cell membrane. In the presence of a Ca^{2+}-channel antagonist, e.g. **nifedipine** or **amlodipine**, Ca^{2+} entry is prevented and vascular smooth muscle is relaxed. This causes vasodilation and reduces BP. The pharmacology of Ca^{2+}-channel blockers is described in more detail on p. 132.

K+-CHANNEL OPENERS

Some vasodilators relax vascular smooth muscle by opening K+ channels in the muscle cell membrane and allowing extra K+ to enter. This reduces the membrane potential (makes it more negative or hyperpolarises it, see Fig. 7.11), pulling it further away from the activation threshold, and the muscle cell relaxes.

Minoxidil

Minoxidil is primarily an arterial dilator. It is well absorbed when given orally and is metabolised in the liver. Its half-life

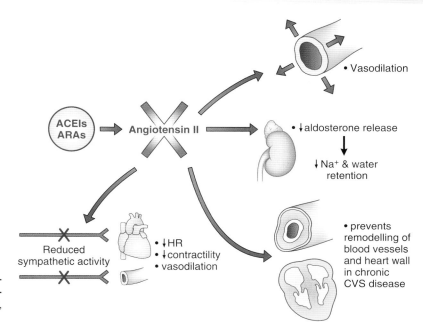

Fig. 7.16 The beneficial effects of angiotensin-converting enzyme inhibitors and angiotensin-receptor antagonists in cardiovascular disease. HR, Heart rate.

is about 4 hours, but its vasodilator effect is potent and long-lasting, which triggers reflex sympathetic compensatory mechanisms. As a result, there is tachycardia and activation of the RAAS with Na^+ and water retention, which usually require additional treatment with a β-blocker and a diuretic, respectively. Minoxidil is therefore not a first-line agent and is used to treat severe hypertension that does not respond satisfactorily to other drugs. One of its metabolites stimulates hair growth, and hirsutism is an unwanted effect, particularly in women, although the drug is used topically to treat male-pattern baldness.

Nicorandil

This vasodilator is given orally to treat angina. It is classed as a K^+-channel opener, but its vasodilator activity is partly due to its action in increasing NO levels in vascular smooth muscle. It dilates both healthy and diseased coronary arteries, improving blood flow to the myocardium, and causes systemic vasodilation, reducing both preload and afterload. It has a short plasma half-life (1 hour), and its main side-effects are similar to those of the nitrates, including headache, hypotension, lethargy, and fatigue. It may also cause GI side-effects, including vomiting.

DRUGS AND THE RENIN–ANGIOTENSIN–ALDOSTERONE SYSTEM

The RAAS has a central role in the control of peripheral resistance and blood volume and is the target of several important drugs used to treat hypertension and IHD.

ANGIOTENSIN-CONVERTING ENZYME INHIBITORS

Examples: captopril, ramipril, lisinopril

The first ACEI, **captopril**, was developed in the 1970s as the product of rational drug design. The structure of the active site of ACE was known, and the drug development programme that produced captopril exploited this understanding to predict which chemical modifications to

their test compounds would produce an effective inhibitor. ACEIs are used to treat hypertension, heart failure, and diabetic nephropathy, as well as to improve prognosis following MI. Because activation of the RAAS affects cardiovascular function in several ways (Fig. 7.16), ACEIs and angiotensin receptor antagonists (discussed below) have more than one mechanism of action. By blocking the production of angiotensin II, they cause vasodilation, mainly of arterioles, although they act also on the venous system; this is the main reason for their very effective antihypertensive activity. Reducing angiotensin II levels also reduces angiotensin II-stimulated aldosterone release, which in turn reduces water and Na^+ absorption by the kidney and reduces circulating blood volume. This contributes to the hypotensive effect, as well as reducing cardiac workload. Because angiotensin II stimulates the sympathetic nervous system, inhibiting its production reduces sympathetic tone in the CVS, reducing heart rate and causing vasodilation. In addition, angiotensin II stimulates the proliferation of smooth muscle cells, and is believed to be one of the factors that promote thickening of blood vessel walls in hypertension and the hypertrophy of cardiac ventricular muscle in heart failure. These structural changes are called remodelling and are compensatory responses of the muscle to increased BP. Initially they help to maintain cardiovascular function but ultimately worsen the situation. Thickened blood vessel walls stretch less and exacerbate rising BP, and hypertrophic cardiac muscle demands more oxygen and interferes with effective pumping. Blocking this action of angiotensin II is likely to help prevent remodelling and to preserve normal cardiovascular structure and function in chronic cardiovascular disease.

ACEIs also have an important place in the treatment of diabetic nephropathy and diabetes-related hypertension. Diabetes mellitus is strongly associated with renal vascular disease, which in turn accelerates the development of hypertension. This further damages the renal vasculature and promotes a cycle of deteriorating kidney function and worsening hypertension. Angiotensin II is a key player in this because its vasoconstrictor action increases BP in the glomerular capillaries and alters the structure of the glomerular filter, making it more permeable and contributing to the proteinuria and structural glomerular damage seen in diabetic people developing kidney impairment. ACEIs and ARAs help to break this vicious circle by blocking the effect of angiotensin II in the glomeruli and are significantly renoprotective in diabetic nephropathy.

ACEIs must be used carefully in people with known renovascular disease because they can cause a dramatic and dangerous fall in glomerular filtration rate (GFR). The afferent arteriole bringing blood into the glomerular capillaries is wider than the efferent arteriole, bringing more blood into the glomerulus than there is room for it to leave, raising pressure in the capillaries and driving filtration across the glomerular membrane (Fig. 7.17A). When afferent arteriolar blood flow falls because of, for example, atherosclerosis, the kidney uses angiotensin II to constrict the efferent arteriole and keep filtration pressure high in the glomerulus to maintain GFR (Fig. 7.17B). By blocking angiotensin II production, ACEIs prevent the kidney from making this compensatory adjustment, the efferent arteriole widens, and filtration pressure falls in the glomerular capillaries (Fig. 7.17C).

Pharmacokinetics
All ACEIs are given orally. Some, e.g. **ramipril** and **enalapril**, are pro-drugs, and rely upon activation in the liver. Half-lives vary considerably; captopril's half-life is only 2 hours, but **enalapril** has a half-life of 35 hours, and its active metabolite enalaprilat is 10 hours. **Lisinopril** is given as an active drug and needs only once daily administration because it has a half-life of 12 hours. Caution is needed when co-administered with a **diuretic**, especially when initiating ACEI treatment, because this can result in a sudden and potentially dangerous fall in BP.

Adverse Effects
ACEIs are contra-indicated in pregnancy because they damage the developing fetal kidney. They can cause a range of side-effects, including allergy, electrolyte imbalances, and significant liver impairment: liver function should be monitored and the drug discontinued if there is evidence of liver problems. In up to 35% of patients, a dry, troublesome cough develops, more commonly in women, which can be bothersome enough to lead to the patient wishing to discontinue treatment. ACEI-induced cough is not dose-related and can arise at any time after initiation of treatment. It is attributed to the accumulation of the irritant inflammatory mediator bradykinin in the airways (Fig. 7.18). In addition to producing angiotensin II, ACE also deactivates bradykinin. Inhibition of ACE activity allows bradykinin levels to rise, causing cough. This adverse effect disappears when the drug is withdrawn. Increased levels of bradykinin may also be the reason why ACEIs can cause urticaria and angioedema (sudden swelling in the deeper layers of the skin). Although these side-effects are much rarer than cough, angioedema is sometimes severe enough to cause dangerous tracheal obstruction.

ANGIOTENSIN-RECEPTOR ANTAGONISTS
Examples: losartan, valsartan

Angiotensin II acts on two different receptor types, AT_1 and AT_2, and from a clinical point of view the AT_1 receptor is the more important because this is the subtype involved in the main cardiovascular actions of angiotensin II. Drugs that block the AT_1 receptor therefore have a very similar range of pharmacological activity to the ACEIs, although they do not cause cough (because ACE is still produced and is still available to break down bradykinin). **Losartan** was the first orally active drug in this group, and although its half-life is short (2 hours), metabolism produces an active metabolite with a half-life of 10 hours, and losartan can be given once daily. As with ACEIs, ARAs should be used carefully in people with renovascular disease and not in pregnancy.

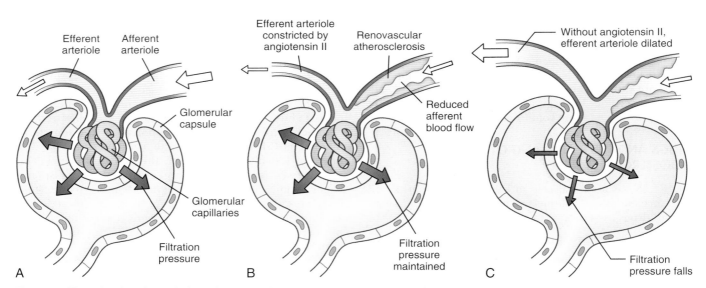

Fig. 7.17   The role of angiotensin in maintaining glomerular filtration rate in renal artery disease. A. The healthy glomerulus: the afferent arteriole is wider than the efferent, maintaining filtration pressure. B. Renovascular disease: the afferent arteriole is narrowed by e.g. atherosclerosis, so to maintain filtration pressure, the efferent arteriole is constricted by angiotensin II. C. Angiotensin-converting enzyme inhibitors (ACEIs) and angiotensin-receptor antagonists (ARAs) block this compensatory adjustment, and filtration pressure falls.

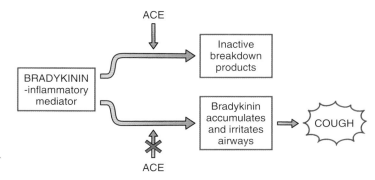

Fig. 7.18 Mechanism of action of angiotensin-converting enzyme inhibitor (ACEI)–induced cough.

RENIN ANTAGONIST

The only renin antagonist currently available is **aliskiren**, licensed for the treatment of hypertension. It binds to renin and prevents it from converting angiotensin I to angiotensin II. Angiotensin II levels therefore fall and its effects are significantly reduced. Aliskiren is given orally, and because of its long half-life (24–40 hours), it is only given once daily and takes up to two weeks to achieve effective steady state plasma levels. As with **captopril**, aliskiren was a product of rational drug design and effectively reduces BP when used as monotherapy. Used alone, it is generally well tolerated, although it can cause diarrhoea and hypokalaemia. However, effective control of hypertension frequently requires concurrent use of two or more drugs, and issues have been identified when aliskiren is combined with ARAs or ACEIs in patients with diabetes, cardiovascular disease, or renal disease. In these patients, the rates of serious side-effects including renal dysfunction and hypotension are high and these drugs should therefore not be used in combination.

ENDOTHELIN-RECEPTOR ANTAGONISTS

Endothelin is a powerful vasoconstrictor released by the endothelial lining of blood vessels and vascular smooth muscle as part of the normal regulation of blood vessel tone. It acts on two receptor types, ET_A and ET_B, and it probably causes prolonged, local vasoconstriction, increases BP, and

activates inflammatory mediators mainly through ET_A receptors. It also stimulates proliferation and fibrosis in the blood vessel wall and in the heart, which may contribute to the remodelling damage seen in the heart and blood vessels in cardiovascular disease and is likely to be involved in the pathogenesis of atherosclerosis. Despite endothelin's well-understood multifunctional role in cardiovascular pathophysiology, endothelin antagonists have so far only proved useful in pulmonary arterial hypertension and in treating finger ulcers in systemic sclerosis. In pulmonary arterial hypertension, endothelin levels are consistently raised, and endothelin-receptor antagonists improve exercise tolerance, reduce mean pulmonary artery pressure, and delay the progression of the disease.

Bosentan

Bosentan was the first endothelin antagonist discovered, licensed in 2001, and it blocks both ET_A and ET_B receptors equally. It is used to treat pulmonary arterial hypertension, is given orally, has a half-life of around 5 hours, and is cleared by the liver and the kidney. It is teratogenic, so is contraindicated in pregnancy, and can cause liver impairment, so hepatic monitoring is important and it should be avoided in all but the mildest degrees of pre-existing liver disease. It commonly causes GI side-effects, and because it is an enzyme inducer, it can increase the clearance rates of a range of other drugs including **warfarin, opioids,** and **Ca^{2+}-channel blockers**.

Focus on: Hypertension

Hypertension is a common disorder in which sustained high BP damages the heart and the arterial system. It is a major risk factor for cardiovascular disease and greatly increases the risk of stroke, myocardial infarction, heart failure, cardiac arrhythmia, and kidney disease. It is a major factor in the development of atherosclerosis (see below) which itself is both a cause and a manifestation of cardiovascular disease. Most cases are primary (essential) hypertension, sustained high BP with no directly identifiable cause. Risk factors for essential hypertension include increasing age, male sex, overweight, obesity, heredity, high salt intake, high alcohol intake, sedentary lifestyle, and low birthweight. Fewer than 10% are directly related to another condition; this is secondary hypertension and causes include pregnancy, renal disease, and a range of endocrine disorders including diabetes.

Regulation of BP in health is a complex process, and a range of factors contribute, including normal RAAS activity, normal endothelial function, cardiac function, balanced sympathetic/parasympathetic activity, insulin resistance, and balanced activity of a large range of hormones, cytokines, and other mediators. There is also evidence for an inflammatory and immunological component, and it has been shown that in hypertension, activated immune cells infiltrate the kidney and blood vessels, both key organs in BP regulation. There is increasing evidence that much of the end-organ damage seen in hypertension—in the kidneys, the brain, the blood vessels, and the heart—is due to ongoing inflammation. Research into precisely which immune cells and which inflammatory mechanisms are involved is ongoing and may lead to novel treatments for hypertension in the future: this would be particularly useful for the

Continued

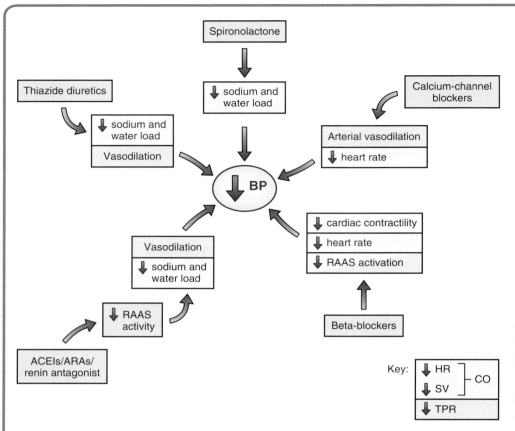

Fig. 7.19 The mechanism of action of the main drugs used to treat hypertension. ACEIs, Angiotensin converting enzyme inhibitors; ARAs, angiotensin receptor antagonists; CO, cardiac output; HR, heart rate; RAAS, renin-angiotensin-aldosterone system; SV, stroke volume; TPR, total peripheral resistance.

substantial subset of hypertensive people for whom conventional antihypertensive treatment does not work.

Considering the multiple processes contributing to BP regulation, it is not surprising that the pathophysiology of essential hypertension is complex. In an ideal scenario, a single drug would be effective in reducing BP to target levels, but often more than one agent is needed. Current treatment options for hypertension usually centre around one or more of the parameters controlling BP as described above: SV, HR, or TPR (Fig. 7.19).

Angiotensin-Converting Enzyme Inhibitors/Angiotensin-Receptor Antagonists

These agents are usually first-line treatment in younger people with hypertension and in diabetes at any age because they slow the development of diabetic nephropathy. They reduce peripheral resistance through their vasodilator action, and they reduce blood volume and cardiac output because they increase water and Na$^+$ excretion.

Thiazide Diuretics

This class of diuretic is usually the preferred choice in hypertension because they have a moderate but sustained effect on Na$^+$ and water excretion. They may be the preferred initial option in older people and those with any degree of heart failure because they reduce oedema and circulating blood volume, which helps to reduce cardiac workload. In longer-term use, diuretics also have a vasodilator action. The mechanism of action of this is not known, but it is likely to contribute significantly to their hypotensive effect, especially in longer-term treatment. Diuretics are considered in more detail in Chapter 9.

Calcium-Channel Blockers

These are usually first-line treatment in older non-diabetic people with hypertension. Their vasodilator action, mainly in the arterial system, reduces peripheral resistance. These drugs may also reduce cardiac contractility and slow the heart, also helping to reduce BP.

Second-Line Agents

If monotherapy is inadequate, other first-line drugs can be added (although **ACEIs** and **ARAs** should never be co-prescribed). If this fails, other antihypertensive agents may be added to the regimen. This may bring clinical benefit, because two or more low-dose drugs used together can reduce side-effects compared with high-dose monotherapy. **Spironolactone**, a K$^+$-sparing diuretic (p. 177), is of proven usefulness in hypertension resistant to standard treatments. It is an aldosterone antagonist and increases Na$^+$ and water excretion, suggesting that Na$^+$ retention is an important factor in resistant hypertension. **β-blockers** are generally not given unless there are additional indications for their use, because they are less effective than the drug groups listed above and have significant adverse effects, including in diabetes. Other possible options may include **α-blockers** and **aliskiren**.

Adjuvant Drugs

Statins (p. 148) are commonly used in hypertension to reduce blood lipid levels and the risk of a cardiovascular event. Low-dose **aspirin** (p. 121) reduces the risk of thrombosis-related cardiovascular events in at-risk patients.

ISCHAEMIC HEART DISEASE

The left ventricle pumps oxygenated blood into the aorta for distribution to all body tissues. The coronary arteries supply the myocardium. Coronary artery disease (also called ischaemic heart disease (IHD)), restricts myocardial oxygen supply because blood flow through the narrowed coronary arteries is inadequate to meet the heart's needs. IHD is the leading cause of death worldwide and is usually caused by atherosclerotic changes in the coronary artery wall.

Atherosclerosis

Atherosclerosis is a chronic inflammatory condition of blood vessels that causes deposition of semi-liquid fatty material within the blood vessel wall and damages and roughens the endothelium. The initial changes take the form of a fatty streak on the endothelium, which enlarges and develops over a period of time to form a mature lesion, called an atherosclerotic plaque, which progressively obstructs the vessel lumen as it expands. The fatty streak is initiated by deposition of a form of cholesterol called low-density lipoprotein (LDL) cholesterol in the arterial wall, which triggers ongoing inflammation that drives ongoing injury. The main pathological features are shown in Fig. 7.20A, and Fig. 7.20B is a photomicrograph of a coronary artery showing the gross appearance of an atherosclerotic plaque. The plaque core is a semi-fluid accumulation of fatty material, including cholesterol and other lipids, and infiltrated with inflammatory cells including lymphocytes. Characteristic of these plaques are foam cells, macrophages that have consumed large quantities of fat, which appear under the microscope as dense foamy bubbles in the cytoplasm. Smooth muscle cells grow into the core, and collagen and other fibrous material is deposited in the plaque. As the plaque grows, the blood vessel lumen becomes progressively narrower and blood flow is obstructed. The whole plaque is covered with a rough fibrous cap, which lacks the smooth surface of healthy endothelium and increases the risk of thrombus formation. The most advanced plaques become calcified and stiff, which makes them more likely to rupture. If the plaque splits, exposing its fatty contents to the bloodstream, a blood clot forms over the area of rupture, because the lipid-rich core is highly thrombogenic. This causes sudden and immediate obstruction of the artery and is the commonest cause of acute myocardial infarction and sudden coronary death. Fragments of this clot can also travel in the bloodstream and lodge elsewhere, e.g. in the pulmonary circulation, which causes a pulmonary embolism.

Risk Factors for Atherosclerosis. Some risk factors are non-modifiable, e.g. age, male sex, and heredity. Modifiable risk factors include smoking, hypertension, hyperlipidaemia, poorly controlled diabetes, and systemic inflammation. Not all blood lipids promote atheroma formation. LDL cholesterol and very-low-density lipoprotein (VLDL) cholesterol, together called non-high-density lipoprotein cholesterol, are strongly associated with atheroma, whereas high-density lipoprotein (HDL) cholesterol transfers cholesterol to the liver for removal from the bloodstream, an anti-atherogenic effect, and reduces the risk of atherosclerosis. Reducing LDL cholesterol blood levels is a standard therapeutic approach, and is proven to reduce cardiovascular events because it reduces deposition of these lipids in arterial walls, but it is also recognised that the total cholesterol:HDL cholesterol ratio is an important indicator of cardiovascular risk. Ideally this ratio should be as low as possible, and values above 6 are considered high.

ISCHAEMIC HEART DISEASE AND MYOCARDIAL INFARCTION

In the early stages of IHD, with mild to moderate coronary artery obstruction, blood flow generally meets the heart's needs at rest or in gentle exercise, but more demanding exercise increases its oxygen needs beyond what can be supplied through the narrowed coronary arteries. The myocardium becomes ischaemic, metabolism shifts from aerobic pathways to anaerobic pathways, and lactate (the physiological form of lactic acid) starts to accumulate. This causes the characteristic pain of angina. When blood flow is below the critical minimum needed for cell survival even at rest, the

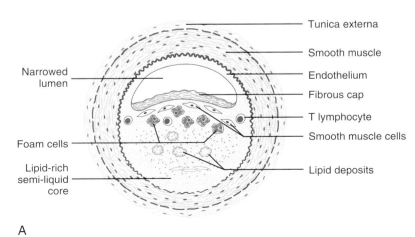

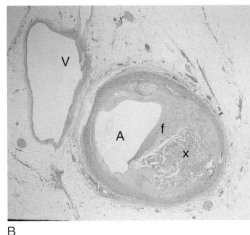

A

B

Fig. 7.20 Atherosclerosis. A. The main features of an atherosclerotic plaque. B. Photomicrograph of a diseased coronary artery. The artery lumen (A) is reduced and the fibrous cap (f) and lipid core (x) are clearly shown. The coronary vein (V) is adjacent. (Modified from Cross S (2019) *Underwood's pathology: a clinical approach,* 7th ed, Fig. 13.4. Oxford: Elsevier.)

muscle cells begin to die. This is infarction, and if a large enough portion of the myocardium is involved, the effective beating action of the heart cannot continue and sudden death may follow.

DRUGS USED TO TREAT ISCHAEMIC HEART DISEASE

A range of lifestyle changes underpins the management of people with IHD, but the aim of drug treatment is to reduce the heart's workload, improve its oxygen supply, improve exercise tolerance, and extend life. Drugs that reduce the heart rate improve coronary artery flow, because during cardiac systole the coronary arteries are compressed by the contracting myocardium. During diastole, however, when the heart muscle relaxes, they open up again. Reducing heart rate increases the length of time spent in diastole and therefore improves coronary artery flow. Drugs that reduce blood lipids, particularly LDL cholesterol, reduce the risk of a first or subsequent coronary event.

VASODILATORS

The pharmacology of the main vasodilators is discussed above, but their usefulness in IHD and angina is threefold:

- they dilate systemic arteries, which reduces afterload and cardiac workload.
- they dilate the coronary arteries, increasing myocardial blood flow.
- they are venodilators, which pool the blood in systemic veins and reduce venous flow to the heart, reducing preload and cardiac workload.

Ca^{2+}-channel blockers, e.g. **amlodipine**, **diltiazem,** and **nifedipine**, as well as **nitrates** and K^+-channel agonists, e.g. **nicorandil,** may all be used.

β-BLOCKERS

The pharmacology of β-blockers is described above. In IHD, they slow the heart and therefore improve coronary artery blood flow by increasing time spent in diastole and reduce contractility and oxygen consumption. This in turn reduces BP, further relieving cardiac effort and alleviating the pain of angina. Cardioselective agents include **atenolol, bisoprolol,** and **metoprolol**. Some β-blockers, e.g. **pindolol** and **carvedilol**, also produce a degree of vasodilation, which reduces afterload and reduces cardiac work. The drugs vasodilate via different mechanisms: pindolol weakly stimulates β-receptors in blood vessels, and carvedilol blocks vascular α-receptors.

STATINS

Examples: simvastatin, atorvastatin, pravastatin

Statins were introduced in the 1980s and inhibit the liver enzyme hydroxymethylglutaryl co-enzyme A (HMG co-A) reductase. This enzyme catalyses a crucial step in cholesterol synthesis, so in the presence of a statin, hepatic cholesterol production is inhibited. This in turn reduces circulating levels of non-HDL ('bad') cholesterol. Statins are used in both primary and secondary prevention of cardiovascular events like myocardial infarction and stroke: that is, in people who have never had a cardiovascular event, and in people who have had one or more such event. They protect against cardiovascular

events even in people whose blood lipid profile is normal and are recommended for use in type 1 diabetes even in the absence of other cardiovascular risk factors. In addition to their effect on blood lipids, statins have additional biological activities, including improving the health of vascular endothelium, stabilising atherosclerotic plaques, and reducing the systemic inflammatory response, all of which may contribute to cardiovascular protection. Statins are also used to treat primary hyperlipidaemias and hypercholesterolemia.

Pharmacokinetics

Statins are given orally and most undergo significant first-pass metabolism. Half-lives vary considerably between these drugs. **Simvastatin** and **pravastatin** have short half-lives of 1–2 hours and are best taken at night because cholesterol synthesis is highest at night. **Atorvastatin** has a much longer half-life of more than 30 hours.

Adverse Effects

Statins are generally well tolerated, even at high doses. Muscle pain is commonly reported, but actual muscle damage caused by statins is rare. This may be due to statin-induced leakage of Ca^{2+} from the endoplasmic reticulum within muscle cells, which may damage the cell. People with pre-existing muscle conditions are more susceptible than those with no such history, and exercise has been shown to reduce its incidence. Statins may also cause liver damage, although there is evidence that certain statins may protect against liver cancer and protect liver function in patients with pre-existing liver disease. They may trigger diabetes in patients with predisposing factors, who should be monitored. They are contra-indicated in pregnancy because fetal abnormalities have been reported.

Additional Lipid-Modifying Drugs

Fenofibrate may be used with statins if blood lipid profiles remain unsatisfactory with statins alone. Fenofibrate reduces blood fatty acid levels by activating fatty-acid transporters in the liver, which increases their removal from the bloodstream. It may also decrease LDL cholesterol levels and increase HDL cholesterol, but this is variable. Fenofibrate has a long half-life of 20 hours and is given once daily. It is a pro-drug, activated by hepatic metabolism, and mainly eliminated in the urine. **Ezetimibe** blocks cholesterol uptake in the small intestine by inhibiting the cholesterol transporter in the duodenal epithelium and reduces absorption of dietary cholesterol by about half. It has a synergistic action when combined with statins, enhancing statin-induced improvement in blood lipid profile, and also further reducing the systemic inflammation seen in atherosclerosis as well as reducing the likelihood of cardiovascular events.

ANTITHROMBOTIC DRUGS

Treatment with antithrombotic drugs reduces the risk of clots forming at the plaque site. Low-dose **aspirin** inhibits platelet activation via blockade of platelet thromboxane A_2 production (p. 152). **Clopidogrel** (p. 152) reduces clotting risk by irreversibly preventing platelet aggregation. Anticoagulant therapy may also be used in for example acutely developing coronary syndromes, in which the risk of thrombosis is significantly elevated. Antithrombotic drugs are discussed in more detail below.

HAEMOSTASIS

Haemostasis, or blood clotting, is the physiological mechanism that converts fluid blood to a firm, semi-solid thrombus. In health, blood remains fluid unless and until clotting is needed to stop blood loss, but inappropriate blood clotting is an important pathophysiological complication in a range of conditions, including myocardial infarction, some cardiac arrhythmias including atrial fibrillation, atherosclerotic vascular disease, serious infections and sepsis, pulmonary embolism, and stroke. There is a range of rare, inherited disorders that increase blood coagulability, but more common factors that increase the risk of thrombosis include pregnancy, varicose veins, smoking, surgery, and malignant disease. Antithrombotic drugs are used when the risks associated with clotting outweigh the risks associated with haemorrhage.

KEY DEFINITIONS

- Antithrombotic:
  a drug that by any mechanism prevents the formation or enlargement of blood clots
- Anticoagulant:
  a drug that prevents blood clotting by inhibiting one or more clotting factors
- Antiplatelet:
  a drug that prevents blood clotting by inhibiting platelet activity
- Fibrinolytic:
  a drug that dissolves an existing blood clot

PLATELETS AND CLOTTING

Platelets, produced in the red bone marrow, are small cell fragments packed with clotting factors including **serotonin** and **ADP**. Platelets also contain the enzyme cyclo-oxygenase (COX, see also p. 119). Healthy blood vessel endothelium constantly produces anticoagulant substances including **prostacyclin** and **nitric oxide** to prevent inappropriate clotting. However, injury to a blood vessel stimulates the endothelial cells to produce adhesion factors, to which platelets stick. Once the platelet is attached to the endothelium, it is activated, becomes sticky, and other platelets stick to it. Ongoing blood clotting is a good example of a positive feedback process, accelerating clot growth and expansion. Platelet adhesion molecules produced by an activated platelet include receptors for fibrinogen, and fibrinogen sticking to platelets via these receptors produces a progressively expanding fibrous network which permanently traps platelets and red blood cells. Over the few minutes following injury, platelets therefore rapidly accumulate and are activated, releasing their clotting factors and activating the blood-clotting cascade. Antiplatelet drugs like **aspirin** and **clopidogrel** block blood clotting by inhibiting platelet activity.

THE BLOOD-CLOTTING CASCADE

A blood clot forms because of the serial activation of a number of clotting factors circulating in the bloodstream. Most clotting factors are enzymes produced in the liver, and to avoid inappropriate clotting they circulate as inactive precursors which are only activated when needed. The final event in thrombus formation is called the final common pathway, in which Factor X (FX) activates prothrombin activator which in turn activates the enzyme thrombin. Thrombin converts fibrinogen to fibrin (Fig. 7.21). Fibrin forms

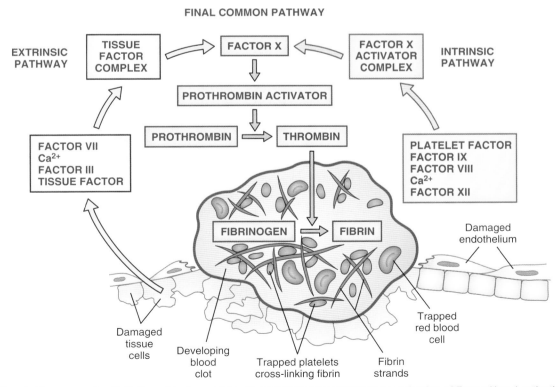

FINAL COMMON PATHWAY

Fig. 7.21 The clotting cascade. Both the extrinsic and intrinsic pathways lead ultimately to activation of Factor X and activation of the final common pathway.

the sturdy framework of the clot, in which red blood cells and platelets are trapped as it grows. Some anticoagulant drugs, e.g. **dabigatran,** directly inhibit thrombin and block fibrin production.

The final common pathway is activated by two related pathways, the intrinsic and extrinsic pathways (Fig. 7.21), which are usually activated simultaneously. Both require Ca^{2+} and both contribute to activating FX. The intrinsic pathway is initiated when inactive clotting factor XII (FXII) in the bloodstream comes into contact with collagen exposed at the blood vessel wall injury site. This activates FXII, which, in co-operation with a platelet-derived factor and clotting factors VIII and IX, produces a substance called FX activator complex. FX activator complex activates FX, which then activates the final common pathway. The other pathway, the extrinsic pathway, is activated when damaged tissues release a substance called tissue factor, also called thromboplastin. Tissue factor, in co-operation with clotting factors III and VII, produces a substance called tissue factor complex, which then activates FX and the final common pathway. Some anticoagulant drugs, including **apixaban**, directly inhibit activated FX.

Vitamin K is required for synthesis of several clotting factors, including factors II (prothrombin), VII, IX, and X. **Warfarin** and **phenindione** are examples of anticoagulant drugs that antagonise vitamin K.

NATURAL ANTICOAGULANTS

Physiological regulation of the clotting cascade involves a few natural anticoagulants which control clotting and normally prevent inappropriate clotting, and which also terminate it once the bleeding episode is resolved. As mentioned above, healthy endothelium produces anticoagulants, important contributors to the prevention of inappropriate clotting. These include antithrombin, an inhibitor of both thrombin and activated FX. The body produces a powerful stimulant of antithrombin activity, **heparin**, which is essential to physiological suppression of the clotting process, and which is in widespread use as an anticoagulant.

ANTICOAGULANTS

Blood flow is slower in veins than arteries, predisposing to thrombosis, and clots that form here have time to develop and are rich in fibrin. Because most anticoagulants directly or indirectly reduce thrombin activation and therefore fibrin production, they prevent thrombus development more effectively in the venous circulation than in the arterial circulation, where clots contain higher proportions of platelets than fibrin. The main side-effect of anticoagulant therapy is haemorrhage, and anticoagulants should therefore be used with great care, if at all, in patients with bleeding disorders and in those at increased risk of haemorrhage, e.g. peptic ulcer disease or hypertension.

VITAMIN K ANTAGONISTS

Examples: warfarin sodium, phenindione

Vitamin K is a co-factor in one key step in the synthesis of clotting factors II, VII, IX, and X. Co-factors are essential participants in a wide range of biochemical reactions, and the body needs only tiny quantities because they are constantly recycled. The vitamin K molecule is deactivated each time

it is used to make a molecule of clotting factor and must be converted back to its biologically active form in order to be used again. Vitamin K antagonists block its reactivation, and so the vitamin remains in its deactivated form and clotting factor synthesis stops (Fig. 7.22). Their anticoagulant effect may take several days to develop, because although clotting factor production is halted, the factors already present in the blood will initially ensure normal clotting.

Warfarin

Warfarin belongs to the coumarin group of anticoagulants. The first coumarin to be discovered, **dicoumarin**, was isolated in 1940 from a fungus that infected cattle fodder and was causing the animals to die from internal bleeding. Warfarin, derived from coumarin, was originally developed as a rat poison, but found a place in clinical medicine in the mid-1950s as a therapeutic anticoagulant. Although warfarin is an effective anticoagulant, its use is in decline because of the development of newer, safer agents including thrombin inhibitors and Factor X inhibitors.

Pharmacokinetics

Unlike **heparin**, the only available anticoagulant at the time the coumarins were being developed, warfarin is given orally. It is well absorbed and very highly bound to plasma proteins, so it has a long half-life of up to 48 hours. A single dose takes effect in 14–16 hours and lasts for four to five days, and at the end of a course of warfarin it takes two or three days for clotting times to return to normal, reflecting the time required to produce adequate levels of new clotting factors. Warfarin crosses the placenta and is both teratogenic and haemorrhagic in the developing baby, so should be avoided where possible in pregnancy. Warfarin is associated with a range of drug interactions. Its antithrombotic effect is additive to that of other anticlotting

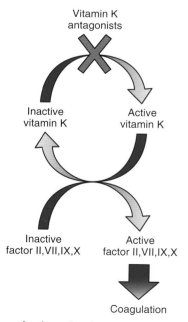

Fig. 7.22 The mechanism of action of the vitamin-K antagonists. (Modified from Padmanabhan S (2014) Handbook of pharmacogenomics and stratified medicine, Fig. 24.1. San Diego: Academic Press.)

drugs, e.g. **aspirin**, increasing bleeding times, and great care must be taken if these drugs are used together. Its action is potentiated by a range of drugs, e.g. **amiodarone** and a range of **antimicrobials**, which inhibit the liver enzymes that metabolise warfarin. Its action is reduced by enzyme inducers such as **alcohol** and **phenytoin**, which enhance the liver enzymes that metabolise warfarin and accelerate its clearance from the bloodstream.

Adverse Effects

The main side-effect is haemorrhage and bleeding times should be routinely monitored. If bleeding times are excessively long with ongoing bleeding or significant risk of dangerous haemorrhage, **vitamin K** (**phytomenadione**) can be given intravenously to restore clotting factor production; it takes up to 6 hours for full effect. Alternatively, blood clotting can be immediately restored to normal by infusion of functional clotting factors.

HEPARIN

Examples: dalteparin, enoxaparin (low-molecular-weight (LMW) heparins), unfractionated heparin

Heparin is the oldest anticoagulant in regular clinical use and is on the World Health Organisation list of essential medicines. It was discovered in 1918 by a medical student called L. Emmett Holt, who named it heparin because he was working with liver extracts, although it is also produced by a range of other tissues including mast cells and lung and blood vessel endothelium. Chemically, heparin belongs to a family of complex sugars called glycosaminoglycans (GAGs), which are joined together to form much larger molecules, the size of which depends on the number of individual GAG molecules used. Heparin can therefore exist in a range of different molecular weights. Unfractionated heparin is extracted from a range of animal sources and contains heparin molecules with a range of molecular weights between 3000 and 30 000 kDa. LMW heparins are separated from unfractionated heparin and contain molecules with MW less than 7000 kDa. The molecular weight of the heparin units affects the pharmacokinetics of the preparation, including absorption.

Heparin exerts its anticoagulant effect by binding to antithrombin. Antithrombin is one of the key natural brakes on clotting and blocks thrombin and FX activity. Heparin binds to antithrombin and greatly enhances its activity, further reducing the action of thrombin, fibrin production, and clot development (Fig. 7.23).

Pharmacokinetics

Heparin must be given by injection because heparin molecules are too large and heavily charged to be absorbed across the wall of the GI tract. It is used intravenously or subcutaneously, but not intramuscularly because of the risk of haematoma formation. LMW heparin is usually given subcutaneously and is well absorbed from injection sites. Its anticoagulant effect is generally predictable when the dose is calculated in relation to body weight, and routine blood clotting monitoring is usually not required. It does not bind significantly to plasma proteins and is cleared from the bloodstream by the liver and the kidneys. Its half-life is longer than unfractionated heparin, and so requires less frequent administration.

Unfractionated heparin's absorption is more variable and less predictable than that of LMW heparin and, depending on dose, its half-life ranges from 30 minutes to 3 hours.

Adverse Effects

Heparin has a narrow therapeutic index. Its main side-effect is haemorrhage, which is potentially fatal. Bleeding caused by excess unfractionated heparin can be rapidly reversed by IV administration of **protamine sulphate**, which binds to heparin in the bloodstream and deactivates it. Protamine sulphate is much less effective in stopping haemorrhage induced by LMW heparin, because it binds to it less strongly.

Another potentially lethal side-effect of heparin develops as the result of an autoimmune reaction against platelets in the presence of heparin. In about 1 in 50 patients, the interaction between heparin and platelets stimulates the production of antiplatelet antibodies that activate platelets and trigger thrombosis. In addition, the widespread activation of platelets leads to their clearance from the circulation and thrombocytopenia. In this situation, heparin must be discontinued and an alternative anticoagulant, such as **danaparoid** or a **direct thrombin inhibitor,** used instead.

Danaparoid

This is a heparin-like agent (a heparinoid) made up of a number of different GAGs related to heparin. As with

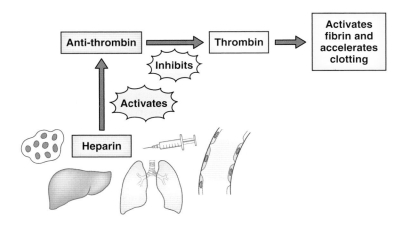

Fig. 7.23   The action of heparin.

heparin, its anticoagulant effect is due to activation of antithrombin. It has a low MW of 5500 kDa and is completely absorbed from subcutaneous administration.

DIRECT THROMBIN INHIBITORS

Examples: argatroban, dabigatran, bivalirudin

Thrombin is the enzyme that releases fibrin from fibrinogen (Fig. 7.21). Drugs that bind to and inhibit thrombin therefore block the terminal stage in the final common pathway. Without sticky fibrin to form the clot framework, clot formation is disrupted.

Dabigatran

This anticoagulant was licensed in 2008 and was the first new anticoagulant in over 50 years. One important advantage claimed by its manufacturer is that unlike **warfarin**, the standard agent in use at the time, monitoring blood levels is unnecessary. Dabigatran is given orally as an inactive prodrug, **dabigatran etexilate**, which is converted to the active form in the liver. Its onset of action is rapid, and its half-life is short, about 40 minutes. Life-threatening dabigatran-induced bleeding can be reversed with **idarucizumab**, an antibody which binds with high specificity and high affinity to dabigatran and prevents it from binding to thrombin. Renal function should be assessed before treatment is begun, because the drug is cleared mainly by the kidney, and monitoring renal function is particularly important in elderly people, who are most at risk of life-threatening bleeds with this drug.

Bivalirudin

The use of leeches in ancient medical practice to bleed patients has been revived in modern medicine in a limited number of clinical situations. Leech saliva contains a powerful anticoagulant called **hirudin**, so that when the leech bites its target for a blood meal, the blood remains fluid to allow the leech to feed. Leeches are sometimes used in plastic surgery or other situations to prevent clotting and maintain blood flow to a tissue. Hirudin is a directly acting thrombin inhibitor, and bivalirudin is a stable, synthetic hirudin analogue with a short half-life of around 25 minutes.

FACTOR Xa INHIBITORS

Examples: apixaban, fondaparinux, rivaroxaban

Activation of FX is the first step in the final common pathway (Fig. 7.21). Inhibiting activated FX (FXa) therefore blocks clotting initiated by both the extrinsic and intrinsic pathways. Routine monitoring of bleeding times is not needed, because their clinical effect correlates very well with dose and so is predictable.

Pharmacokinetics

These agents are given orally and are incompletely absorbed from the GI tract. Their half-lives are around 12 hours, but the onset of anticoagulant action is quick. They are only partially metabolised, and much of the administered drug is excreted unchanged in the faeces and urine.

Adverse Effects

Haemorrhage and anaemia are common but less so than with warfarin. **Rivaroxaban** can cause nausea.

ANTIPLATELET DRUGS

Antiplatelet drugs are most useful in conditions where there is inflammatory endothelial damage, primarily atherosclerosis, which triggers platelet activation. The endothelium of arteries is exposed to considerably more shear stress than veins because blood flow and pressure is much higher in the arterial than the venous system, and so arterial endothelial damage is more common than venous endothelial damage. Clots that form in arteries are therefore rich in platelets, and antiplatelet drugs are more effective in preventing arterial thrombosis than venous thrombosis.

ASPIRIN

Although aspirin has traditionally been a standard anti-inflammatory drug, its antiplatelet action has led to its widespread use to reduce thrombotic events in cardiovascular disease, as well as in primary prevention of thromboembolism in people without overt disease but with significant risk factors. Aspirin inhibits platelet activation by irreversibly inhibiting platelet COX, the enzyme that produces prostaglandins. Platelets synthesise a prostaglandin called thromboxane A_2 (TXA_2), which activates the platelet and causes local vasoconstriction by contracting vascular smooth muscle. TXA_2 is therefore a pro-clotting substance, and by inhibiting platelet COX and preventing TXA_2 production, aspirin suppresses blood clotting and increases bleeding times (see also p. 152).

Low-dose aspirin, i.e. aspirin concentrations significantly lower than required for an anti-inflammatory effect, achieves effective antithrombotic action. The standard maintenance antiplatelet dose is 75 mg aspirin daily, compared to up to 2.4 g daily as an analgesic/anti-inflammatory. This is mainly because aspirin irreversibly destroys platelet COX, permanently abolishing its clotting action, so that restoring full platelet activity requires the synthesis of brand-new platelets. After a single dose of aspirin, platelet TXA_2 generation recovers slowly, at the rate of about 10% per 24 hours, as new platelets are released into the bloodstream from the bone marrow to replace the defunct ones.

Pharmacokinetics

Aspirin (acetylsalicylic acid) has a short plasma half-life of about 20 minutes and is broken down by plasma esterases to release the active ingredient, salicylic acid, which diffuses passively into platelets.

Adverse Effects

Because prostaglandins have a wide range of physiological functions in healthy tissues, COX inhibitors have a range of unpleasant side-effects. The low dose used in cardiovascular prevention means that it is usually well tolerated, but it may still cause, for example, GI irritation and should be avoided in people with active peptic ulcer disease or a history of the same. Haemorrhage and allergy are also common side-effects. The side-effects of COX inhibitors are discussed in more detail on p. 120.

ADENOSINE-RECEPTOR ANTAGONISTS

Examples: clopidogrel, ticagrelor, prasugrel

ADP is an important pro-clotting factor released by platelets. ADP promotes and accelerates platelet activation by acting on the P2Y$_{12}$ receptor found on the platelet membrane. The more platelets are activated, the more ADP is released to activate more platelets, a very good example of a positive feedback system. Adenosine-receptor antagonists bind to the platelet P2Y$_{12}$ receptors and block them, preventing adenosine from attaching and activating the platelet (Fig. 7.24). Precursors of the current group of agents were identified in the 1970s as ADP antagonists only by chance, because researchers were actually screening for anti-inflammatory drugs, and further work produced **clopidogrel** in 1998. Adenosine-receptor antagonists are often used with **aspirin** in a range of thromboembolic disorders including ischaemic heart disease and acute coronary syndromes because the antiplatelet effects of the combination are additive.

Pharmacokinetics

Clopidogrel and **prasugrel** are pro-drugs and require activation in the liver. Both bind irreversibly to the platelet ADP receptors, and so their action is long-lasting even though clopidogrel's active metabolite has a half-life of only around half an hour. Adenosine-receptor inhibitors are given orally, sometimes with an initial loading dose to ensure rapid onset of action.

Adverse Effects

Care should be taken when co-prescribing with other drugs that have an antiplatelet effect: this list includes nonsteroidal anti-inflammatory drugs as well as perhaps less obvious agents such as **fluoxetine and sertraline** (p. 58). **Clopidogrel** and **ticagrelor** commonly cause GI upset and skin reactions. All agents in this group can cause haemorrhage.

DIPYRIDAMOLE

Dipyridamole is used orally, sometimes with aspirin and sometimes as a modified-release formulation. Its mechanism

of action is not entirely clear, and it may inhibit platelets in several ways: for example, it has been shown to inhibit TXA$_2$ synthesis, and it enhances the antiplatelet action of prostacyclin.

FIBRINOLYTIC DRUGS

Examples: streptokinase, alteplase, tenecteplase

Clot-dissolving (fibrinolytic) drugs are used to break down a formed clot and restore blood flow through an occluded vessel. Rapidly restoring blood flow through an artery following thrombosis, e.g. in a cerebral or a coronary artery, can make the difference between life and death for a patient, or the difference between significant disability and complete recovery. Fibrinolytics are used in a range of situations, including deep venous thrombosis, pulmonary embolism, myocardial infarction, or blocked in-situ cannulas or stents. The main hazard with using these drugs is haemorrhage. Fibrinolytic drugs are more effective the younger the clot, because as a clot matures, its fibrin content steadily increases and it becomes denser, more compact, and less susceptible to drug action. Treatment outcomes are therefore significantly better when drug infusion is begun as soon as possible after the onset of symptoms.

THE FIBRINOLYTIC SYSTEM

Following clotting, controlled dissolution of a blood clot (fibrinolysis) is an essential step in tissue healing and restoring blood flow. The key enzyme responsible for dissolving the blood clot is plasmin, which is converted from its inactive form plasminogen by two enzymes: thrombin and plasminogen activator (tPA). Plasmin digests fibrin and breaks the clot up (Fig. 7.25). It may seem counter-intuitive that thrombin, a key accelerator of clotting, also promotes fibrinolysis, but this is one of the key checks and balances in regulation of clotting and helps to ensure that the clotting cascade does not run away with itself.

Streptokinase

Streptokinase was discovered by chance in 1933 when it was observed that streptococcal bacteria dissolved blood clotted in test tubes used for an unrelated experiment. The active enzyme was isolated and named streptokinase as a nod to its microbial origin. It is now known that streptokinase activates

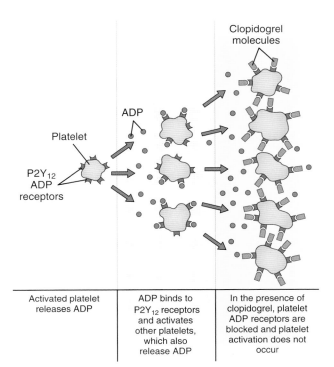

Fig. 7.24 The antiplatelet action of the adenosine-receptor antagonists.

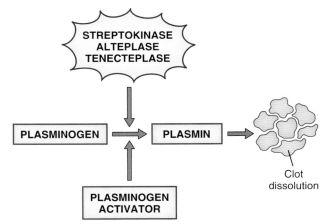

Fig. 7.25 The mechanism of action of fibrinolytic drugs.

plasminogen, i.e. it acts like naturally occurring tPA to release clot-dissolving plasmin, but its mechanism of action was not worked out until the 1940s, when plasmin and plasminogen themselves were isolated. To clear a blocked coronary artery in myocardial infarction, it is recommended that treatment starts within 12 hours of the onset of symptoms, but the earlier the better, because early treatment correlates directly with reduced mortality and improved cardiac function post-infarction.

Pharmacokinetics

Streptokinase is a highly efficient and fast-acting thrombolytic with a half-life of around 25–30 minutes and is given by IV infusion.

Side-Effects

Allergy is common, probably because streptokinase is derived from bacterial sources. In addition, streptokinase can trigger an immunological response with the generation of anti-streptokinase antibodies. These antibodies can persist for years and will neutralise streptokinase if given again. Because of this, streptokinase is only used on one occasion and if thrombolysis in the same patient is required in the future, a different agent is chosen. A range of cardiovascular adverse effects, including cardiac arrest, hypotension, heart failure, and cardiac ischaemia, are all common.

Alteplase and Tenecteplase

Alteplase and tenecteplase are human tPA produced by recombinant DNA technology, and therefore do not have the antigenicity associated with streptokinase. Both are given intravenously and metabolised in the liver. **Alteplase** has a shorter half-life (less than 5 minutes) and must be given by infusion, followed up with maintenance anticoagulant therapy to prevent re-occlusion of the artery with a new clot. **Tenecteplase** has higher affinity for fibrin than alteplase and a longer half-life (23 minutes), so it is given as a single bolus.

HAEMOSTATIC DRUGS

Haemostatic drugs promote clotting and stop haemorrhage. Purified clotting factor preparations are available for the treatment of conditions associated with deficiency; for example, **purified factor XIII** is used to treat haemophilia A.

Tranexamic Acid

Tranexamic acid is a synthetic antifibrinolytic used in general surgery and in trauma to reduce the risk and extent of bleeding and the need for transfusions. It is used to reduce blood loss in women with very heavy menstrual periods, to stop prolonged nosebleeds, and to control prolonged bleeding following dental surgery. It works by stopping plasminogen activation, and so reduces plasmin production and protects the developing fibrin clot (Fig. 7.25). It is also used to treat hereditary angioneurotic oedema (HAE), a rare condition caused by a deficiency of a key inhibiting enzyme that restrains the action of several enzyme cascades, including complement and clotting. Although not licensed in all countries, there is some evidence that tranexamic acid can reduce the severity of the attacks of swelling that characterise HAE.

It is given orally or intravenously, and is generally well tolerated, although there is a risk of seizures with higher doses. It is a small molecule and is excreted unchanged in the urine, so care must be taken if kidney function is reduced. Its half-life is around 2 hours, but this is extended in renal impairment.

REFERENCES

Awtry, E.H., Loscalzo, J., 2000. Aspirin. Circulation 101 (10), 1206–1218.

Echt, D.S., Ruskin, J.N., 2020. Use of flecainide for the treatment of atrial fibrillation. Am. J. Cardiol. 125 (7), 1123–1133.

Lei, M., Wu, L., Terrar, D.A., et al., 2018. Systematic review: modernised classification of cardiac antiarrhythmic drugs. Circulation 138 (17), 1879–1896.

Marsh, N., Marsh, A., 2000. A short history of nitroglycerine and nitric oxide in pharmacology and physiology. Clin. Exp. Pharmacol. Physiol. 27 (4), 313–319.

Norlander, A.E., Madhur, M.S., Harrison, D.C., 2018. The immunology of hypertension. J. Exp. Med. 215 (1), 21–33.

Ruggenenti, P., Cravedi, P., Remuzzi, G., 2010. The RAAS in the pathogenesis and treatment of diabetic nephropathy. Nat. Rev. Nephrol. 6 (6), 319–330.

Sirtori, C.R., 2014. The pharmacology of statins. Pharmacol. Res. 88, 3–11.

ONLINE RESOURCES

Florek, J.B., Lucas, A., Girzadas, D., 2023. Amiodarone. In: StatPearls [Internet]. StatPearls Publishing, Treasure Island. Available from: https://www.ncbi.nlm.nih.gov/books/NBK482154/.

Ornelas, A., Zacharias-Millward, N., Menter, D.G., et al., 2017. Beyond COX-1: the effects of aspirin on platelet biology and potential mechanisms of chemoprevention. Cancer Metastasis. Rev. 36 (2), 289–303.

Drugs and the Respiratory System

INTRODUCTION

The respiratory system, conventionally divided into upper and lower parts, brings atmospheric air into the lungs, from which it extracts oxygen and into which it excretes waste carbon dioxide. The epithelia lining the respiratory passageways and the alveoli are constantly exposed to the external environment via this inhaled air, so that respiratory infections are very common, especially if normal respiratory defence mechanisms are compromised in some way. Antimicrobial agents are described in Chapter 11.

THE RESPIRATORY SYSTEM

The main respiratory structures and organs of the upper and lower respiratory tracts are shown in Fig. 8.1A. Air inhaled through the nose or mouth travels through the trachea, which splits into the right and left primary bronchi to direct air into the right or left lung, respectively. Within each lung, the primary bronchus divides into secondary bronchi, which through progressive and extensive branching produce 30,000 tiny terminal bronchi which direct air into a total of around 450 million microscopic air sacs called alveoli (Fig. 8.1B). Alveolar walls are only one epithelial cell thick, and each alveolus is wrapped in a dense network of capillaries, the walls of which are also only one cell thick. Because the membrane formed between the fused alveolar and capillary walls is so thin, gas exchange is rapid and efficient; oxygen is absorbed by diffusion from the alveolar air into the bloodstream and carbon dioxide diffuses from the bloodstream into the alveoli, to be excreted in exhaled air.

THE STRUCTURE OF THE RESPIRATORY PASSAGEWAYS

The respiratory passageways are lined with epithelium, which varies in structure depending on the location. The epithelium lining the pharynx is stratified, because this part of the system is shared with the gastrointestinal (GI) system; the upper layers of cells can be safely rubbed off by swallowed food and drink because they are constantly being replaced with cells from the lower layers. The trachea and the larger airways are lined with ciliated epithelium (see Fig. 8.5) and contain numerous goblet cells for mucus production. The sticky mucus blanket lining the upper airways traps inhaled particles and is constantly moved towards the mouth by the beating action of the cilia. This so-called mucociliary escalator (see below) is an important pulmonary defence mechanism. The epithelium of the alveoli is composed of thin, flattened squamous cells to allow rapid gas exchange.

The walls of the larger airways are supported with embedded rings or plates of cartilage, preventing them from partial or complete collapse when air pressures change, and the lungs expand and recoil during normal respiration. The smaller airways and the alveoli have no cartilage, but they are kept open by the elastic fibres of the lung, which exert constant tension on their walls and prevent them from collapse.

Smooth Muscle of the Respiratory Passageways

Under the control of the autonomic nervous system, smooth muscle within the walls of the respiratory passageways regulates airway diameter and so controls air flow in the lung. Sympathetic fibres supplying the muscle release **noradrenaline**, which acts on β_2-adrenoceptors on the muscle cells (see Fig. 4.5) and relaxes it, opening the airways and increasing airflow. Parasympathetic fibres release **acetylcholine**, which acts on M_3 muscarinic receptors on the bronchial smooth muscle (see Fig. 4.8) to contract it, causing bronchoconstriction and reducing air flow. There is very little smooth muscle in the larger airways and, in any case, there is a substantial amount of cartilage in their walls, holding them open and preventing obstruction. However, the walls of the small- to medium-sized airways contain substantial amounts of smooth muscle, allowing significant adjustment to their diameter and permitting the lungs to direct air flow to areas of the lung receiving good blood supply.

DRUG-INDUCED PULMONARY TOXICITY

The lungs have a generous blood supply because they receive the entire output of the right ventricle, and so receive high concentrations of circulating drugs. Over 600 drugs in all fields of medicine and some recreational drugs have been associated with pulmonary toxicity, which is generally an idiosyncratic adverse effect and not usually dose-related. Risk factors include increasing age, genetic predisposition, and pre-existing lung disease or damage. Any respiratory structure or tissue may be involved, including the supporting elastic tissue of the lung, the pulmonary vasculature, the pleura, the muscles of respiration, the airways, or the alveoli. Fig. 8.2 shows the histology of **bleomycin**-induced lung damage compared to healthy tissue. The healthy lung

tissue shows thin-walled, interconnected alveolar spaces. The damaged lung is infiltrated with inflammatory cells, and the alveolar epithelium is thickened with loss of normal alveolar architecture. Drug-mediated lung damage may be due to a range of pathological changes (Table 8.1), and toxicity may be acute or chronic. Stopping the drug may reverse the changes, but in some cases the lung damage is permanent.

DRUGS AND PULMONARY DEFENCE MECHANISMS

The total surface area in the alveoli exposed to inhaled air, with all its suspended contaminants and micro-organisms, is thought to be around 70 m^2. One of the main functions of the upper respiratory tract is, therefore, to clean this air and protect the lungs from damage and infection.

CILIATED EPITHELIUM

The trachea and large airways are lined with ciliated columnar epithelium (Fig. 8.5). Cilia are present on the epithelial lining deep into the respiratory tree, to the level of the terminal bronchioles. They are thread-like motile structures anchored in the epithelial cell membrane. Through a coordinated beating action, they clear mucus and other secretions, along with particles trapped on their sticky surface, from the respiratory passageways and carry them towards the throat for swallowing. This is called the mucociliary escalator.

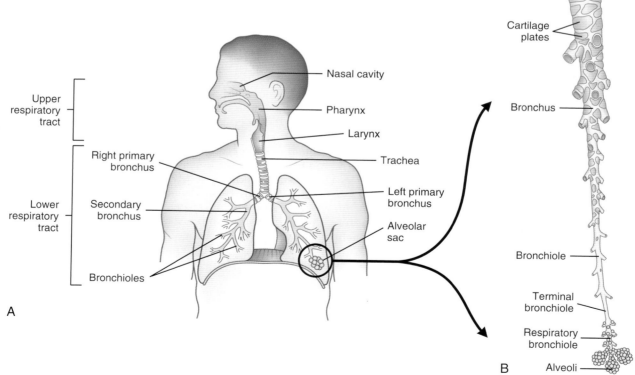

Fig. 8.1   The main structures and organs of the respiratory system. A. The upper and lower respiratory tracts. B. Progressive divisions of the bronchial tree and the alveoli. (Modified from (A) Thibodeau G and Patton K (2016) Anatomy and physiology, 9th ed. St Louis: Mosby and (B) www.Netter.com: Illustrations 155 (bronchus, acinus) and 191 (circulation). Elsevier.)

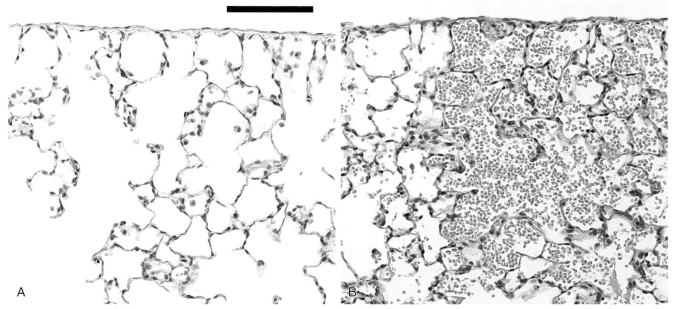

Fig. 8.2 Histology of lung tissue. A: Healthy alveoli. B: Bleomycin-induced lung damage. (Modified from Miller DL (2016) Mechanisms for induction of pulmonary capillary hemorrhage by diagnostic ultrasound: review and consideration of acoustical radiation surface pressure. *Ultrasound in Medicine & Biology*, 42(12), pp. 2743-2757.)

Table 8.1   Some Examples of Drugs that Cause Pulmonary Toxicity

Toxic Effect	Drug(s)
Inflammation and fibrosis of the lung substance	Amiodarone; azathioprine; bleomycin; chlorambucil; methotrexate; oxygen; nitrofurantoin; phenytoin; statins; sulphasalazine
Capillary leak syndrome: the pulmonary capillaries become increasingly permeable, causing pulmonary oedema	Cocaine; cyclophosphamide; diamorphine; iodine-containing radiographic contrast agents; methotrexate
Hypersensitivity (allergy)	β-blockers; methotrexate; nitrofurantoin
Bronchospasm	Aspirin and other non-steroidal anti-inflammatory drugs; amiodarone; amphotericin B; β-blockers; dipyridamole; nitrofurantoin; penicillamine
Pleural injury	Amiodarone; bleomycin; carmustine; cyclophosphamide; methotrexate; nitrofurantoin; phenytoin

MUCUS

Mucus is produced by goblet cells present in the columnar epithelial lining of the upper airways and forms a thin blanket overlying the cilia. Mucus is a viscous water-based gel containing mucins, which are complex sugar/protein molecules, and particles present in inspired air adhere to mucus layer and are trapped. The consistency of mucus is normally thin enough to allow the ciliary escalator to transport it without difficulty and clear it efficiently from the respiratory passageways; however, in respiratory infection or irritation, mucus production increases, and the mucus often becomes thicker and stickier. This makes the job of the ciliary escalator more difficult and increases the need to cough to help clearance.

In some situations, mucus viscosity significantly affects clearance. The parasympathetic nervous system promotes secretion of a fluid mucus that is easily moved by ciliary action.

Antimuscarinic drugs such as **hyoscine** are used to reduce the volume of respiratory secretions, e.g. before surgery. However, they thicken the mucus, which hampers normal clearance and can cause mucus pooling, airway obstruction, and increased risk of infection. In some respiratory conditions, such as cystic fibrosis, continual production of thick mucus leads eventually to failure of ciliary action.

Mucolytics and Expectorants

Mucolytics are agents that liquefy mucus and facilitate its clearance from the airways. Simple measures such as steam inhalation, which may be used with menthol or eucalyptus, hydrate and soften mucus and can be helpful. Drugs such as **acetylcysteine** and **carbocisteine** disrupt the binding of the mucins within mucus, increasing its water content and thinning it. In addition, there is evidence that acetylcysteine reduces mucus production and may have some

Focus on: Drug Delivery Via Inhalation in Respiratory Disorders

Drugs given to treat airway disorders are often administered by inhalation. This route delivers the drug directly to the target tissue, achieving high pulmonary drug concentrations and a rapid onset of action. The dose delivered can therefore be reduced compared to the systemic dose, reducing the incidence and severity of adverse effects.

Drugs for inhalation are formulated specially for this delivery route. Drug formulations include dry powder preparations, aerosols, or suspensions, which are then administered using an appropriate inhaler device. It is important to choose an appropriate device to meet the patient's needs. Table 8.2 summarises key features of the main inhaler devices available.

Less than 10% of an inhaled dose of drug reaches the smaller airways. Most is deposited in the inhaler device and in the mouth, throat, and upper airways, from where it is cleared by the mucociliary escalator and swallowed. The swallowed drug is absorbed into the bloodstream from the gastrointestinal tract and liver; in addition, some drug is absorbed across the bronchial walls. In this way, a proportion of an inhaled dose reaches the systemic circulation (Fig. 8.3). This may contribute to the drug's clinical effect but may also cause systemic side-effects. The likelihood of this happening increases with the drug dose, dosing frequency, and the chemical characteristics of the drug. For example, if the drug is very fat-soluble, it will be readily absorbed into the blood, or if it is very potent then even small circulating quantities may cause side-effects.

It is desirable that inhaled drugs given for a local effect (e.g. bronchodilators in asthma) that reach the circulation should be rapidly cleared, for example by liver metabolism, to minimise systemic side-effects.

Factors Affecting Inhaled Drug Access to the Airways

Whereas a dose of drug given orally or by parenteral routes can be accurately calculated, drug delivery by inhalation cannot be easily quantified because the amount of drug reaching the airways depends upon a range of factors. One of these is the action of the mucociliary escalator. Healthy mucociliary function efficiently but variably clears inhaled particles, including drug molecules, and it is not possible to measure this in individual patients. Another is the drug formulation, which is important because the size of the drug particle determines how far it may travel into the respiratory tree, which in turn determines which clearance mechanisms contribute (Fig. 8.4). Large particles (10 μm or more in diameter) are heavy and do not travel far when inhaled: they land on the membranes of the mouth, throat, and large airways and are swallowed or cleared by mucociliary action. However, if the particles are very small (1 μm or less), they are so light that they remain suspended in the air and are breathed back out again, never reaching their target tissue. Drug deposition in the small airways is optimal when the drug particle size falls in the range 2–5 μm, and this can be maximised if the patient holds their breath for several seconds after

Table 8.2   Key Features of Inhaler Devices

Inhaler Device	Comments	Disadvantages
Manually activated pressurised metered dose inhaler	A pre-calculated dose of aerosolised drug is driven from the inhaler under pressure by a propellant substance when the inhaler is manually activated.	Requires good co-ordination of inhalation and inhaler activation, which is difficult in many people including children and the elderly. Requires adequate inspiratory effort, potentially a problem in children and the elderly and when airway obstruction is present
Breath-activated pressurised metered dose inhaler	As above, but drug release is triggered by inhalation.	Requires good inspiratory effort; difficult in children, frail elderly, and when airflow is obstructed
Spacer devices	This is a plastic chamber attached to the inhaler mouthpiece. Released drug disperses into the air in the spacer and is breathed in over a period of time. It is very useful for children and those unable to effectively use metered dose inhalers alone.	Spacers are bulky, inconvenient, and cannot be used with breath-activated inhalers because sufficiently high airflow rates cannot be achieved on inhalation.
Dry powder inhalers	The drug is delivered as particles into the airway.	Requires good inspiratory effort and the ability to hold the breath for at least 10 seconds following activation
Nebulisers	The drug is delivered into the airways as a fine mist, produced by bubbling pressurised air or oxygen through a solution of the drug. High doses can be delivered rapidly and comfortably in acute attacks.	Equipment is bulky and may not be available outside of healthcare settings.

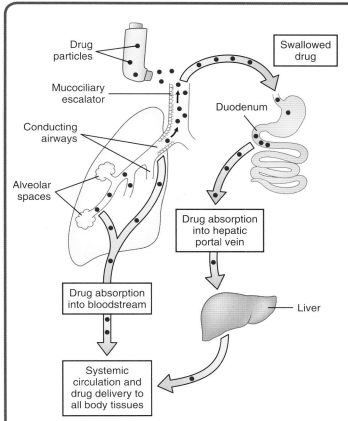

Fig. 8.3   Routes of access into the systemic circulation following drug inhalation.

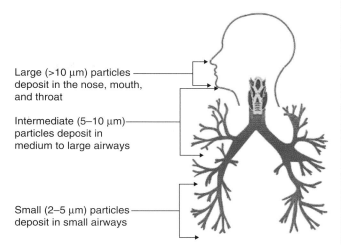

Fig. 8.4   Drug penetration into the airways depends upon particle size. Large particles deposit in the upper tract. The optimal size for deposition in the small airways is 2–5 µm in diameter. (Modified from Tekade RK (2020) Drug delivery systems, Fig. 11.8. St. Louis: Academic Press.)

inhalation; this gives the drug particles more time to fall by gravity and adhere to the airway epithelium. Drug particles depositing in the alveoli can be removed and destroyed by alveolar macrophages.

A range of inhalation devices is available, but effective drug delivery with all of them depends very much on pa-tient technique. If inhalation of drug triggers coughing, most will be immediately expelled and therefore ineffec-tive. If the patient's respiratory effort is poor, e.g. in chil-dren or frail elderly people, less drug reaches the target airways. In addition, drug penetration into the respirato-ry tree is reduced if the airways are narrowed by inflam-mation or bronchoconstriction; this means that during exacerbations of the disease, inhaled drugs may be con-siderably less effective than normal.

Alternative Routes to Inhalation

During exacerbations, drugs can be given orally or intra-venously to ensure that high concentrations reach the lung tissues via the bloodstream. This of course means that the risk and incidence of side-effects are increased.

anti-inflammatory action. An expectorant is an agent that helps the movement of material, including mucus, out of the airways. Traditional expectorants include **squill** and **guaifenesin**, which may be added to proprietary cough preparations, but there is no evidence that they have any benefit.

Dornase Alfa

Dornase alfa is a synthetic form of human deoxyribonu-clease, the enzyme that breaks down DNA in the body. It is given by nebuliser in cystic fibrosis. The thick mucus produced in this condition is rich in neutrophils, because of the repeated infections, and when these cells break down, they release their DNA along with other cellular constituents. The very long DNA molecules are highly vis-cous, and dornase alfa snips them up into much smaller segments, thinning the mucus and facilitating clearance. Fig, 8.6A shows sputum from a patient with cystic fibro-sis stained for DNA. The elongated DNA molecules are clearly seen. Fig. 8.6B shows the effect of dornase alfa: the DNA polymers have been effectively degraded, greatly reducing the viscosity of the sputum.

Mannitol

Inhaled mannitol powder is thought to liquefy mucus by generating an osmotic gradient between the mucus layer

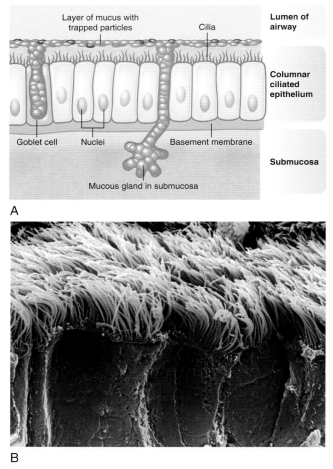

Fig. 8.5   **The epithelial lining of the trachea and large airways.** (From Waugh A and Grant A (2018) Ross & Wilson anatomy and physiology in health and illness, 13th ed, Fig 10.12. Oxford: Elsevier.)

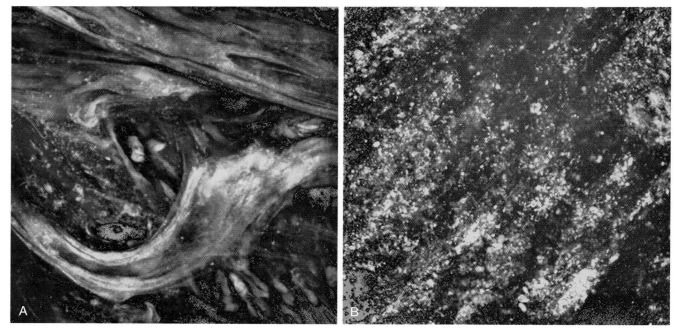

Fig. 8.6   **The effect of dornase alfa on cystic fibrosis sputum stained for DNA.** A. In untreated sputum, the elongated DNA molecules are clearly seen. B. Dornase alfa digests and degrades the DNA polymers, reducing mucus viscosity. (From Gardenhire DS (2012) Rau's respiratory care pharmacology, 8th ed, Fig. 9.9. St. Louis: Mosby.)

and the epithelial cells lining the airway. Mannitol is not absorbed and increases the osmolarity of the mucus. This osmotic gradient pulls water from the airway tissues into the mucus, hydrating it. This is also the basis of its activity as an osmotic diuretic (p. 174) and in reducing cerebral oedema by pulling water from brain tissue into the bloodstream. It

can cause airway irritation, cough, haemoptysis, and sore throat.

Ivacaftor
Ivacaftor was licenced in 2012 for use in cystic fibrosis (see Focus on: Tailored Genetic Therapy in Cystic Fibrosis box).

Focus on: Tailored Genetic Therapy in Cystic Fibrosis

Cystic fibrosis (CF) is the most common inherited autosomal recessive disease in Caucasians. Because the faulty gene causing this disorder is recessive, an affected individual must inherit a faulty gene from both parents for the disease to manifest; people with one faulty gene and one normal gene are clinically healthy but can pass the gene to their children (they are carriers). CF is caused by a faulty ion channel in the membranes of secretory epithelial cells, including the lungs, pancreas, and genitourinary tract. This channel, called the cystic fibrosis transmembrane conductance regulator (CFTR), allows the cell to export chloride ions through its plasma membrane, pulling water with them and hydrating respiratory and gastrointestinal secretions. Fig. 8.7 shows the production of CFTR proteins and their role in chloride ion secretion. The code for the protein is transcribed from the *CFTR* gene into a molecule of mRNA, which is then read by a ribosome in the cytoplasm to synthesise the CFTR

protein. It travels to the cell surface and is inserted into the membrane; this process is called trafficking. When the CFTR channel function is abnormal or inadequate, chloride secretion is decreased or absent, reducing water transport out of the cell. This dehydrates and thickens secretions. The lungs are normal at birth, but the viscous secretions are rapidly colonised with a range of microorganisms, and repeated infections cause inflammation and progressive destruction of the lung tissue. Respiratory failure is usually the cause of death. Fig. 8.8 summarises the pathophysiology of CF. Treatment plans include physiotherapy to mobilise thick secretions and help airway clearance, aggressive antibiotic management of infections, oral replacement of digestive enzymes, and exercise plans to optimise physical fitness. Even so, CF remains a life-limiting disease, and development of new therapies is a key research focus.

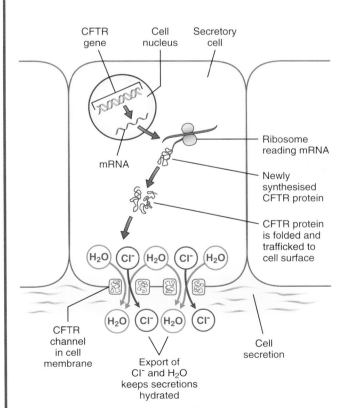

Fig. 8.7 The production and function of cystic fibrosis transmembrane conductance regulator protein.

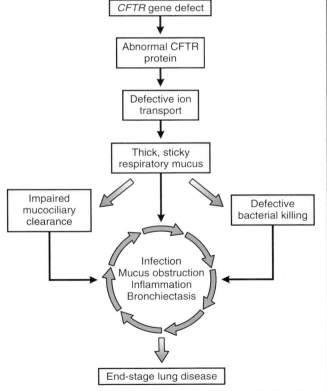

Fig. 8.8 **The pathophysiology of cystic fibrosis.** (Modified from Broaddus VC, Ernst JD, King TE Jr, et al. (2022) Murray & Nadel's textbook of respiratory medicine, 7th ed, Fig. 67.4. St. Louis: Elsevier.)

Continued

The gene that codes for the CFTR channel is found on chromosome 7, and it is a large gene, increasing the number of possible mutations that may occur within its genetic sequence. In fact, there are around 2000 different mutations in this gene, each of which changes the code in a different way and so produces a wide range of abnormal amino-acid sequences in the final CFTR protein. Different mutations interfere with channel production or function at different stages in the process, and this opens the possibility of designing drugs to specifically target individual channel abnormalities: a pharmacogenetic approach. The most common mutation in American and northern European patients is called the F508del mutation and involves the loss of only one amino acid from the CFTR protein, but even this slight change means that the protein cannot fold into the correct shape, and the cell destroys it instead of trafficking it to the cell surface. Nearly 90% of patients with CF have at least one copy of this common mutation. Other mutations produce channels that cannot open correctly or do not stay open long enough, or lead to reduced production of the CFTR protein.

CFTR Modulators

These new agents are low-molecular-weight molecules which target a specific defect in the CFTR channel and improve its function. Re-establishing correct chloride flow rehydrates mucus, improves pulmonary clearance, and reduces the likelihood of obstruction in other systems including the gastrointestinal tract. Identifying the specific mutation in the patient's *CFTR* gene identifies the nature of the defect in the CFTR protein, and an appropriate CFTR regulator can be prescribed to improve channel function.

There are three types of CFTR modulators: potentiators, correctors, and amplifiers. Not all are available in all countries.

- Potentiators, e.g. **ivacaftor,** increase the length of time that the CFTR channel remains open, allowing movement of additional chloride.
- Correctors, e.g. **lumacaftor** and **elexacaftor** (the latter not currently available in the UK), allow the CFTR protein to assume the right shape for it to be trafficked to the cell surface and incorporated into the cell membrane, increasing the number of channels at the cell surface.
- Amplifiers increase production of CFTR protein and are currently in development.

Understanding the genetic basis of the faulty protein allows tailored therapy to be offered to patients with certain mutations. For instance, **ivacaftor** alone is not effective in patients with the common F508del mutation, because this mutation results in unstable CFTR protein that is quickly broken down and so little reaches the cell surface to benefit from the action of ivacaftor. However, using **ivacaftor** and **lumacaftor** together can significantly improve pulmonary function, because lumacaftor increases the amount of CFTR protein reaching the cell surface, and ivacaftor keeps the new channels open for longer.

Pharmacokinetics and Adverse Effects

The currently available CFTR modulators are given orally and may be given in combination: **ivacaftor** and **lumacaftor** are used together in the UK and other combinations are used in other countries. **Ivacaftor** has a half-life of around 12 hours following oral administration, and its absorption is enhanced if taken with fat-containing foods. Regular monitoring of liver enzyme levels is recommended because it can increase liver transaminase levels. It is metabolised by the cytochrome (CYP) 3A family of liver enzymes, and so interacts with drugs that induce or inhibit these enzymes. For example, a range of antimicrobials including the **azole antifungals** and **macrolide antibiotics**, which are CYP3A inhibitors, can significantly increase ivacaftor blood levels.

COUGH

Coughing is an essential reflex mechanism for clearing the airways of accumulated mucus, accidentally inhaled materials, or other obstructions. It is controlled by the cough centre in the brain stem. Irritation of the respiratory epithelium triggers sensory impulses that travel to the cough centre via the vagus nerve. The cough centre responds by activating the respiratory and abdominal muscles to produce the sequence of events of cough. There is an initial deep inspiration, to bring enough air into the lungs for an effective cough. The vocal cords in the larynx are then pulled together (closing the glottis), and the abdominal muscles, diaphragm, and intercostal muscles contract sharply. This generates a rapid rise in intrathoracic pressure. Then the glottis opens, and the high intrathoracic pressure generates fast, high-volume airflow out of the airways. A persistent cough should always be investigated, and the cause identified and treated where possible.

Antitussives

Antitussives are drugs that suppresses cough and are used to relieve the discomfort and disturbance caused by persistent dry cough. The cough reflex is suppressed by central nervous system (CNS) depressants, including **alcohol** and **sedating antihistamines**. This can be clinically helpful, e.g. to treat a dry cough that disturbs sleep, but the potential for compromising the airway in vulnerable individuals by interfering with this important protective reflex should always be considered. **General anaesthetics** depress cough and can compromise the airway during induction of and recovery from anaesthesia unless the airway is carefully protected. Antitussives are not used when the cough is productive, because they predispose to mucus accumulation in the airways and increase the risk of obstruction and infection.

Opioids

Opioids (Ch. 6) are the most effective antitussive medications currently available and suppress cough at sub-analgesic doses. They act on μ (mu) receptors in the cough centre in the brainstem and reduce their sensitivity. Weak opioids such as **codeine** and **pholcodine** have fewer side-effects and are less likely to cause dependence than more powerful opioids like **morphine**. However, **morphine** and **diamorphine** are used in palliative care in patients with lung cancer, in whom a persistent, exhausting, and distressing cough is a frequent symptom. Side-effects include constipation and respiratory depression. Opioids also thicken sputum and depress ciliary action, and so care is needed, for example, in chronic obstructive pulmonary disease (COPD).

OBSTRUCTIVE AIRWAYS DISEASE

Obstructive airways disease is a general term encompassing mainly asthma and COPD. In both these conditions, there are chronic inflammatory changes in the airways which cause varying degrees of airflow limitation, although the aetiology and progression of the disorders are different.

ASTHMA

Asthma is characterised by reversible airway obstruction, with periods of good lung function interspersed with episodes of deteriorating function, airway narrowing, and airflow obstruction. It is frequently associated with allergy, which stimulates mast cells and basophils in the airway to release a range of inflammatory mediators and cytokines, including leukotrienes, platelet-activating factor, and interleukins (ILs). Fig. 8.9 shows the main inflammatory mediators and cytokines involved, and also shows the targets of the main drugs used in asthma. The smooth muscle tissue in the bronchial walls is thickened and hyperreactive and responds inappropriately with exaggerated bronchoconstriction to a range of triggers. The smaller airways, whose walls contain a lot of smooth muscle and have no cartilage to keep them open, are disproportionately affected. Bronchodilators, including β$_2$-agonists, **leukotriene-receptor antagonists**, and **theophylline** help reverse bronchoconstriction and improve airflow.

Inflammation is a key feature, and the airway wall is swollen and infiltrated with a range of inflammatory and

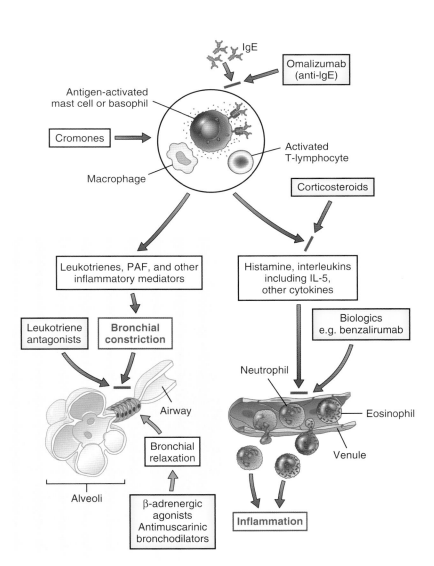

Fig. 8.9 The main inflammatory mediators and cytokines involved in asthmatic airway inflammation. The sites of action of the main drugs used to treat asthma are also shown. (Modified from Abbas AK, Lichtman AH, and Pillai S (2021) Cellular and molecular immunology SAE, 10th ed, Fig. 20.10. New Delhi: Elsevier.)

immune cells including macrophages, mast cells, eosinophils, and T-lymphocytes. Activated T-lymphocytes release a wide range of pro-inflammatory cytokines, including **Interleukins**. The ongoing inflammatory response damages the epithelium, causing patchy desquamation and exposing the basement membrane, which contributes to the ongoing airway hypersensitivity. Goblet cells are hypertrophic, and mucus production increases. Loss of the ciliated epithelium decreases mucus clearance, so mucus accumulates and plugs airways. With time, the chronic inflammation leads to structural changes and permanent remodelling of the airway wall. **Glucocorticoids** are the mainstay of anti-inflammatory treatment in asthma. Fig. 8.10 shows the main pathological features of an asthmatic airway compared with normal.

The cause of asthma is not known, although it is likely to be multifactorial. There is often an inherited component with a strong familial tendency. Allergy is a common and important component in asthma, and asthma often co-exists with other allergic conditions such as hay fever and eczema.

BRONCHODILATORS

These drugs reduce airflow obstruction by relaxing bronchial smooth muscle and opening the airways. They are usually used to relieve symptoms, although sometimes they are useful prophylactically, for example, before exercise if exercise is a trigger factor. Because of this, they are sometimes called relievers or rescue agents.

B_2-Agonists

Examples: salbutamol, terbutaline, salmeterol

The use of sympathetic drugs to improve symptoms in asthma dates to 3000 BC, when physicians in ancient China used extracts of the plant *Ephedra equisetina* to treat dyspnoea. The active agent, **epinephrine (adrenaline)**, was isolated in 1897, and the first β-agonist drug, **isoprenaline**, was synthesised in 1940. It was used in the treatment of asthma, but it is not selective for β_2-receptors and has significant activity on β_1-receptors too, including those in the heart (see Fig. 4.5). This meant that even when used in the relatively

small doses needed by inhalation to improve asthma symptoms, enough was absorbed into the systemic circulation to cause unwanted cardiovascular side-effects including hypertension and arrhythmias. The discovery of β_1 and β_2 subtypes and their distribution in the respiratory and cardiovascular systems led to the development of drugs relatively selective for β_2-receptors, which cause bronchodilation with minimal activity on the heart. The first β_2-selective agonist, **salbutamol**, is 29 times more active on the β_2-receptor than the β_1-receptor and was introduced in the late 1960s. Since then, a range of similar agents have been produced including the longer-acting agents **formoterol** and **salmeterol**. β_2-agonists bind to and activate sympathetic β_2-receptors on smooth muscle cells in the airway wall. They mimic the action of the sympathetic nervous system, which prepares the body for stress or activity, and relax bronchial smooth muscle by reducing calcium entry into the smooth muscle cells. Because calcium is essential for activation of the contractile proteins in the muscle cell, this leads to bronchodilation, increases air flow, and maximises oxygen intake. In addition, they improve ciliary function and have an anti-inflammatory action. β_2-agonists and glucocorticoids have a synergistic effect (see later and Fig. 8.11).

Pharmacokinetics

β_2-agonists are given by inhalation for occasional use in well-controlled asthma and may also be given orally or by intramuscular or intravenous injection if required. Short-acting agents, e.g. **salbutamol** and **terbutaline**, usually take effect within 5 minutes of inhalation, and their duration of action is usually between 4 and 6 hours. **Salmeterol** has a duration of action of around 12 hours, so is useful for managing night-time symptoms and takes up to half an hour to begin working. **Formoterol's** duration of action can be up to 24 hours, and its onset of action is within 2–3 minutes. Overuse of these drugs, however, downregulates β_2-receptor numbers and reduces their effectiveness.

Long-acting agents have been associated with increased mortality rates in severe asthma; the reasons for this are

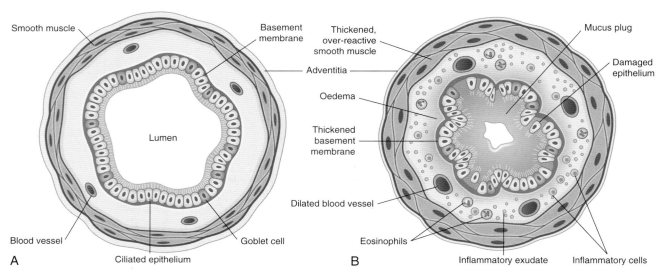

Fig. 8.10 The normal and asthmatic airway. A. Structural features of the healthy airway. B. Pathological changes in asthma. (From Waugh A and Grant A (2018) Ross & Wilson anatomy and physiology in health and illness, 13th ed, Fig 10.12. Oxford: Elsevier.)

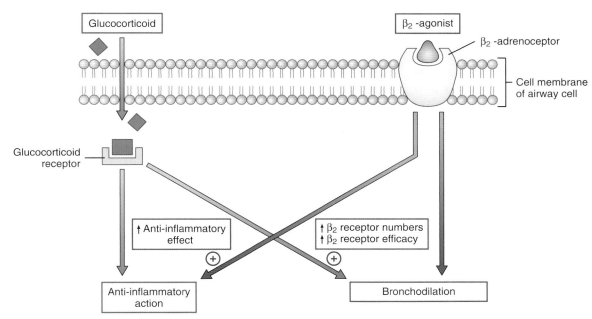

Fig. 8.11   Positive synergism between glucocorticoids and β₂-agonists in the asthmatic airway.

unclear. Current advice is that they should only be used in conjunction with an anti-inflammatory steroid and should only be added into therapy if adequate control is not achieved with shorter-acting agents. Patients taking these agents should be reviewed regularly and the drug withdrawn if no clinical benefit is observed.

Adverse Effects

Significant systemic side-effects can occur if circulating drug levels are high enough, including from high doses of inhaled drug. At higher doses, β₂-agonists also activate β₁-receptors: i.e. their selectivity at the subtypes of the β-receptor is dose-dependent. This includes cardiac β₁-receptors, leading to tachycardia, palpitations, hypertension, and arrhythmias. A fine tremor can occur, due to stimulation of β₂-receptors on skeletal muscle. They can cause hypokalaemia by shifting potassium from the blood into cells via an action on the sodium–potassium pump in the cell membrane. Hypokalaemia in turn can cause potentially fatal cardiac arrhythmias, and care should be taken in people who are at risk of hypokalaemia, including concurrent use of **theophylline** in severe asthma. Because they reduce blood potassium levels, these drugs are also used to treat hyperkalaemia. They may cause hyperthyroidism because sympathetic stimulation increases release of thyroid hormone from the thyroid gland. They increase blood glucose levels, because sympathetic stimulation increases glycogen breakdown in the liver, releasing glucose into the bloodstream, which may interfere with blood glucose control in diabetes.

Theophylline

Theophylline is a methylxanthine, a family of chemicals that includes **caffeine**; strong coffee was recommended in 1786 for asthma in a letter written by William Withering (of **digoxin** fame, p. 133). As a group, xanthines have bronchodilator, diuretic, and anti-inflammatory properties, although their exact mechanism of action is unclear. They act at several

targets in human cells and probably produce their pharmacological action via more than one pathway. One potential mechanism of action is via their blockade of adenosine receptors on airway smooth muscle cells. Adenosine triggers bronchoconstriction, so antagonism at their receptor may account at least in part for the bronchodilator action of the xanthines. In addition, they inhibit one form of the enzyme phosphodiesterase (PDE), which breaks down cyclic AMP (cAMP) inside cells, including smooth muscle cells. This increases cAMP levels and relaxes bronchial smooth muscle, inducing bronchodilation. Other types of PDE inhibitors are used to treat heart disease (p. 133). They may also have a central effect and stimulate the respiratory centre in the brainstem. Finally, the anti-inflammatory effect of xanthines may be due to their ability to increase the activity of anti-inflammatory genes and suppress the activity of inflammatory cells. Xanthines are usually used to manage acute, severe exacerbations of asthma.

Pharmacokinetics

Theophylline is given orally. It is well but unpredictably absorbed from the GI tract, giving fluctuating plasma levels which could increase the risk of side-effects; modified release preparations are preferred, which are absorbed at a steadier rate and help to stabilise plasma levels over extended periods. **Aminophylline** is a preparation of theophylline and **ethylendiamine**. Ethylenediamine has no pharmacological activity, but it makes theophylline much more soluble in water, giving a formulation suitable for intravenous injection. Once in the body, it releases theophylline, which is responsible for its pharmacological effects. The plasma half-life of theophylline is 4–8 hours, and it is heavily plasma protein-bound.

Adverse Effects

Theophylline has a wide range of potentially serious side-effects because it affects such a wide range of cellular targets important in a range of body tissues. It has a narrow therapeutic index, and side-effects become increasingly common at plasma levels at the upper end of the therapeutic range and above. Therapeutic drug monitoring is helpful in managing dosing. Adverse effects include cardiac arrhythmias, probably due to adenosine antagonism and seizures due to CNS stimulation, both of which can be fatal. Gastric acid secretion is increased and so is GI motility, with GI pain, gastro-oesophageal reflux, diarrhoea, and increased risk of peptic ulcers. Hypokalaemia can occur, especially when theophylline is used with $β_2$-agonists. Theophylline is metabolised in the liver, and its effects are decreased in the presence of enzyme inducers, including smoking, **alcohol**, **phenytoin**, and **St. John's wort**. Enzyme inhibitors can reduce theophylline clearance and increase circulating levels: these include **isoniazid**, **interferons**, and **carbamazepine**.

Antimuscarinic Bronchodilators

Examples: aclidinium, ipratropium, tiotropium

The parasympathetic nervous system causes bronchoconstriction via the action of acetylcholine on M_3 receptors in bronchial smooth muscle (see Fig. 4.8). Drugs that block M_3 receptors therefore cause bronchodilation and are used to relieve bronchospasm in obstructive airway disease, including asthma and COPD.

Pharmacokinetics

Ipratropium is given by inhalation in maintenance treatment of asthma and in the management of acute asthma. Its peak action occurs 30–60 minutes after administration, and it is effective for 3–6 hours. It is also given intranasally to reduce rhinorrhoea, for example, in hay fever. It is a large, highly charged molecule, so is poorly absorbed into the bloodstream, and so is generally not associated with systemic side-effects, although care must be taken not to contaminate the eye directly because of the risk of glaucoma (see below). Longer-acting agents include **aclidinium** (duration of action, 8 hours) and **tiotropium** (64 hours).

Adverse Effects

Antimuscarinic drugs can cause a range of systemic antimuscarinic side-effects (see p. 51) by blocking muscarinic receptors throughout the body and antagonising the 'rest and digest' functions of the parasympathetic nervous system. Care is needed in people with glaucoma or at risk of glaucoma because these drugs can increase intraocular pressure (see Fig. 4.11). Antimuscarinic agents can also block the effects of the parasympathetic nervous system on the heart and predispose to tachycardia and arrhythmias: the risk is increased if antimuscarinics are used in conjunction with **β-agonists**.

ANTI-INFLAMMATORY DRUGS

Preventing or reversing the inflammatory changes associated with the asthmatic airway alleviates the signs and symptoms of the disorder and improves airway function. They should be used on a regular basis even when the asthma is not troublesome to suppress airway inflammation, and so they are sometimes referred to as preventers.

Glucocorticoids

Examples: budesonide, beclometasone, fluticasone

Glucocorticoids are the mainstay of anti-inflammatory treatment in asthma. They are superior to other anti-inflammatory medications in the management of recurrent and chronic disease and prevent or reduce the rate of asthma exacerbations. They block the activity and proliferation of inflammatory cells in the airway wall and prevent the production of a wide range of inflammatory mediators and cytokines. Their mechanism of action is discussed on p. 111. Because they can cause a wide range of potentially severe side-effects, they should be used at the lowest effective dose and given systemically only when required to manage severe disease and for as short a period as possible.

Glucocorticoids and $β_2$-agonists demonstrate therapeutic synergism when used together in asthma. Glucocorticoids increase the number and efficacy of $β_2$-receptors in the airways, and therefore improve the bronchodilator response to $β_2$-receptor agonists. $β_2$-agonists in turn have an anti-inflammatory action and enhance the airway response to glucocorticoids (Fig. 8.11).

Pharmacokinetics

Maintenance glucocorticoid therapy is delivered by inhalation wherever possible to minimise side-effects. However, because steroid molecules are small and fat-soluble, they are readily absorbed across the airway wall and can reach physiologically active levels in the bloodstream if used in high doses to manage severe asthma or used excessively. For this reason, it is desirable that they are quickly cleared from the circulation by hepatic metabolism. Bioavailability and half-lives of the commonly used steroids vary significantly. **Fluticasone, budesonide, mometasone, and ciclesonide** are quickly removed from the bloodstream by first-pass metabolism, and any swallowed drug from an inhaled dose is rapidly cleared. **Beclometasone** is metabolised much more slowly and so has a longer plasma half-life. Liver impairment can therefore increase circulating levels of any inhaled glucocorticoid. Water-soluble drugs, for example **budesonide**, dissolve in the watery mucus lining the airways and are more efficiently cleared by the mucociliary escalator. More lipid-soluble drugs, including **fluticasone** and **beclomethasone,** enter the airway tissues and remain there for extended periods, extending the duration of their activity.

Adverse Effects

Local side-effects from deposition of inhaled glucocorticoid in the mouth and throat include hoarseness from the build-up of drug on the vocal cords, and oral thrush because glucocorticoids suppress local immune defences. It is good practice to rinse the mouth and/or brush the teeth after inhalation. If the drug reaches physiologically active levels in the circulation, either because of high inhaled doses or oral/parenteral use in severe disease, any of the wide range of side-effects may be seen, including growth suppression in children, osteoporosis, cataract, and adrenal suppression (Cushing's syndrome, see Fig. 6.16).

Cromones

Cromones (**nedocromil sodium** and **sodium cromoglicate**) are add-on options in the treatment of asthma and are used as antiallergy medications in some other situations, e.g. food allergy. They are not helpful in acute asthma, but they may benefit some patients, particularly children, in maintenance therapy. Their anti-inflammatory action is less effective than glucocorticoids, and their mechanism of action is not fully understood. They stabilise mast cells and reduce mast cell release of inflammatory mediators including **histamine**, which may be their main mechanism of action in allergy treatment. They also suppress the activity of a range of inflammatory cells including neutrophils, eosinophils, and macrophages and reduce the release of a range of inflammatory mediators and cytokines. **Nedocromil sodium** is given only by inhaler, because it is a large, electrically charged molecule not absorbed across the wall of the GI tract, but **sodium cromoglicate** can be given orally or by inhaler.

Leukotriene Receptor Antagonists

Leukotrienes are synthesised by the enzyme lipoxygenase from arachidonic acid, an important constituent of the cell membrane, which is released from the cell membrane if the cell is injured or exposed to a range of potentially damaging stimuli. Leukotrienes are closely related to the prostaglandins (p. 167); their biosynthesis and main activities are summarised in Fig. 8.12. They contribute to the pathophysiological changes in asthma via a range of actions: they recruit and activate inflammatory cells including mast cells, neutrophils, and macrophages; they increase vascular permeability and cause oedema in the airway wall; they constrict bronchial smooth muscle; they stimulate mucus production; and they damage the epithelial lining of the airway, which in turn increases airway sensitivity and destroys the cilia. Drugs that either block leukotriene synthesis (lipoxygenase inhibitors) or block their receptors (leukotriene-receptor antagonists) are used as second-line drugs in conjunction with steroids and bronchodilators to optimise asthma control.

Lipoxygenase Inhibitors

These agents are not available in the UK but are used in other countries including the US and India. **Zileuton** was the first agent approved for the treatment of asthma and is given orally. Its most significant side-effect is elevation of liver enzymes.

Leukotriene Receptor Antagonists

Examples: montelukast, zafirlukast

These agents do not prevent leukotriene synthesis, but block leukotrienes from attaching to and activating their receptors on airway tissues (Fig. 8.12). Used regularly as adjunct therapy with glucocorticoids, they can improve airway function and reduce symptoms, and seem to be particularly useful in children and in exercise-induced bronchoconstriction. They are taken by mouth and are generally well tolerated. Common side-effects include GI upset and headache. Rarely, they have been associated with Churg–Strauss syndrome, an autoimmune response in which intense systemic vasculitis can cause widespread damage to a range of body tissues including the nervous system and the heart. Withdrawal or reduction of glucocorticoid treatment may increase the risk.

Immunosuppressants

The use of monoclonal antibodies against the cells and mediators involved in the pathophysiology of asthma is the most recent development in asthma treatment. They are used under specialist care in severe asthma only because suppression of the immune and inflammatory responses can cause serious side-effects.

Omalizumab

Omalizumab is an antibody to IgE, the immunoglobulin associated with allergy. In severe allergic asthma, IgE triggers and promotes airway inflammation. By binding to IgE in the blood and in body tissues, omalizumab prevents it from

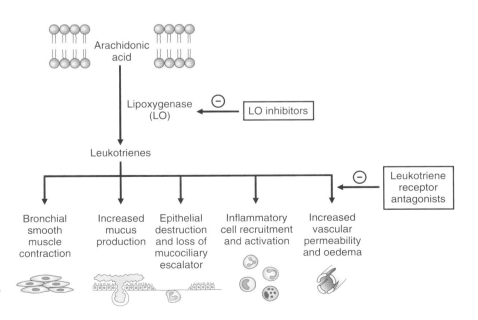

Fig. 8.12 Biosynthesis and activity of the leukotrienes.

binding to mast cells and triggering histamine release and the resultant allergic response. It is therefore used in severe persistent allergic asthma, as well as certain other allergic conditions. It is given by subcutaneous injection and the dose is calculated according to the patient's IgE levels and bodyweight. It is generally better tolerated than other biologics, although it can cause a range of side-effects including skin reactions and has been associated with Churg–Strauss syndrome (see above).

Benralizumab

IL-5 is an important inflammatory mediator in asthma. It is released by T-lymphocytes in the asthmatic airway and binds to its receptors on other inflammatory cells including eosinophils, which are of particular importance in allergic asthma. IL-5 promotes eosinophil maturation, activity, and survival, and therefore enhances the allergic inflammatory reaction. Benralizumab is an antibody to the IL-5 receptor. By blocking IL-5 receptors on eosinophil cell membranes, benralizumab reduces eosinophil activity and survival, depletes eosinophil numbers, and suppresses allergic inflammation (Fig. 8.13). Because eosinophils are an important part of the body's defence against helminthic infections, it is important to treat any such infection before beginning benralizumab treatment in asthma.

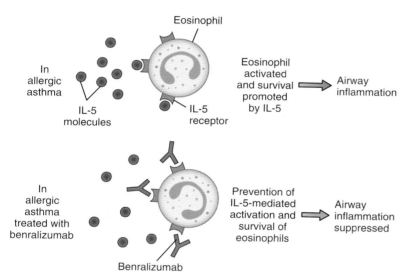

Fig. 8.13 The mechanism of action of benralizumab. IL-5, Interleukin-5.

CHRONIC OBSTRUCTIVE PULMONARY DISEASE

Chronic obstructive pulmonary disease (COPD) is associated with persistent and progressive airflow obstruction and is usually caused by tobacco smoking, although chronic exposure to lung irritants such as air pollution may also be responsible. It is usually understood to comprise chronic bronchitis and emphysema, which is irreversible destruction of alveoli and their supporting tissue, leaving large nonfunctional spaces in the lung. The chronic irritation caused by exposure to cigarette smoke sets up a progressive inflammatory response, with infiltration and activation of inflammatory cells and the release of inflammatory mediators and cytokines. Neutrophils in the inflammatory exudate release proteases, which digest and destroy the protein structure of lung tissue, including the elastic fibres that allow the lungs to recoil during expiration. This means the lungs gradually expand and the total lung capacity increases, although the lung's ability to exchange gases is progressively lost because of alveolar destruction. The airway walls become swollen, and mucus glands hypertrophy and produce increased quantities of mucus. The ciliated epithelium lining the airways is progressively destroyed by the ongoing inflammation, and so mucus is retained in the airways, leading to plugging and regular infections. Prompt and aggressive antibiotic treatment of infection is important to minimise airway damage.

Bronchodilators

β_2-agonists and antimuscarinic agents (see above) may both help relieve bronchospasm, especially in acute exacerbations, although in general they are less helpful in COPD than in asthma.

Glucocorticoids

Generally, the inflammatory changes in COPD airways respond poorly to inhaled steroids, and if these drugs are tried in a patient, the response should be monitored and the drug withdrawn if they do not help.

Phosphodiesterase Inhibitors

Roflumilast is a PDE inhibitor specific for PDE4, the form of the enzyme found in the lung. PDE breaks down the important intracellular messenger cAMP. Inhibition of the enzyme

Focus on: The Stepwise Principles of Asthma Treatment

Asthma management aims to minimise symptoms, prevent or minimise acute flare-ups, and optimise physical and psychological health. Current guidelines follow a stepwise approach to drug treatment, with patients maintained on the lowest doses of as few drugs as possible to give optimal control with minimal side-effects, but with the flexibility to step up or step down treatment as needed. There are slight differences between guidelines depending on the issuing body, but the fundamental principles remain consistent. Guidelines are available for different age groups, and it is important to follow the correct algorithm depending on the age of the patient. Fig. 8.14 shows the 2019 British Thoracic Society/Scottish Intercollegiate Guidelines Network (BTS/SIGN) algorithm for the stepwise treatment of asthma in adults. In very mild or intermittent asthma, or in suspected asthma, a short-acting bronchodilator, usually a β_2-agonist, should be prescribed. Inhaled glucocorticoids may be trialled to see if they make a difference. If there are nocturnal symptoms, or if there are daytime symptoms occurring more than three times a week or if the bronchodilator needs to be used more than three times a week, a regular glucocorticoid inhaler should be added. If control is still not achieved, and the prescriber is confident that the existing treatment regime is being adhered to, the next addition is a long-acting bronchodilator. From there, the next step is an increase in glucocorticoid dose or adding in second-line agents, e.g. a leukotriene-receptor antagonist. In more severe disease, specialist management should be sought; this may include regular oral steroids or the addition of biologics such as **omalizumab**.

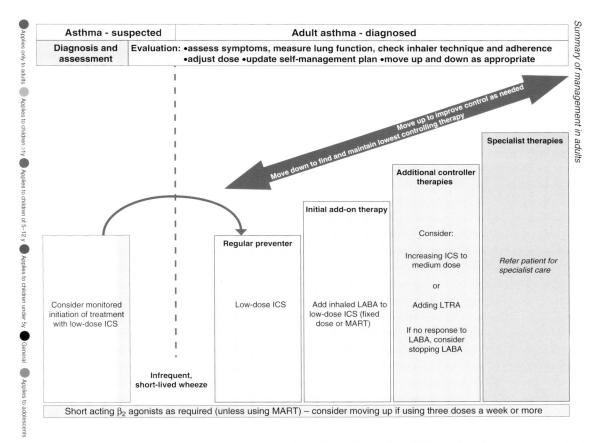

Fig. 8.14   British Thoracic Society/Scottish Intercollegiate Guidelines Network guidelines for the management of asthma (2019). ICS, Inhaled corticosteroid; MART: maintenance and reliever therapy, formulations containing both a glucocorticoid and a bronchodilator; LABA, long-acting β_2-agonist; LAMA, long-acting muscarinic antagonist; LTRA, leukotriene-receptor antagonist. (From British Thoracic Society and Scottish Intercollegiate Guidelines Network's 'British Guideline on the Management of Asthma' (2019), with permission.)

increases cAMP levels in lung tissues, and this has a range of anti-inflammatory actions, including preventing neutrophil accumulation of neutrophils and eosinophils in the airway wall, reducing the inflammatory action of the inflammatory cells present, and improving the survival of the ciliated epithelium lining the airway. Roflumilast is given orally and is a pro-drug, converted to its active form by liver enzymes. This means that any change in liver enzyme activity, either by other drugs that induce or inhibit them or in liver impairment can affect its action. It should be avoided in moderate to severe liver impairment and with inducers including **rifampicin** and a range of **anticonvulsants**.

REFERENCES

Borghardt, J.M., Kloft, C., Sharma, A., 2018. Inhaled therapy in respiratory disease: the complex interplay of pulmonary kinetic processes. Can. Respir. J. J. Can. Thorac. Soc. 2018,2732017.

Chauhan, B.F., Ducharme, F.M., 2012. Anti-leukotriene agents compared to inhaled corticosteroids in the management of recurrent and/or chronic asthma in adults and children. Cochrane Database Syst. Rev. 2014 (5), CD002314.

Derichs, N., 2013. Targeting a genetic defect: cystic fibrosis transmembrane conductance regulator modulators in cystic fibrosis. Eur. Respir. Rev. 22 (127), 58–65.

Hatipoglu, M.K., Hickey, A.J., Garcia-Contreras, L., 2018. Pharmacokinetics and pharmacodynamics of high doses of inhaled dry powder drugs. Int. J. Pharm. 549 (1–2), 306–316.

Matera, M.G., Rinaldi, B., Calzetta, L., et al., 2019. Pharmacokinetics and pharmacodynamics of inhaled corticosteroids for asthma treatment. Pulm. Pharmacol. Therapeut. 58,101828.

O'Reilly, R., Elphick, H.E., 2013. Development, clinical utility and place of ivacaftor in the treatment of cystic fibrosis. Drug Des. Dev. Ther. 7, 929–937.

ONLINE RESOURCES

Camus, P., 2024. Pneumtox online. Available at: https://www.pneumotox.com/drug/index/.

Condren, M.E., Bradshaw, M.D., 2013. Ivacaftor: a novel gene-based therapeutic approach for cystic fibrosis. J. Pediatr. Pharmacol. Therapeut. 18 (1), 8–13 Available at: http://doi.org/10.5863%2F1551-6776-18.1.8.

Scottish Intercollegiate Guidelines Network, 2024. British guideline on the management of asthma. Available at: https://www.sign.ac.uk/sign-158-british-guideline-on-the-management-of-asthma.

Renal and Genitourinary Drugs

INTRODUCTION TO THE URINARY SYSTEM

The main organs of the urinary system are the kidneys and the bladder. The kidneys control the composition and volume of body fluids by regulating excretion of wastes, water, electrolytes, and other substances: this includes drugs and their metabolites, and impaired renal function can cause drug toxicity. Unwanted and excess substances leave the kidneys as urine, which travels to the bladder through the ureters to be stored until it is convenient to excrete it, at which time it passes to the exterior via the urethra. Additional roles of the kidney include production of erythropoietin, the hormone that regulates red blood cell production, and activation of vitamin D. Because it controls the body's fluid load, the kidney also plays a key role in blood pressure regulation and releases renin, the enzyme which activates the renin–angiotensin–aldosterone system (RAAS, see also Fig. 7.15).

STRUCTURE AND FUNCTION OF THE KIDNEY

The kidney is a bean-shaped organ enclosed in a robust protective capsule. Internally there are three distinct regions: a dark outer layer called the cortex, an inner layer called the medulla, and a cavity called the renal pelvis, into which urine drains and which opens into the ureter (Fig. 9.1). The functional unit of the kidney is called the nephron, and each kidney contains around 1.5 million nephrons.

THE NEPHRON

Each nephron is essentially a long, folded tubule, with an expanded end called the glomerular capsule and the other end opening into a network of drainage tubes called collecting ducts (CDs), which drain urine towards the renal pelvis. Fig. 9.2 shows the structure of a typical nephron.

The Regions of the Nephron

The glomerular capsules are located in the cortex. Each capsule contains a tuft of glomerular capillaries supplied by an afferent arteriole, and water and low-molecular-weight substances are filtered out of the blood here, forming a fluid called filtrate. Filtrate flows from the capsule into the first part of the tubule, called the proximal convoluted tubule (PCT), which leads into the loop of the nephron (loop of Henle). The loop forms a hairpin bend dipping into the medulla before returning to the cortex and forming the final section, the distal convoluted tubule (DCT). The distal convoluted tubule in turn empties into the collecting ducts, which drain urine into the renal pelvis.

Filtration in the Glomerulus

Filtration through the glomerular capillary walls is driven by the hydrostatic (blood) pressure generated by the difference in diameter of the afferent and efferent arterioles. The afferent arteriole is wider than the efferent arteriole, and so blood pressure in the glomerular capillaries is around 55 mmHg (compare with standard capillary pressure, which is only around 25 mmHg). This higher-than-average blood pressure in the glomerular capillaries drives filtration out of the blood and into the glomerular capsule. Low-molecular-weight molecules including water, ions, glucose, urea, and other substances are filtered out of the blood and enter the glomerular capsule. Higher molecular-weight substances, including plasma proteins and some drugs, are too large to pass through the pores in the glomerular filter and remain in the bloodstream (Fig. 9.3).

Glomerular Filtration Rate
This is the volume of filtrate produced every minute, and in health, is an impressive 125 mL/min, equivalent to 180 L every 24-hour period, or around 78 times the total plasma volume every day.

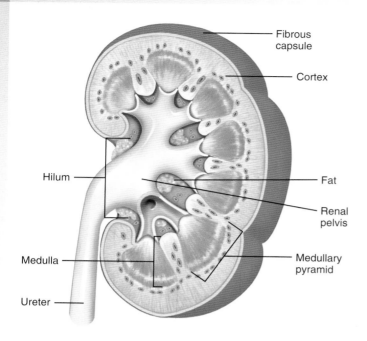

Fig. 9.1 The internal structure of the kidney. (Modified from Patton K and Thibodeau G (2020) Structure & function of the body, 16th ed, Fig. 18.2. St. Louis: Elsevier.)

URINE FORMATION

KEY POINTS

Three processes contribute to the formation of urine (Fig. 9.4).
- Filtration: Water and small molecules are filtered out of the glomerular capillaries into the glomerular capsule, forming filtrate.
- Reabsorption: As the filtrate passes through the nephron, water, organic nutrients, electrolytes, and other key substances are reabsorbed from the filtrate back into the bloodstream.
- Secretion: Unwanted materials, including drugs, hydrogen ions, and other waste products, are actively pumped out of the bloodstream and into the filtrate for excretion.

Fig. 9.5 shows the main sites of sodium (Na^+), chloride (Cl^-), and potassium (K^+) reabsorption in the nephron, and also indicates the region of the nephron where the main diuretics exert their effect.

Reabsorption and Secretion in the Different Regions of the Nephron

The efferent arteriole opens into a second network of capillaries that wrap around the nephron for efficient reabsorption from the filtrate into the blood. Additionally, unwanted substances including excess hydrogen (H^+) ions, creatinine, and molecules too large to be filtered in the glomerulus can be actively secreted out of the blood into the filtrate for excretion.

Reabsorption of materials from the filtrate occurs along the length of the nephron, the walls of which contain a number of pumps and transport mechanisms. As electrolytes and

other solutes, for example glucose and Na^+ ions, travel from the filtrate back into the bloodstream, this creates an osmotic gradient between these fluids: that is, the bloodstream becomes more concentrated than the filtrate. As a result, water travels passively from the filtrate and is reabsorbed into the bloodstream. The quantity of solutes reabsorbed is therefore a major determinant of water reabsorption by the nephron. Na^+ reabsorption in particular is an important factor in water reabsorption: the more Na^+ reabsorbed into the blood, the more water is reabsorbed, reducing urine volume.

Around 99% of the filtrate is reabsorbed into the blood as it travels through the nephron, and the end product, urine, contains waste and unwanted substances concentrated in a relatively small volume of water.

Reabsorption and Secretion in the Proximal Convoluted Tubule

The PCT is equipped with a range of carrier mechanisms for active reabsorption, and to increase available surface area for this, it is lined with simple epithelium with a brush border of microvilli. Sixty to seventy percent of the filtrate volume is reabsorbed into the peritubular capillaries here, including Na^+, K^+, bicarbonate, and Cl^- ions. Ninety-nine percent of organic nutrients, including glucose, amino acids, and free fatty acids, are actively reabsorbed in the PCT; water follows passively by osmosis. The PCT is also an important site for secretion of unwanted materials that are too large to be filtered in the glomerulus, including **diuretics** and other drugs, and of the waste products, uric acid and ammonium compounds. H^+ ions are also secreted here in exchange for Na^+: as H^+ ions are pumped into the filtrate, Na^+ ions are reabsorbed (Fig. 9.5.1).

Reabsorption in the Loop of the Nephron

Filtrate entering the loop is at the same osmotic pressure as (isotonic to) the filtrate formed in the glomerular capsule. The descending limb is permeable to water, so water is reabsorbed here, concentrating the filtrate. However, the ascending limb is impermeable to water but possesses a co-transporter complex called the $Na^+/K^+/2Cl^-$ co-transporter (Fig. 9.5.2) which reabsorbs these three ions. Loop diuretics such as **furosemide** act here. As the filtrate travels through the ascending limb, it therefore becomes progressively more dilute, because electrolytes are reabsorbed but water cannot follow.

Reabsorption and Secretion in the Distal Convoluted Tubule

Only about 10% of the volume of the original filtrate arrives in the DCT, because 90% has already been reabsorbed. The walls of the DCT contain pumps and channels that reabsorb Na^+ and Cl^- (Fig. 9.5.3); water follows passively by osmosis. These pumps exchange Na^+ for K^+, so as Na^+ is retained, K^+ is lost and vice versa. Thiazide diuretics, such as **bendrofluazide**, act here. The mineralocorticoid hormone **aldosterone** increases the number of pumps and channels here, increasing Na^+ and water reabsorption and enhancing K^+ loss. The DCT is also the main site of calcium (Ca^{2+}) reabsorption; **parathyroid hormone** acts here to increase Ca^{2+} reabsorption (see Fig. 9.9) and decreases Ca^{2+} loss in

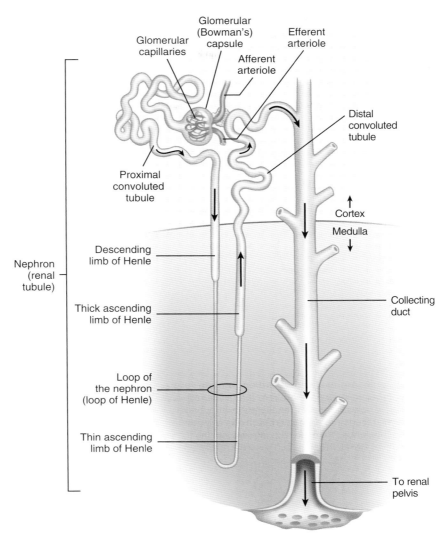

Fig. 9.2 The structure of a typical nephron. (Modified from Thibodeau G and Patton K (2019) Anatomy and physiology, 10th ed, St Louis: Mosby; and Applegate E (2011) The anatomy and physiology learning system, 4th ed. Philadelphia: Elsevier.)

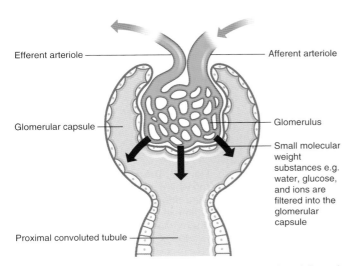

Fig. 9.3 Glomerular filtration. (Modified from Waugh A and Grant A (2020) Ross & Wilson anatomy and physiology in health and illness, 14th ed, Fig. 13.9. Oxford: Elsevier.)

the urine. Secretion of H$^+$ ions, K$^+$ ions, and some drugs also takes place here.

Reabsorption in the Collecting Duct
Aldosterone increases the number of Na$^+$ pumps and channels in the walls of the CD, increasing reabsorption of Na$^+$ and water. **Anti-diuretic hormone** (ADH) increases the number of aquaporins (water channels) in the walls of the CD, increasing water reabsorption and reducing urine volume. **Amiloride** and **spironolactone** act here.

DIURETICS

Diuretics increase urine production and promote the loss of water and electrolytes, mainly Na$^+$, from the body. Most work by a direct action on tubular Na$^+$ transport mechanisms and increase the Na$^+$ content of the filtrate, increasing its osmolarity, which in turn reduces water reabsorption and increases urine volume. In addition, diuretics may affect renal handling of other electrolytes because many of the transport mechanisms in the renal tubule exchange or

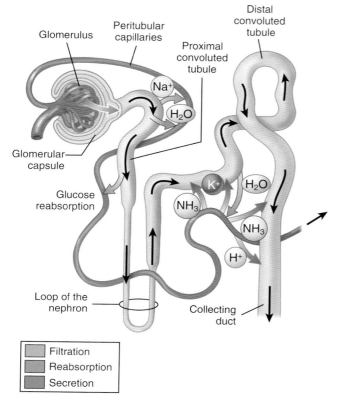

Fig. 9.4 Filtration, reabsorption, and secretion in urine formation. The green arrow represents filtration from the glomerular capillaries. The turquoise arrows represent reabsorption of substances from the filtrate into the bloodstream. The purple arrows represent secretion of unwanted substances from the bloodstream into the filtrate. (Modified from Patton KT, Bell FB, Thompson T, et al. (2022) Anatomy & physiology, 11th ed, Fig. 42.17. St. Louis: Elsevier.)

co-transport more than one ion. Diuretic therapy can therefore lead to excessive or deficient levels of other electrolytes, most significantly K^+, Cl^-, and Ca^{2+}.

Most diuretics must be present in the filtrate in order to work because most target a Na^+-transport mechanism on the epithelium lining the tubule. However, most are heavily plasma protein-bound, and so are too large to be filtered in the glomerulus and can only reach the filtrate by active secretion into the tubule by transporters in the PCT (Fig. 9.6). These transporters secrete a range of substances into the filtrate and have a finite working capacity. This means that once the diuretic drug plasma concentration is high enough to saturate these transporters, no additional drug will reach the filtrate, and increasing the drug dose will have no further therapeutic effect. It also means that if there is another drug in the bloodstream which is also secreted into the filtrate using the same transporters, the two drugs will compete at the transporter and reduced levels of the diuretic may reach the filtrate. This can reduce diuretic action.

Diuretics are useful in cardiovascular disease to reduce circulating blood volume and blood pressure and are used to reduce fluid load in situations associated with oedema or fluid retention, like raised intracranial pressure, pulmonary oedema, liver disease, and nephrotic syndrome. However, in conditions that reduce renal blood flow, e.g. heart failure, drug delivery to the kidney is reduced and this can reduce drug effectiveness.

OSMOTIC DIURETICS

Example: mannitol

Osmotic diuretics do not directly interfere with renal ion transport mechanisms, but their presence in body fluids increases the osmotic pressure of that fluid and so influences water movement between body compartments. The sugar mannitol is the prototype agent in this group, but other

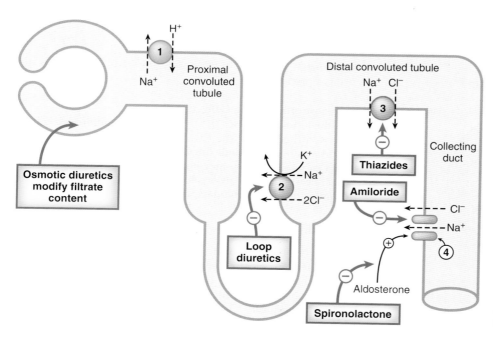

Fig. 9.5 The main regions of the nephron where sodium, chloride, and potassium are reabsorbed, and the sites of action of the main groups of diuretic drugs. (Modified from Ritter JM, Flower RJ, Henderson G, et al. (2020) Rang & Dale's pharmacology, 9th ed, Fig. 30.4. Oxford: Elsevier.)

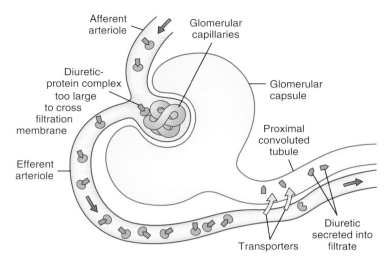

Fig. 9.6 Secretion of diuretics into the filtrate in the proximal convoluted tubule. Diuretics are heavily plasma protein-bound and so do not filter out of the blood in the glomerulus. Transporter mechanisms in the wall of the proximal convoluted tubule actively extract them from the bloodstream and pump them into the filtrate. Once in the filtrate, they inhibit their target sodium-transport mechanism.

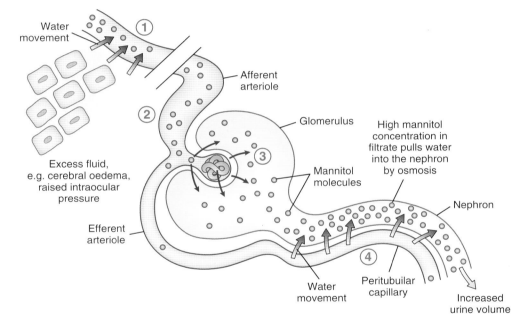

Fig. 9.7 The mechanism of action of mannitol: osmotic diuresis. 1. Mannitol in the bloodstream pulls water out of the tissues. 2. Increased blood volume increases filtration rates in the glomerulus. 3. Mannitol is filtered but not reabsorbed. 4. Mannitol increases the osmotic pressure of the filtrate and pulls water from the bloodstream into the nephron.

substances with similar actions include urea and isosorbide. High levels of other solutes in the urine, e.g. glucose, also produce an osmotic diuresis.

Mannitol is given intravenously to reduce intracranial pressure, relieve cerebral oedema, and reduce intraocular pressure. It does not leave the bloodstream, so it increases the osmotic pressure of the blood, which pulls fluid from the tissues into the circulation and therefore reduces oedema. This increases blood volume and blood flow to the kidney, increasing glomerular filtration and the amount of filtered Na^+, which itself may increase urine volume. Mannitol is filtered in the glomerulus but is not reabsorbed, so it remains in the filtrate, increasing its osmotic pressure. This generates an osmotic gradient between the tubule filtrate and the fluid outside the tubule and reduces water reabsorption, increasing urine volume (Fig. 9.7). Its plasma half-life is around 2 hours, although this is extended if renal function is poor.

Adverse Effects

Initially, because mannitol in the blood draws fluid from the tissues into the circulation and increases circulating blood volume, it can precipitate heart failure. Once diuresis commences, however, there can be hypovolaemia and hypotension, and pre-existing heart failure may be exacerbated by depleting circulating blood volume. Cardiovascular function should therefore be assessed before beginning treatment.

LOOP DIURETICS

Examples: bumetanide, ethacrynic acid, furosemide, torasemide

Loop diuretics are the most potent diuretics available because they inhibit the $Na^+/K^+/Cl^-$ co-transport complex in the ascending limb of the loop of the nephron (Fig. 9.8), which normally reabsorbs around 25% of the filtrate's Na^+ content. This complex pumps Na^+, K^+, and Cl^- from the filtrate into the epithelial cells of the nephron, and the ions are

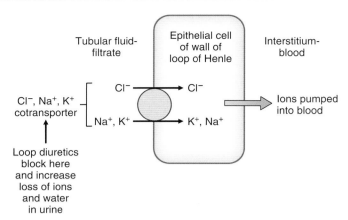

Fig. 9.8 The sodium/potassium/chloride co-transporter complex of the ascending limb of the loop of the nephron. (Modified from Shanbhag TV, Shenoy S, and Nayak V (2021) Pharmacology for dentistry, 4th ed, Fig. 5.3. New Delhi: Elsevier India.)

then pumped out the other side of the cells into the bloodstream, taking water with them. Loop diuretics bind to the Cl-transporting unit of the complex but are too large to travel through the transporter, and so they block it. This increases Na$^+$ and Cl$^-$ loss in the urine, which increases its osmolarity and reduces water reabsorption. Loop diuretics have vasodilator activity, which may be helpful in certain circumstances: for example, in heart failure because it reduces afterload, and in hypertension because it reduces blood pressure. In general, however, loop diuretics are not the optimal choice in hypertension because their duration of action is too short and the diuresis they produce is excessive. They are usually the diuretic of choice to relieve pulmonary oedema and fluid retention secondary to heart failure and in renal disease.

Pharmacokinetics

Bumetanide and **torasemide** are better and more reliably absorbed when given orally than **furosemide**, and all can be given intravenously if rapid diuresis is needed; intravenous administration gives peak effect within half an hour. **Furosemide's** plasma half-life is 1.5–2 hours, and with oral administration its effects last around 6 hours; about 50% is metabolised in the kidney, and the remainder is excreted unchanged. **Bumetanide** has a plasma half-life of 1 hour and is metabolised by the liver and kidney. **Torasemide** has a half-life of 3–4 hours and is mainly metabolised in the liver. Loop diuretics are tightly bound to plasma albumin and so are not filtered in the glomerulus, but reach the filtrate by secretion in the PCT; if this is compromised by poor renal function, diuretic action can be reduced. Several drugs, including **non-steroidal anti-inflammatory drugs** and some **antimicrobials**, inhibit the transporters that secrete loop diuretics into the filtrate and so impair their actions.

Adverse Effects

As with any diuretic, there may be urinary frequency and urgency, nocturia, and incontinence. Hypokalaemia is a common occurrence, because blocking Na$^+$ reabsorption in the loop means that the filtrate arriving in the DCT contains high Na$^+$ levels; this stimulates renin release, which in turn stimulates aldosterone secretion from the adrenal cortex (the RAAS, see Fig. 7.15). This increases activity of the

DCT's Na$^+$/K$^+$ pumps, which reabsorb Na$^+$ in exchange for K$^+$, and K$^+$ is lost in the urine. Hypokalaemia is potentially dangerous because it can predispose to cardiac arrhythmias. Diuretic-induced hypokalaemia increases the arrhythmogenic action of certain anti-arrhythmic drugs, e.g. **digoxin,** a clinically important interaction. Other electrolyte imbalances include hyponatraemia and hypomagnesaemia. Ca^{2+} excretion is increased, and loop diuretics may be used to bring plasma Ca^{2+} down in hypercalcaemia. Uric acid secretion is impaired, and blood uric acid levels rise. The loop diuretics, especially **furosemide**, can produce dose-related ototoxicity, giving deafness, tinnitus, and vertigo, because they affect the delicate hair cells of the inner ear responsible for hearing and balance; function usually returns to normal when the drug is withdrawn.

Excessive water and Na$^+$ loss can reduce the circulating blood volume and cause hypotension. If renal blood flow falls, renal function can be impaired.

THIAZIDE DIURETICS

Examples: chlorothiazide, bendrofluazide, hydrochlorothiazide; chlortalidone, indapamide, and metolazone have thiazide-like activity but are not structurally related to thiazides.

The original drug in this group, **chlorothiazide**, was first introduced to the market in 1957, and the agent most commonly used today, **bendrofluazide**, was introduced in 1960. Thiazides are used mainly in hypertension and heart failure. They are heavily plasma protein-bound, and so are not filtered in the glomerulus and reach the filtrate via active secretion in the PCT (Fig. 9.6). Thiazides inhibit the Na$^+$ pump in the DCT, reducing Na$^+$ reabsorption and therefore increasing Na$^+$ and water excretion. This has a knock-on effect on Ca^{2+} excretion. Blocking Na$^+$ reabsorption in the tubular epithelial cell reduces Na$^+$ levels in the cell. This activates a Na$^+$/Ca^{2+} transporter in the basolateral membrane which exchanges Na$^+$ for Ca^{2+}. When activated, this transporter imports Na$^+$ into the cell in exchange for Ca^{2+}, which is transported into the bloodstream (Fig. 9.9). Thiazide-induced reduction in Na$^+$ reabsorption therefore reduces urinary Ca^{2+} and increases circulating blood Ca^{2+} levels: this is why thiazides are sometimes used to reduce Ca^{2+} excretion (and therefore urinary Ca^{2+} concentration) in people prone to urinary stones. Elevating blood Ca^{2+} can also be helpful in people at risk of osteoporosis. In long-term use, they have a vasodilator effect, which contributes significantly to their therapeutic use in hypertension.

Pharmacokinetics

Thiazides are less potent than loop diuretics and have a slower onset of action, but their duration of action is longer. For example, bendrofluazide has a plasma half-life of 3–4 hours but is active over 12–24 hours.

Adverse Effects

As with any diuretic, there may be urinary frequency and urgency, nocturia, and incontinence. There is a significant risk of hypokalaemia because the filtrate arriving in the distal section of the DCT and the CDs contains high Na$^+$ levels; this stimulates the RAAS as described for the loop diuretics above, which increases Na$^+$ reabsorption at the expense of K$^+$, which is lost in the urine. Electrolyte imbalances including hypokalaemia and hyponatraemia are more frequent with thiazides than loop diuretics because thiazides have a considerably longer duration of action. In higher doses, thiazides can cause erectile dysfunction, which is reversible on stopping the drug; sometimes reducing the dose can resolve the problem. They compete with uric acid for the transporter which secretes them into the tubule, so they increase blood levels of uric acid; for this reason, they should be used with caution in people with, or at risk of, gout.

Thiazides impair glucose tolerance and can cause hyperglycaemia, thought to be secondary to thiazide-induced hypokalaemia. Low blood K^+ levels reduce the ability of pancreatic β-cells to release insulin in response to falling blood

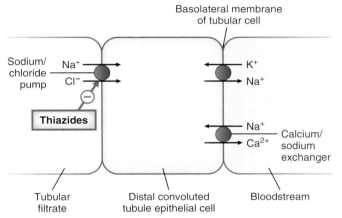

Fig. 9.9 Thiazides increase sodium loss in the urine and calcium retention. 1. Thiazides inhibit the sodium/chloride pump in the distal tubule, increasing the loss of these ions and water in the urine. 2. Falling sodium concentrations in the cell activate a sodium-calcium pump on the basolateral membrane, which imports sodium from the blood in exchange for calcium. Blood calcium levels therefore rise. (Modified from Hemmings H and Egan T (2013) Pharmacology and physiology for anesthesia, Fig. 34.8. Philadelphia: Saunders.)

glucose levels. As a result, blood glucose rises. Thiazides should therefore be used with care in diabetes.

POTASSIUM-SPARING DIURETICS

Examples: amiloride, eplerenone, spironolactone, triamterene

K^+-sparing diuretics act at the distal portion of the DCT and CD, the walls of which contain pumps and channels that reabsorb Na^+ and Cl^- in exchange for K+. They are weak diuretics because most electrolyte reabsorption has already taken place: the DCT and CD are the sites of any final adjustments to Na^+ reabsorption, and relatively small quantities of Na^+ are reabsorbed here. However, they may be usefully combined with a loop or thiazide diuretic to reduce the risk of hypokalaemia. Although all the K^+-sparing diuretics block this mechanism, preventing Na^+ reabsorption and so retaining K^+, their mechanisms of action are slightly different.

Spironolactone and **eplerenone** are aldosterone antagonists. Aldosterone, the main mineralocorticoid from the adrenal cortex, binds to DNA in the tubular cell and increases production of Na^+ pumps and channels in the DCT and CD and so enhances Na^+ reabsorption, with water following passively (Fig. 9.10A). Spironolactone prevents aldosterone from binding to its receptor and so reduces Na^+ pump and channel pump production. With fewer pumps and channels available, less Na^+ is reabsorbed, increasing Na^+ and water loss in the urine (Fig. 9.10B). Because Na^+ reabsorption increases K^+ loss, the diuresis and increased Na^+ loss seen with spironolactone is accompanied by K^+ retention.

Amiloride and **triamterene** bind directly to Na^+ channels in the DCT and CD, preventing Na^+ reabsorption, increasing urinary Na^+ and water loss, and retaining K^+.

Pharmacokinetics

These drugs are given orally and are generally well absorbed with the exception of **amiloride**, whose oral bioavailability is only around 50%, and less if there is food in the gastrointestinal (GI) tract. **Spironolactone** is a pro-drug and is

Fig. 9.10 The mechanism of action of spironolactone. A. The steroid hormone aldosterone enters the distal convoluted tubule/collecting duct cells and binds to its receptor in the cytoplasm. The hormone–receptor complex then binds to DNA and stimulates production of sodium pump protein. This increases sodium reabsorption and reduces sodium and water loss in the urine. B. Spironolactone (as its active metabolite canrenone) binds to and blocks aldosterone receptors. This prevents sodium pump synthesis. Sodium and water loss in the urine therefore increases but without additional potassium loss.

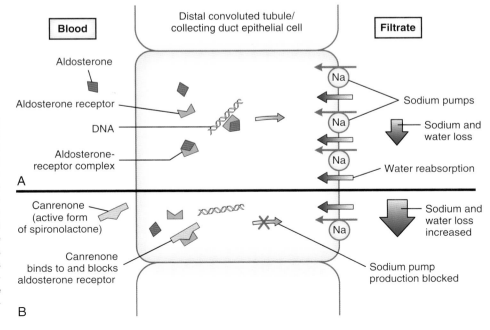

metabolised in the wall of the GI tract and the liver to the active metabolite **canrenone** (Fig. 9.10B), which has a longer half-life than spironolactone (16 hours to spironolactone's 90 minutes). Both **triamterene** and **amiloride** are secreted into the tubule in the PCT. As with steroid drugs in general, **spironolactone** and **eplerenone** can take several days to achieve full therapeutic effect; triamterene and amiloride, on the other hand, have a rapid onset of action.

Adverse Effects

These drugs can cause hyperkalaemia, and care is needed if there is already a predisposition to raised K^+ levels, for example in renal failure or with co-administration of **β-blockers**, **angiotensin-converting enzyme inhibitors,** or **angiotensin-receptor antagonists**, all of which can increase plasma K^+. The aldosterone-receptor antagonists are structurally related to steroids (otherwise they would not be able to bind to steroid receptors) and can block steroid receptors elsewhere in the body, including oestrogen, progesterone, and testosterone receptors. **Spironolactone** is more likely than **eplenerone** to cause such side-effects; it may cause gynaecomastia, menstrual irregularities, and testicular atrophy. Due to its anti-androgen effect, **spironolactone** can be used to treat hirsutism in women with polycystic ovary disease and male pattern baldness.

CARBONIC ANHYDRASE INHIBITORS

Examples: acetazolamide

The enzyme carbonic anhydrase is found in the cells along the length of the nephron but is present in particularly high concentrations in the PCT, which is therefore the main site of action of these agents. Inside the tubule cell, carbonic anhydrase catalyses the conversion of carbon dioxide and water into carbonic acid, which then rapidly dissociates into a H^+ ion and a bicarbonate ion. The H^+ ions produced are then exchanged for Na^+ ions across the wall of the tubule: H^+ ions are secreted into the filtrate and Na^+ ions reabsorbed (Fig. 9.11). Blocking the enzyme therefore reduces the availability of H^+ ions for exchange, and less Na^+ can be reabsorbed. This Na^+ is then lost in the urine, taking water with it. Along with increased Na^+ loss, bicarbonate ion excretion is also increased, producing an alkaline urine and

a mild acidosis. This mild acidosis stimulates respiration and is the basis for the use of acetazolamide in altitude sickness: by increasing respiratory effort, it helps to counteract the hypoxia caused by the reduced oxygen content of the atmosphere at altitude.

However, the diuretic action of carbonic anhydrase inhibitors is weak and short-lived. One reason for this is that the H^+/Na^+ exchange mechanism in the PCT accounts for a relatively small proportion of total tubular Na^+ reabsorption, so the impact of inhibiting it is fairly minor. In addition, the PCT cells respond to the inhibition of carbonic anhydrase by simply producing more enzyme, restoring its activity. With more effective diuretics available, the use of acetazolamide is now generally restricted to reducing intraocular pressure in people with glaucoma, as well as its more specialised use in altitude sickness as explained above.

MALE SEXUAL FUNCTION

To achieve penetration in sexual intercourse, the penis must become rigid (erect). The internal structure of the penis is shown in Fig. 9.12. In section, the penis is seen to

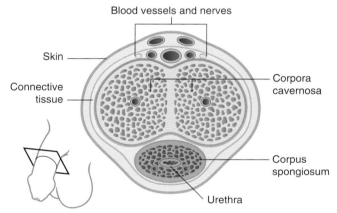

Fig. 9.12 Cross-section showing the internal structure of the penis. (From Waugh A and Grant A (2020) Ross & Wilson anatomy and physiology in health and illness, 14th ed, Fig. 13.9. Oxford: Elsevier.)

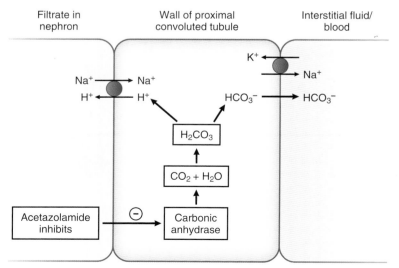

Fig. 9.11 The mechanism of action of carbonic anhydrase inhibitors. (Modified from Hemmings H and Egan T (2013) Pharmacology and physiology for anesthesia, Fig. 34.8. Philadelphia: Saunders.)

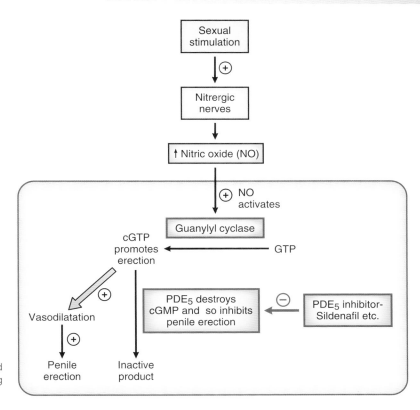

Fig. 9.13 Mechanism of action of sildenafil. (Modified from Ritter JM, Flower RJ, Henderson G, et al. (2012) Rang & Dale's pharmacology, 7th ed, Fig. 34.6. Oxford: Elsevier.)

be constructed from three columns of tissue running the length of the organ. The corpus spongiosum encloses the urethra. The two corpora cavernosa (singular: corpus cavernosum) run laterally to each other. Each is supplied by a deep artery of the penis, and they are rich in sinusoids, spaces that fill with blood during erection. Parasympathetic stimulation of these arteries during sexual excitement causes vasodilation, increasing blood flow, engorging the sinusoids, and stiffening the penis.

ERECTILE DYSFUNCTION

The inability to achieve or maintain an erection sufficient for sexual intercourse (erectile dysfunction) is common, and prevalence increases with age. There is often a psychological component, but a range of conditions that may interfere with vascular or neurological function may be responsible. There is a strong correlation between erectile dysfunction and cardiovascular disease, including ischaemic heart disease, stroke, and hypertension. Other recognised risk factors include obesity, diabetes mellitus, neurological disease such as multiple sclerosis, testosterone deficiency, and benign prostatic hypertrophy. A wide range of drugs, including recreational substances such as **alcohol** and **marijuana**, can cause erectile dysfunction: the most common include **benzodiazepines**, **selective serotonin re-uptake inhibitors**, **thiazide diuretics**, **β-blockers**, and **tricyclic antidepressants**.

PHOSPHODIESTERASE INHIBITORS

Examples: avanafil, sildenafil, tadalafil

The phosphodiesterases (PDEs) are a family of enzymes which break down the important intracellular signalling molecules cyclic AMP (cAMP) and cyclic guanosine

monophosphate (cGMP) (p.33). Sexual arousal increases the levels of nitric oxide in the tissues of the penis, which activates guanylyl cyclase and increases cGMP production. cGMP relaxes the smooth muscle in the erectile tissue of the corpora cavernosa and the arteries that supply them, increasing blood flow into the penis and facilitating engorgement and erection. PDE_5 breaks cGMP down, reducing cGMP levels and so reducing engorgement. Sildenafil and the other drugs in this category inhibit PDE_5, increasing cGMP levels, which increases blood flow into the penis and promotes and prolongs erection (Fig. 9.13). Sildenafil and tadalafil are also used in pulmonary hypertension: by relaxing pulmonary artery smooth muscle, these drugs reduce pulmonary artery pressure.

In conjunction with non-pharmacological measures (e.g. reducing alcohol consumption, stopping smoking, and weight loss if indicated), PDE inhibitors are the mainstay of erectile dysfunction management.

Pharmacokinetics

Sildenafil is rapidly absorbed from the GI tract and has a duration of action of 3–5 hours, so a single dose must be taken within a relatively short timeframe in advance of anticipated sexual activity. Tadalafil has a longer duration of action (17–24 hours) and can be taken as a regular daily dose to allow for spontaneous activity and/or when sexual activity is regular. PDE_5 inhibitors are primarily metabolised by CYP3A4 enzymes in the liver, which metabolise a range of other drugs. As a result, enzyme inhibitors such as the **azole antifungals** (e.g. **ketoconazole**), **Ca²⁺-channel blockers** (e.g. **verapamil**), **grapefruit juice**, and **macrolide antibiotics** (e.g. **erythromycin**) are likely to increase PDE_5 inhibitor levels and precipitate toxicity, and enzyme inducers including some **anticonvulsants** (e.g. **carbamazepine** and **phenytoin**) and **St. John's wort** increase the clearance of PDE$_5$ inhibitors and decrease their effectiveness.

Adverse Effects

Although the PDE$_5$ inhibitors are relatively selective for this form of the enzyme, they may also inhibit other members of the PDE family in other tissues, giving a range of side-effects. PDE$_5$ inhibitors relax vascular smooth muscle and can cause systemic vasodilation, reducing blood pressure and affecting systemic haemodynamics. They should therefore be used with care, if at all, in individuals with cardiovascular disease or compromise, including hypotension, heart failure, a history of heart attack or stroke, or ischaemic heart disease. In addition, they have clinically important interactions with other hypotensive agents, including **nitrates** and **α-blockers** and can cause a potentially dangerous fall in blood pressure. Rarely, priapism (sustained and painful erection) occurs. By an action on PDE$_6$ in the rods and cones of the retina, these drugs can cause vision problems; this is more likely with high-dose **sildenafil** than with the other PDE$_5$ inhibitors.

ALPROSTADIL

Natural prostaglandins (PGs) have very short half-lives, usually too brief to be clinically useful, and so stable synthetic analogues are often more suitable. PGE is an important vasodilator in normal physiological regulation of cardiovascular function, and the synthetic PGE$_1$ analogue alprostadil is used to relax penile arterial smooth muscle and increase penile engorgement in the diagnosis and treatment of erectile dysfunction, usually as a second-line treatment if a PDE$_5$ inhibitor cannot be used because of side-effects or a contra-indicating factor. Alprostadil can be applied topically to the penis tip, given as an intra-urethral pellet, or injected directly into the corpus cavernosum. The main side-effects include painful erection, and if enough drug escapes into the circulation, there may be headache and dizziness from systemic vasodilation.

REFERENCES

Koeppen, B., & Stanton, B. (2018). Renal physiology, 6th ed. Oxford: Elsevier.

ONLINE RESOURCES

Arumugham, V.B., Shahin, M.H., 2021. Therapeutic uses of diuretic agents. In: StatPearls [Internet]. StatPearls Publishing, Treasure Island. Available from: https://www.ncbi.nlm.nih.gov/books/NBK557838/.

Ellison, D.H., 2019. Clinical pharmacology in diuretic use. Clin. J. Am. Soc. Nephrol. 14 (8), 1248–1257. Available at: https://cjasn.asnjournals.org/content/14/8/1248.

Drugs and the Gastrointestinal Tract 10

FOCUS ON

THE STRUCTURE AND FUNCTION OF THE GASTROINTESTINAL SYSTEM

The gastrointestinal (GI) tract is essentially a long tube, open at both ends, adapted for the ingestion, digestion, and absorption of fluids and nutrients, and the excretion of unwanted solid materials. Foodstuffs and fluids enter the tract at the mouth and are subjected to both mechanical and chemical change as they pass through the tract, with wastes excreted via the anus. Mechanical digestion includes the grinding and crushing action of the teeth in chewing, as well as the mixing and churning that takes place in the stomach, and chemical digestion is carried out by a range of enzymes which are added to the contents of the tract at various stages. Several important organs associated with the tract, including the liver, pancreas, and gallbladder, release hormones and enzymes that regulate and contribute to healthy GI function. GI side-effects are associated with a wide range of drugs. For example, **antibiotics** alter GI flora and motility, and may cause diarrhoea, nausea and vomiting, and more seriously, antibiotic-induced colitis, caused by overgrowth of *Clostridium difficile*. A wide range of drugs affect autonomic nervous system function either adversely or as their main therapeutic action and alter motility and secretory activity of the tract: for example, **first-generation antihistamines** have antimuscarinic side-effects and commonly cause dry mouth due to reduced salivary secretion and constipation by inhibiting tract motility. Drugs that irritate the tract, e.g. **non-steroidal anti-inflammatory drugs** (NSAIDs), can cause ulceration, bleeding, or perforation. GI side-effects may be more severe if, as is commonly the case, the medication is taken orally, but because the tract receives a generous blood supply, drugs given parenterally can still affect its function. It follows that impaired GI function may affect absorption and excretion of drugs taken orally; this is discussed in more details in Chapter 2.

THE MAIN GASTROINTESTINAL ORGANS

The main organs of the GI tract are shown in Fig. 10.1. Foodstuffs enter the tract via the mouth, where chewing begins the process of mechanical digestion and mixes them with saliva. Saliva lubricates the food and contains amylase, a digestive enzyme that begins to digest any carbohydrate present. From the mouth, food is propelled by peristaltic waves sweeping down the muscular oesophagus to the stomach. The highly acidic gastric juices have significant antimicrobial action, but also stop the action of salivary amylase. The only significant chemical digestion in the stomach is performed by pepsin, secreted by chief cells in the gastric lining and which begins protein digestion. The stomach

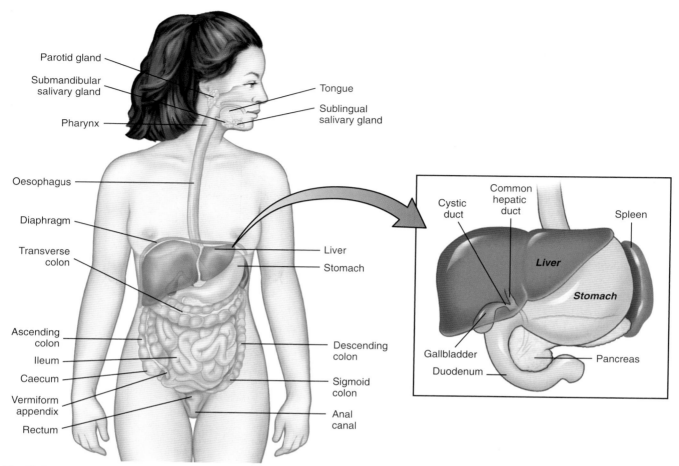

Fig. 10.1   The main organs of the gastrointestinal tract. (From Patton K and Thibodeau G (2020) Structure & function of the body, 16th ed, Fig. 16.1. St. Louis: Elsevier.)

walls contain three layers of smooth muscle whose fibres run in different directions to each other: regular, rhythmical, and co-ordinated contraction of these layers mixes and churns the stomach contents, producing a liquid called chyme. The next section of the tract, the small intestine, has three segments, the duodenum, the jejunum, and the ileum, and is around 7 m (22 feet) long in total. Most digestion and absorption take place here. Digestive enzymes are secreted into the small intestine by intestinal glands and the epithelial cells lining the tract, and fluids containing digestive enzymes from the pancreas and the gallbladder are emptied into the duodenum. These include lipases, which digest fats, proteases which digest proteins, and maltases, sucrases, lactases, and amylases which digest carbohydrates. The pancreatic juices and bile from the gallbladder are very alkaline, which rapidly increases the pH of the acidic chyme arriving in the duodenum from the stomach and protects the duodenum from acid damage.

The small intestine is coiled within the abdominal cavity, anchored to the posterior abdominal wall by folds of the peritoneum, and opens into the large intestine (the colon) at the ileocaecal valve. The colon arches over the small intestine and opens into the rectum. The opening from the rectum to the exterior, the anus, is normally under voluntary control in the adult and ensures faecal continence.

NERVOUS CONTROL OF THE GASTROINTESTINAL TRACT

Healthy GI function depends upon the muscle found in the wall of the tract all the way from the mouth to the anus. Except for the tongue and the muscle of the throat and external anal sphincter, which are composed of voluntary muscle, the tract walls contain smooth muscle. This regulates forward propulsion of the tract contents by peristalsis, as well as mixing and churning activity in the stomach and intestines. GI smooth muscle is under the overall control of the autonomic nervous system, but much of its activity is controlled locally by reflexes, local hormones, and changing conditions: for example, **histamine** stimulates gastric acid secretion, and stretching of the walls of the intestine stimulates peristalsis. The walls of the intestines contain two dense networks of nerves (plexuses), together called the enteric nervous system (Fig. 10.2). The myenteric plexus is sandwiched between the two layers of smooth muscle in the tract wall, and its main function is regulation of intestinal motility. The submucosal plexus lies between the mucosal lining of the tract and the smooth muscle layer, and its main functions are regulation of blood flow and control of the quantity and composition of secretions. The enteric nervous system is innervated by the autonomic nervous system, but also contains much shorter neurones

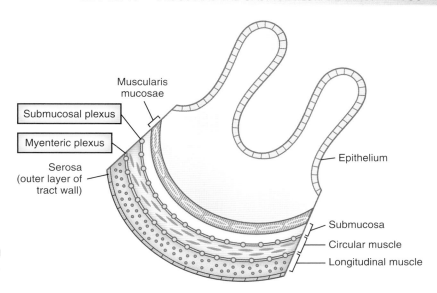

Fig. 10.2 The enteric nervous system. (Modified from Costanzo L (2022) Costanzo physiology, 7th ed, Fig. 8.1. Philadelphia: Elsevier.)

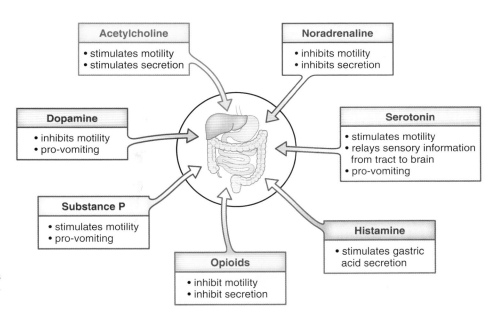

Fig. 10.3 The main neurotransmitters and hormones affecting gastrointestinal motility and secretion.

internal to the plexus giving reflexive local control independent of autonomic control: for example, these are the neurones which stimulate contraction when the wall of the tract is stretched, and which adjust the volume and composition of secretions in response to different foodstuffs travelling through.

Neurotransmitters in the Gastrointestinal Tract

A wide range of neurotransmitters are released by nerves supplying the glands and smooth muscle of the GI tract and regulate its function (Fig. 10.3). **Acetylcholine** (ACh), released by parasympathetic nerves and acting on muscarinic receptors, is the main stimulator of GI motility and secretion, including gastric emptying and intestinal peristalsis. On the other hand, **noradrenaline** from sympathetic nerves shuts the tract down; in a fight-or-flight situation, digesting a meal is not a priority. **Enkephalins**, members of the endogenous opioid family, act on mu (μ) receptors on myenteric nerves, inhibiting contraction and secretion. This is the reason why **morphine** and other opioids have a powerful

constipating action. Ninety-five percent of the body's **serotonin** (5-hydroxytryptamine, 5-HT) is found in the GI tract, where it stimulates motility and secretion by acting on 5-HT$_4$ receptors. Serotonin also activates sensory neurones, sending sensory impulses such as pain, nausea, and stretch from the GI tract to the brain, primarily by acting on 5-HT$_3$ receptors on these afferent nerves. The development of drugs with selective action on these subtypes has been of significant clinical use: 5-HT$_4$-receptor agonists such as **prucalopride** are used to treat constipation, whereas 5-HT$_3$-receptor antagonists, e.g. **ondansetron,** inhibit sensory impulses travelling to the vomiting centre (VC) in the brain and are effective anti-emetics. **Substance P** is a powerful stimulant of intestinal contraction and stimulates neurokinin 1 (NK$_1$) receptors on sensory fibres, sending impulses from the GI tract to the brain, including to the VC. **Aprepitant**, an NK$_1$ antagonist, is an effective anti-emetic. **Dopamine** (DA) inhibits GI motility and is an important neurotransmitter in vomiting pathways: dopamine antagonists such as **metoclopramide** are widely used to manage nausea and vomiting.

DRUGS AND GASTRIC FUNCTION

Swallowed food and drink arrive in the stomach, which acts as a reservoir, storing the food and regulating its delivery into the small intestine. Food can stay in the stomach for extended periods, depending on the quantity and composition of the meal and on gastric motility. In this time, it is well churned and mixed with gastric juices, and the liquid chyme is squirted into the duodenum through the pyloric sphincter.

GASTRIC ACID SECRETION

The gastric mucosa contains parietal cells, which secrete hydrochloric acid (HCl) into the stomach, keeping gastric pH very low, usually between 1 and 2. This highly acidic environment contributes to the breakdown of hard-to-digest materials such as plant cell walls and connective tissue in meat, and kills or damages most microbes.

The parietal cell does not synthesise HCl within its own intracellular fluid, because this would destroy the cell. Instead, it pumps chloride ions (Cl⁻) and hydrogen ions (H⁺) separately into the stomach lumen. The mechanisms by which it does this are shown in Figure 10.4. Within the parietal cell, H⁺ ions are generated when carbonic acid (H_2CO_3), which is very unstable, breaks down into H⁺ and a bicarbonate ion (HCO_3^-). This H⁺ is then pumped into the stomach by an ATPase pump called the proton pump, which exchanges the H⁺ for potassium (K⁺). Proton-pump inhibitors (PPIs) like **omeprazole** are first-line treatments in managing conditions associated with excessive acidity. Cl⁻ is pumped into the

parietal cell from the blood by a pump which swaps Cl⁻ for HCO_3^- produced when H_2CO_3 breaks down. K⁺ imported into the parietal cell by the proton pump is then pumped back out into the gastric fluids, co-transported with Cl⁻. In this way, [H⁺] and [Cl⁻] are kept much higher in stomach fluids than in other body tissues and fluids: [H⁺] is three million times more concentrated in gastric juice than in blood. Conditions associated with excessive acidity or failure of the normal physiological measures in place to protect the stomach and duodenum from the corrosive stomach juices are common and include peptic ulceration and gastro-oesophageal reflux disease (GORD).

Mechanisms Protecting the Gastric Mucosa

The tissues of the stomach wall use a range of measures to protect themselves from their own corrosive juices. Mucous glands produce a protective layer of mucus, which is resistant to the corrosive action of both gastric acid and the protein-digesting activity of gastric pepsin: it forms an effective barrier lining the stomach and prevents direct contact between the gastric epithelium and stomach contents. In addition, HCO_3^- produced by the gastric epithelium is pumped into the mucus lining; this keeps the mucus alkaline and helps to neutralise any acid diffusing into the mucus layer. Gastric blood flow is high, helping to wash away any H⁺ ions which manage to diffuse through the mucus layer into the stomach wall. Prostaglandins, particularly **PGE₂** and **PGI₂** (prostacyclin), are important cytoprotective agents in the stomach and are continuously produced in gastric tissues, mainly by cyclo-oxygenase (COX-1, see Ch. 6). They are important vasodilators, ensuring a good blood flow especially in gastric

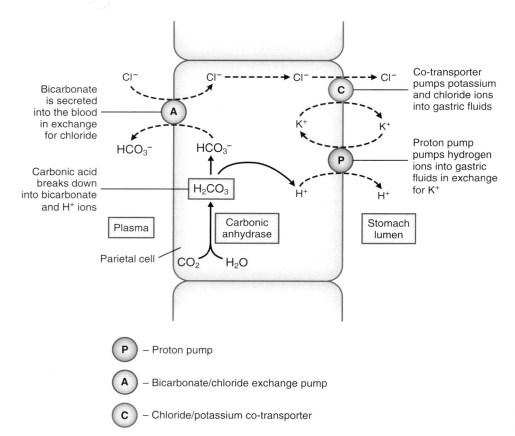

P – Proton pump

A – Bicarbonate/chloride exchange pump

C – Chloride/potassium co-transporter

Fig. 10.4 The proton pump and parietal cell secretion of H+ and Cl- ions into the stomach. (Modified from Ritter JM, Flower RJ, Henderson G, et al. (2020) Rang & Dale's pharmacology, 9th ed, Fig. 31.1. Oxford: Elsevier.)

inflammation; they stimulate HCO_3^- and mucus production and act directly on parietal cells to inhibit acid production by the proton pump (Fig. 10.5). **NSAIDs** block COX and inhibit gastric prostaglandin production, the basis of their gastric irritant effect. Synthetic prostaglandins used to treat acid-related conditions include **misoprostol**.

Stimulants of Gastric Acid Secretion

There are three main physiological stimulants of gastric acid secretion (Fig. 10.5).

Histamine
Histamine is released by enterochromaffin-like (ECL) cells in the gastric mucosa. It is an important stimulant of gastric acid secretion and binds to H_2 receptors on parietal cells, which in turn activates the proton pump and increases acid secretion. H_2-receptor blockers, e.g. **cimetidine**, are widely available to treat conditions associated with excess acid.

Acetylcholine
ACh released by parasympathetic nerves supplying the stomach acts on M_3 receptors on parietal cells, activating the proton pump and increasing acid secretion. This promotes digestive function when the body is resting, and parasympathetic activity ('rest and digest') predominates over sympathetic ('fight or flight'). Antimuscarinic drugs, e.g. **hyoscine** and **atropine**, block M_3 receptors and reduce gastric acid secretion as part of their more widespread inhibitory effects on digestive function.

Gastrin
The hormone gastrin is released into the bloodstream by G cells in stomach glands in response to stretching of the stomach wall and the presence of protein-rich foods in the stomach. It does not directly stimulate parietal cells: instead, it binds to receptors on ECL cells and increases histamine production, which in turn activates the proton pump.

DRUGS THAT REGULATE GASTRIC pH

Conditions associated with excess stomach acid are common and range from the occasional episode of heartburn after a rich or heavy meal to the continual misery of chronic peptic ulceration associated with, for example, *Helicobacter pylori* infection (see Focus on: Treatment of Peptic Ulcers box) or long-term use of **NSAIDs**.

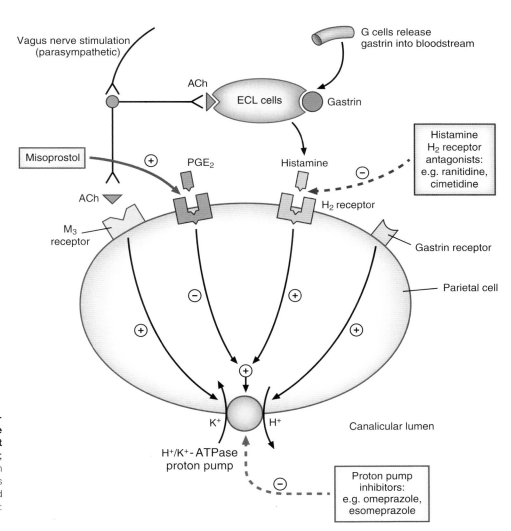

Fig. 10.5 The main agents stimulating gastric acid secretion by the parietal cell, and some drugs that block them. ACh, Acetylcholine; PGE_2, prostaglandin E_2 (Modified from Waller DG, Sampson A, and Hitchings A (2022) Medical pharmacology and therapeutics, 6th ed, Fig. 33.1. Oxford: Elsevier.)

ANTACIDS

Antacids are weak bases, usually prepared as liquid formulations or chewable tablets, which neutralise gastric acid. They are freely available over the counter and are widely used on a non-prescription basis to self-manage upper GI tract disorders. The rise in gastric pH also inhibits pepsin, which works best at pH 2–3.5. Antacids contain calcium, magnesium, or aluminium salts, which react with and neutralise HCl, increasing gastric pH. For example, calcium carbonate ($CaCO_3$) reacts with HCl to form H_2CO_3 and neutral calcium chloride ($CaCl_2$) according to the following reaction:

$$CaCO_3 + 2HCl \rightarrow H_2CO_3 + CaCl_2$$

H_2CO_3 quickly breaks down into water (H_2O) and carbon dioxide (CO_2) gas, which causes the belching associated with $CaCO_3$ use.

Antacids are best taken with food because gastric emptying is much faster on an empty stomach, shortening the duration of action of the drug. Sometimes the thickening agent **alginic acid** is used with an antacid to increase the viscosity of the gastric fluids and help retain the drug in the stomach, and/or **simeticone**, an anti-foaming agent.

Adverse Effects

Taken occasionally and according to manufacturer's instructions, antacids are generally well tolerated. There may be significant absorption of calcium, magnesium, or aluminium which can cause problems particularly in people with impaired renal function who cannot clear the excess. Magnesium salts can cause diarrhoea and aluminium salts can constipate, but using a combination can help minimise any disruption to bowel function. Some antacid preparations contain significant amounts of sodium and should be avoided in people on salt-restricted diets.

Antacids may increase or decrease absorption of a wide range of co-administered drugs by several mechanisms (Fig. 10.6). Antacids may chelate other drugs in the GI tract; that is, the metal ions in the antacid bind to them and form insoluble complexes, reducing their bioavailability: for example, **tetracycline**, **digoxin,** and **quinolone antibiotics** are chelated by antacids, significantly reducing absorption. Some drugs, e.g. **itraconazole**, are formulated to be released from the drug preparation in the acid environment of the stomach, and increasing gastric pH can reduce the amount of free drug reaching the duodenum for absorption, reducing circulating drug levels and drug efficacy. The coating of enteric-coated formulations is pH sensitive, formulated to remain intact in the stomach and break down in the higher pH of the duodenum; if gastric pH rises, this enteric coating may break down in the stomach, exposing acid-sensitive drugs to gastric fluids and reducing the quantity of active drug reaching the duodenum for absorption. On the other hand, the absorption of other drugs may be facilitated by increasing gastric pH. Whenever possible, it is therefore generally advised to separate administration times of antacids and other drugs.

PROTON-PUMP INHIBITORS

Examples: esomeprazole, lansoprazole, omeprazole

The proton pump is the final common mechanism for all stimulants of gastric acid production. The first PPI, **omeprazole**, was introduced in 1989 and is still in widespread use today. Because these agents reduce gastric acid production irrespective of the stimulus (histamine, alcohol, smoking, caffeine, etc.) and have proved to be well tolerated and highly effective, they have become the mainstay of management in acid-related disorders. Globally they are among the most widely consumed drugs and are included on the World Health Organisation's list of essential medicines. They are usually given orally and are absorbed into gastric parietal cells from the bloodstream. Here, they bind irreversibly to one of the subunits of the proton pump, permanently deactivating it (Fig. 10.5). It can take the parietal cell up to 36 hours to synthesise a new pump to replace it, and the irreversible nature of the binding means that the biological

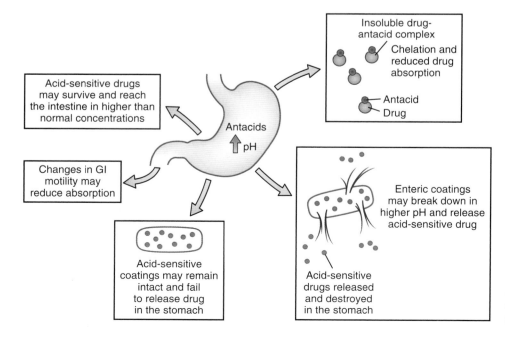

Fig. 10.6 The main mechanisms of antacid-mediated drug interactions. GI, gastrointestinal.

effect of PPIs far exceeds the plasma half-life, and once daily dosing is adequate. Both basal secretion and feeding-stimulated secretion are inhibited. The effectiveness of PPIs improves with repeated administration and is maximal after 5 days of daily dosing. This is because only around a third of proton pumps are activated when a meal is eaten. Over the course of the next few days and meals eaten, more and more of the inactive pumps are recruited in an attempt to maintain acid secretion; after about 5 days, all available pumps are blocked, and acid production is maximally reduced.

Pharmacokinetics

In general, these drugs have short plasma half-lives; **omeprazole's** plasma half-life is 30–60 minutes, **esomeprazole's** is between 60 and 90 minutes, and **lansoprazole's** is around 90 minutes. However, because they irreversibly inhibit the proton pump, their acid-suppressant action is highly effective: a single dose reduces acid production by up to 90% over a 24-hour period. They are acid-sensitive and oral preparations are enteric-coated to protect the drug on its passage through the stomach. The increase in gastric pH reduces absorption of azole antifungals including **itraconazole** (see also **Antacids** above) and some other drugs whose solubility falls at higher pH values, including some **antiviral agents**. They are highly plasma protein-bound and all are metabolised to inactive products in the liver by cytochrome P450 enzymes. This can cause interactions with other drugs also metabolised by members of this family, including **selective serotonin re-uptake inhibitors**, whose plasma levels are increased when taken with a PPI.

Adverse Effects

PPIs may cause a range of GI symptoms including nausea, vomiting, abdominal pain, and diarrhoea. There is evidence linking PPI use to increased risk of GI infections, likely due to improved microbial survival in the less hostile gastric environment. Additionally, changing gastric pH affects the bowel microbiome, the populations of microbes inhabiting the tract, which may help pathogenic species establish themselves. The rise in gastric pH may reduce absorption of calcium and magnesium, and long-term use of PPIs has been associated with increased risk of osteoporosis, fracture, and magnesium deficiency. Compared to H_2-receptor blockers, PPIs have been shown to slightly increase the risk of gastric cancer, and the risk increases with dose and duration of treatment. The reason for this is unclear and it is likely that more than one mechanism is involved. One possible factor may relate to gastrin levels. When gastric pH rises, which would normally happen after eating because food and fluids dilute stomach fluids, gastrin secretion increases in response to aid digestion; gastrin also acts as a growth factor and may stimulate hyperplasia in stomach tissues. PPI use may also mask the symptoms of a pre-existing gastric cancer.

H_2-RECEPTOR ANTAGONISTS

Examples: cimetidine, famotidine, ranitidine

Histamine stimulates gastric acid secretion by stimulating H_2 receptors on gastric parietal cells and activating the proton pump (Fig. 10.5). James Black, a Scottish pharmacologist, identified the subtype of histamine receptors found in the stomach and named them H_2 receptors because H_1 receptors, which mediate the inflammatory and allergic actions of histamine, had already been named. Standard antihistamines such as **chlorphenamine** had been used to treat allergic inflammation since the early years of the 20th century, but recognising that these drugs did not reduce histamine-induced gastric acid secretion, Black reasoned that there must be more than one subtype of histamine receptor and spent several years looking for an agent that would selectively block histamine's action on the stomach. The result was **cimetidine**, which blocked histamine-induced gastric acid secretion but had no anti-inflammatory action, and which came on the market in 1976. Black had already had significant research success in the newly emerging field of receptor subtypes: he had also led the group that in the early 1960s produced the β_2-selective antagonist **propranolol** (p. 131), a highly significant step in the treatment of cardiovascular disease; he shared the 1988 Nobel Prize in Physiology and Medicine for his contribution to pharmacological research.

The use of H_2-receptor antagonists has steadily fallen since the development of PPIs, but they are effective suppressants of both basal and stimulated gastric acid secretion: they reduce 24-hour gastric acid secretion by around 70%. **Ranitidine** was withdrawn from global markets in 2019/2020 following concerns that an impurity in its formulation, called nitrosodimethylamine, a known human carcinogen, could be linked to increased risk of cancer.

As with PPIs, regular use of histamine-receptor antagonists can mask the symptoms of stomach cancer.

Pharmacokinetics

H_2-receptor antagonists are taken orally and have short plasma half-lives, ranging from 1–3 hours. **Famotidine** is the most potent member of the group. **Cimetidine** is a potent inhibitor of hepatic cytochrome P450 enzymes and can reduce the metabolism of a range of other medications, including **anticoagulants** and **tricyclic antidepressants**. H_2-receptor antagonists are mainly eliminated unchanged by the kidney and doses may need to be reduced in people with poor renal function.

Adverse Effects

H_2-receptor antagonists are usually well tolerated. Common side-effects include GI upsets such as diarrhoea or constipation and skin reactions, headache, and myalgia. Rarely, they can cause acute liver injury. **Cimetidine** has weak anti-androgenic activity and blocks testosterone receptors; this can cause gynaecomastia and impotence.

MISOPROSTOL

Misoprostol is a stable synthetic analogue of PGE_1 with gastroprotective actions and is used to treat or prevent peptic ulcer disease: it is also given to prevent or minimise NSAID-induced GI toxicity. Naturally produced gastric PGs are cytoprotective in the stomach as described above (see also Fig. 10.3) but are too unstable to be useful: oral misoprostol has a plasma half-life of around 40 minutes and is metabolised in the liver. It stimulates GI smooth muscle and can cause abdominal cramps, diarrhoea, nausea, and vomiting. It also stimulates uterine smooth muscle, causing uterine cramping and potentially uterine rupture. For this reason, it should not be used in peptic ulcer disease in pregnancy. It has an alternative therapeutic use in termination of pregnancy and induction of labour.

Focus on: Drugs Used in Peptic Ulcer Treatment

Peptic ulcers are caused by exposure of the gastric or duodenal tissues to acid. Risk factors include increasing age, **non-steroidal anti-inflammatory drug** use, smoking, **alcohol** intake, and *Helicobacter pylori* infection, which alone increases the risk of peptic ulcer up to 10-fold. *H. pylori*

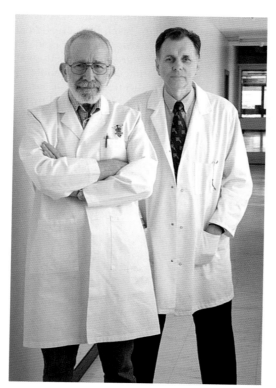

Fig. 10.7 J. Robin Warren and Barry J. Marshall, co-discoverers of the role of *Helicobacter pylori* in peptic ulcer disease and joint winners of the 2005 Nobel Prize for this work. (Photo courtesy of Drs Warren and Marshall, University of Western Australia, Adelaide, Australia.)

infection is also a significant risk factor in gastric carcinoma, the rates of which have fallen since eradication therapy became standard practice in the management of peptic ulcers.

Triple/Quadruple Therapy

H. pylori is associated with 95% of duodenal ulcers and up to 80% of gastric ulcers, and the discovery of the relationship between this bacterium and peptic ulcer disease earned Barry J. Marshall and J. Robin Warren (Fig. 10.7) the Nobel Prize for Medicine in 2005. The incidence of peptic ulceration has steadily decreased since this association was recognised and antibiotic treatment introduced as part of the treatment regime. *H. pylori* is a flagellated bacterium (Fig. 10.8) which burrows into the gastric mucosa and survives in the acid conditions by producing ammonia, which neutralises HCl, and in this way generates a protective pH neutral bubble around itself. Although *H. pylori* infection is common, with up to half the population infected by the age of 50, in most it causes no more than a mild gastritis with little or no increase in gastric acid production. However, in up to 10% of people, it increases gastric acid secretion and inhibits HCO_3^- production, predisposing to peptic ulcers. Although treatment with proton-pump inhibitors **(PPIs)** and **H_2-receptor antagonists** alone can heal an ulcer even in the presence of infection, recurrence is inevitable and cure depends on eradication of *H. pylori*. Currently, triple or quadruple therapy is the standard treatment in *H. pylori*-positive people. In triple therapy, two different **antibiotics** are used, usually for a period of up to 2 weeks, along with high-dose PPI, usually with a cure rate of 80%–90%. Depending on antibiotic resistance, a typical antibiotic regimen includes two from **amoxicillin**, **metronidazole**, and **clarithromycin**. A **tetracycline** or other antibiotic may be substituted if these first-line agents are ineffective. In quadruple therapy, **bismuth** (see below) is added.

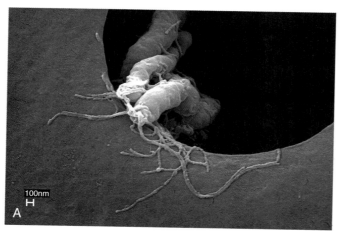
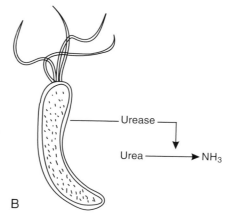

Fig. 10.8 A. Photomicrograph of *Helicobacter pylori*. B. Schematic of *H. pylori*, showing its ability to produce an ammonium cloud around itself due to urease production. (From (A) Photo by Christina Nilsson, Karolinska Institutet, and (B) Shanbhag TV, Shenoy S, and Nayak V (2017) Pharmacology for dentistry, 3rd ed, Fig. 8.6. New Delhi: Elsevier India.)

Bismuth

Bismuth subsalicylate is an antacid with antimicrobial activity. Given orally, it breaks down to release bismuth, which is toxic to a range of gastrointestinal pathogens including *Escherichia coli* and *Clostridium difficile* but is thought to have minimal effects on normal gut flora. It is available over the counter to treat the symptoms of acid reflux and the relief of other gastrointestinal upsets including nausea, flatulence, and diarrhoea. It is the fourth component of quadruple therapy in peptic ulcer disease; it blocks the ability of *H. pylori* to attach to the gastric epithelium and inhibits some of its key enzymes, including the urease it uses to synthesise its protective ammonia cloud. At therapeutic doses, less than 1% of bismuth is absorbed, but systemic side-effects include blackening of the tongue and faeces, encephalopathy and deteriorating mental status, insomnia, and seizures. Bismuth is excreted very slowly via the kidneys, so care is needed in renal impairment.

Sucralfate

Sucralfate is a complex of sucrose sulphate and aluminium hydroxide, which in the acidic environment of the stomach forms a thick gel which coats the ulcer and forms a physical barrier between it and the gastric juices. Because gel formation depends on low pH, it is less effective if stomach acid has been neutralised or reduced by other treatments, so dosing should be appropriately spaced out. In addition, it inhibits pepsin and increases HCO_3^- secretion, reducing tissue damage and promoting healing. Activated sucralfate possesses multiple negatively charged groups, which are responsible for binding to the protein-rich exudate from the ulcer and essential for its activity, but which may also bind a range of drugs including **digoxin, tetracyclines, phenytoin**, and **quinolone antibiotics** and reduce their absorption. The most common side-effect is constipation. Rarely, sucralfate may consolidate into a hardened mass called a bezoar, which can obstruct the tract.

DRUGS AND DISORDERS OF GASTROINTESTINAL MOTILITY

A wide range of neurotransmitters (Fig. 10.3) are released by GI nerves, offering a number of potentially very useful targets for drug action in conditions involving either hypermotility or hypomotility of the GI tract. Other drugs may affect GI motility by interfering directly or indirectly with smooth muscle function.

DRUGS THAT REDUCE GASTROINTESTINAL TONE AND/OR MOTILITY

Increased GI motility and reduced intestinal transit time are usually due to enteric infections or inflammatory conditions such as irritable bowel syndrome (IBS). GI spasm is painful, and sustained increased motility can cause diarrhoea, defined as the passage of three or more watery stools in a 24-hour period. As with increased motility, diarrhoea is also associated with increased intestinal secretion. This potentially pours litres of fluid into the tract in a 24-hour period, exceeding the capacity of the tract to reabsorb it, and which if prolonged can cause life-threatening electrolyte loss and dehydration, especially in children and frail people.

OPIOIDS

Via their action on μ (mu) opioid receptors (MORs) on enteric nerves, opioids decrease the motility of GI smooth muscle, delaying gastric emptying, inhibiting forward peristaltic movement, and halting the propulsion of materials through the tract. Constipation is a troublesome side-effect when opioid drugs such as **morphine** and **codeine** are used as analgesics. Opioids increase intestinal transit time, allowing more time for water absorption and reducing faecal volume.

Loperamide

Loperamide is a synthetic opioid widely available as a constituent of over-the-counter antidiarrhoeal preparations:

it has 50 times the antidiarrhoeal effect of **codeine** and is more potent than **diphenoxylate** (see below). It is taken orally and subject to significant first-pass metabolism, so its bioavailability is very low, usually in the order of 2%. At doses recommended for the treatment of diarrhoea, very little crosses the blood–brain barrier, so loperamide lacks the central action associated with most opioid drugs. It has a high affinity for MORs on nerves of the myenteric plexus and is absorbed directly from the tract into the wall of the intestine: its onset of action is usually within an hour and it is effective for up to 24 hours. In addition to its action on intestinal smooth muscle, it increases absorption of water and electrolytes, although it reduces absorption of nutrients such as glucose. Adverse effects include constipation and nausea. At high doses, loperamide is sometimes used as a recreational agent to achieve euphoria and relieve the unpleasant symptoms of opioid withdrawal; supra-therapeutic doses have been associated with serious cardiac arrhythmias including QT prolongation, torsades de pointes, and cardiac arrests. **Naloxone** is an effective reversal agent.

Diphenoxylate/Atropine

Diphenoxylate is an opioid with the expected antimotility action of this group of drugs, but it crosses the blood-brain barrier in greater quantities than **loperamide**, so its potential for abuse is higher. To discourage abuse, it is used with **atropine**, an antimuscarinic agent: atropine itself has antimotility action because it blocks parasympathetic activity in the tract, but it causes a range of other unpleasant antimuscarinic side-effects, including dry mouth and eyes, nausea, and bloating. Even at therapeutic doses, the atropine component of the preparation can cause antimuscarinic side-effects including tachycardia and closed-angle glaucoma.

Racecadotril

This is a pro-drug and is metabolised in the liver to **thiorphan**. Thiorphan is not a directly acting MOR agonist like **loperamide** or **diphenoxylate**, but it increases the concentrations

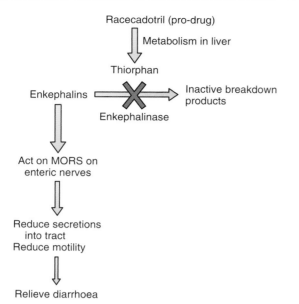

Fig. 10.9 The mechanism of action of racecadotril. MORS, μ opioid receptors.

of endogenous opioids in the GI tract by blocking the enzyme that breaks them down. In the tract, endogenous **enkephalins**, acting on MORs on enteric nerves, contribute to the regulation of gut function. They are broken down by enkephalinase, terminating their action. Thiorphan inhibits enkephalinase, prolonging enkephalin action (Fig. 10.9). Its main therapeutic action in the treatment of diarrhoea seems to be by reducing excessive intestinal secretory activity rather than reducing gut motility: this drug does not reduce transit times, and constipation is therefore not one of its side-effects. Another clinical advantage of not reducing gut motility is that in infection, the drug does not increase retention time and so does not increase the length of time infective products are in contact with the GI wall. Thiorphan acts quickly (within half an hour), and because it does not cross the blood-brain barrier, it does not have central side-effects. Racecadotril is available in many countries worldwide including India and several European countries but not currently in the UK.

ANTIMUSCARINIC AGENTS

Examples: atropine, hyoscine butylbromide, propantheline

Because antimuscarinic drugs have widespread effects on multiple body systems by blocking the action of ACh released by parasympathetic stimulation, their use as antimotility agents is limited. However, antimuscarinic agents may be used for their antispasmodic properties in the GI tract in GI infections, IBS, and other disorders associated with smooth muscle spasm. They cause a range of predictable antimuscarinic adverse effects including dry mouth, tachycardia, constipation, bronchoconstriction, blurred vision, and urinary retention. **Atropine** and **hyoscine** are closely related naturally occurring substances found in a range of poisonous plants including deadly nightshade and henbane. **Atropine** crosses the blood-brain barrier and so has central antimuscarinic side-effects such as sedation as well as peripheral antimuscarinic activity. It is mainly used topically in ocular preparations and in premedication, although it is combined with **diphenoxylate** (see

above) to discourage inappropriate use of this drug. **Hyoscine butylbromide** is the formulation of hyoscine usually used to relieve smooth muscle spasm; it is a quaternary ammonium derivative, which reduces its lipid solubility and means that it is poorly absorbed orally and does not cross the blood-brain barrier. It therefore lacks central nervous system-depressant effects and should not be confused with **hyoscine hydrobromide**, which does cross the blood-brain barrier and is used mainly as an anti-emetic (see below). Hyoscine hydrobromide is also used to reduce respiratory secretions in palliative care. Most of an oral dose is excreted in the faeces because it is poorly absorbed, and the plasma half-life is 5 hours.

SMOOTH-MUSCLE RELAXANTS

Examples: alverine citrate, mebeverine, peppermint oil

Drugs that directly relax smooth muscle may be used in GI disorders associated with spasm.

Alverine Citrate

Serotonergic nerves supplying the GI tract release serotonin (5-HT) which acts on $5-HT_{1A}$ receptors on GI smooth muscle to stimulate contraction and cause pain. Alverine citrate blocks $5-HT_{1A}$ receptors, and so relieves pain and spasm in GI disorders; it also effectively relieves the pain of dysmenorrhoea. Side-effects include headache, dizziness, and nausea.

Mebeverine

Mebeverine is a direct-acting smooth-muscle relaxant used mainly in IBS. It is taken orally, but little reaches the circulation because it is extensively cleared by first-pass metabolism in the liver. It is well tolerated with few significant side-effects. Its mechanism of action is not clear, although it may have antimuscarinic activity. It blocks sodium channels in the smooth muscle cell membrane and reduces calcium levels within smooth muscle cells, both of which promote muscle relaxation and relieve intestinal spasm. Side-effects include skin reactions and facial oedema.

Peppermint Oil

Peppermint oil is the essential oil obtained from the plant *Mentha piperita* and has been used for hundreds of years in traditional medicine as an anti-inflammatory, antispasmodic, and expectorant. It is commonly used to treat the symptoms of IBS. The major constituent of peppermint oil is **menthol**, thought to be responsible for its therapeutic action. Menthol blocks calcium channels in the smooth muscle cells of the GI tract, reducing calcium influx and inhibiting contraction. In addition, peppermint oil has antimicrobial, anti-inflammatory, and anaesthetic properties, all of which may contribute to its therapeutic action. Capsules are enteric-coated to prevent their dissolution in the stomach, because menthol relaxes the sphincter between the oesophagus and the stomach and causes acid reflux.

DRUGS THAT INCREASE GASTROINTESTINAL MOTILITY

The frequency of defaecation varies from individual to individual, but usually falls somewhere between three times daily to once every 3 days. Several disorders impair the co-ordinated contractile activity of the GI tract, leading to increased transit times, constipation, and potentially obstruction. Hypomotility disorders of the tract include achalasia (loss of oesophageal contractility) and GORD, but many systemic disorders impacting on neurological or smooth muscle function, including multiple sclerosis, Parkinson's disease, diabetes, thyroid disease, and systemic lupus erythematosus, also affect GI motility. GI motility is also reduced in pain.

Constipation

Constipation is the passage of stools less frequently than an individual's normal pattern, and the faeces is usually dry, hard, and difficult to expel. It is a common problem, and while it may be a feature of a range of diseases as described above, it is often due to lifestyle factors including insufficient physical exercise, a low-fibre diet, and inadequate fluid intake. It may also be a side-effect of a wide range of drugs, including **opioids**, **antimuscarinic** agents, and **iron supplements**. Because **progesterone** relaxes smooth muscle, constipation is also common in pregnancy. Wherever appropriate, lifestyle advice regarding dietary modifications, drinking more fluid, and taking regular exercise should be the first approach to managing constipation.

LAXATIVES

Laxatives promote defaecation, usually either by softening or lubricating the stool or by stimulating intestinal motility and are used to treat constipation. If laxative use is required for short-term management, their use should be for as limited a time as possible. Laxatives may also be used to cleanse the bowel in preparation for endoscopy, surgery, or radiological procedures. They should not be used in GI obstruction. Laxatives are classified into four main groups (Fig. 10.10).

Bulk-Forming Laxatives

Examples: bran, ispaghula husk, methylcellulose, sterculia

These are all bulky, indigestible plant extracts which retain fluid and soften and expand faecal volume. This stretches the intestinal walls, which stimulates reflexive contraction of its smooth muscle and propels its contents forward. It is important to ensure an adequate fluid intake with these agents to avoid obstruction. They may take 2–3 days to work, but their action is gentle and they are generally well tolerated, although they can cause bloating and flatulence.

Softening Laxatives

Examples: arachis oil, docusate sodium, liquid paraffin

These agents coat and soften the faeces, lubricating their passage through the tract. **Arachis oil** is given as an enema and **liquid paraffin** is given orally; both can cause unpleasant and itchy anal seepage. Accidental inhalation of liquid paraffin can cause aspiration pneumonia. **Docusate sodium** can be given orally or rectally, and has an additional direct stimulant effect on intestinal smooth muscle.

Stimulant Laxatives

Examples: bisacodyl, dantron, glycerol, senna, sodium picosulfate

Stimulant laxatives stimulate enteric nerves, which triggers contraction of intestinal smooth muscle and stimulates water and electrolyte secretion into the tract, promoting

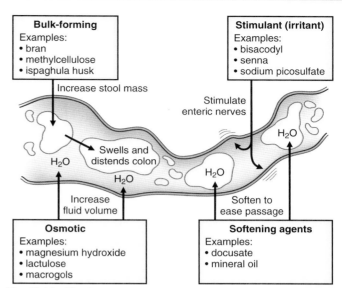

Fig. 10.10 The four groups of laxative drugs. (Modified from Mariotti A, Johnson B, and Dowd FJ (2017) Pharmacology and therapeutics for dentistry, 7th ed, Fig. 28.4. St. Louis: Mosby.)

peristalsis. Because of this, they can cause painful abdominal cramps. Overuse desensitises the enteric nerves and reduces the efficacy of the drugs, which can lead to increased laxative consumption. This further desensitises the nerves, establishing a vicious circle of laxative overuse and deteriorating bowel function, potentially causing an atonic bowel. In general, stimulant laxatives exert their effects rapidly, usually within 12 hours.

Dantron is used only in palliative care, because it is potentially carcinogenic and causes skin irritation: it discolours the urine red, blue, or green. **Co-danthrusate** is dantron formulated with **docusate**, and **co-danthramer** is dantron formulated with a synthetic polymer called a poloxamer, which helps to attract water into the stool. **Glycerol** is given as an enema and stimulates evacuation by irritating rectal nerves and lubricating the rectal contents. **Bisacodyl** can be given orally or rectally. **Senna** is given orally, and is broken down to the active agent **rheinanthrone**, which has the dual action of stimulating enteric nerves and triggering peristalsis, and reducing water absorption from the faeces, softening and expanding it. **Sodium picosulfate** is given orally and is sometimes found as an ingredient in bowel cleansing preparations.

Osmotic Laxatives

Examples: lactulose, macrogol, salt solutions

These agents are concentrated preparations of substances which are not absorbed from the intestines, creating an osmotic gradient between the contents of the tract and the walls of the tract. This osmotic gradient draws fluid into the intestinal contents and traps it there, expanding and softening faeces and stimulating peristalsis. **Lactulose** is a semisynthetic disaccharide which is converted in the colon to organic acids including lactic acid, acetic acid, and formic acid, as well as methane gas, which can cause flatulence. **Macrogols** are large-molecular-weight polymers of ethylene glycol and may be combined with magnesium or phosphate salts in bowel cleansing preparations or with a stimulant

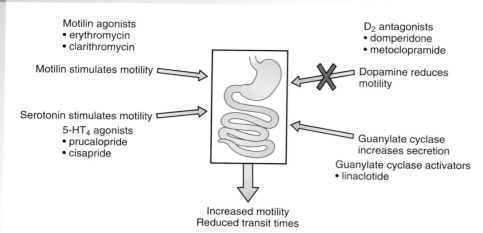

Motilin agonists
• erythromycin
• clarithromycin

Motilin stimulates motility

Serotonin stimulates motility

5-HT$_4$ agonists
• prucalopride
• cisapride

D$_2$ antagonists
• domperidone
• metoclopramide

Dopamine reduces
motility

Guanylate cyclase
increases secretion

Guanylate cyclase activators
• linaclotide

Increased motility
Reduced transit times

Fig. 10.11   The main mechanisms of action of pro-kinetic drugs.

laxative such as **sodium picosulfate.** Macrogol 3350 (3350 is the molecular weight) is taken orally and used both in constipation and to relieve faecal impaction, and can cause abdominal pain and flatulence.

OPIOID-RECEPTOR ANTAGONISTS

Examples: methylnaltrexone, naldemedine, naloxegol

Peripherally acting MOR antagonists are used to block MORs on enteric nerves to prevent **opioid**-related constipation, generally when standard laxatives are inadequate. The molecular structure of these drugs is based on the opioid reversal agent **naltrexone,** but they are chemically modified to reduce lipid solubility and increase electrical charge, which prevents them from crossing the blood-brain barrier and blocking the analgesic and other centrally mediated actions of opioids. **Methylnaltrexone** is given by injection, has a half-life of around 10 hours, and is excreted largely unchanged in the urine and faeces. **Naldemedine** and **naloxegel** are given orally and have half-lives in the order of 11 hours. Their most common side-effects are GI-related, including abdominal pain, nausea, vomiting, and diarrhoea.

PRO-KINETIC DRUGS

Pro-kinetic drugs increase the strength and frequency of GI smooth muscle contraction and shorten transit times (Fig. 10.11).

Dopamine Receptor Antagonists

Examples: domperidone, metoclopramide

In the biosynthetic pathway which produces adrenaline, dopamine is converted to noradrenaline, which in turn is converted to adrenaline (see Fig. 4.12). Dopamine released by enteric nerves has sympathetic activity of its own, and like adrenaline and noradrenaline, inhibits GI motility. The GI tract contains significant quantities of dopamine, which acts on D$_2$ receptors on the intestinal smooth muscle. D$_2$-receptor antagonists are widely used to increase oesophageal, gastric, and small intestinal motility, as well as being effective anti-emetics (see below for more detailed discussion of their pharmacology). They stimulate gastric emptying in conditions such as diabetic gastroparesis and gastroesophageal reflux, and may be used to hasten the movement of barium through the tract in a barium meal. In migraine, gastric emptying is significantly delayed, which contributes to the associated nausea and vomiting, and the use of a D$_2$ antagonist not only helps to relieve this but also speeds the passage of oral analgesia into the

duodenum for absorption. New D$_2$-receptor antagonists currently in clinical trials include **trazpiroben.**

Macrolide Antibiotics

Motilin is a hormone secreted by glandular cells mainly in the duodenum. It stimulates gastric and intestinal motility via action on motilin receptors on GI smooth muscle: it is most active in the stomach. The macrolide antibiotics, including **erythromycin**, **azithromycin**, and **clarithromycin**, act as motilin-receptor agonists at doses lower than required for their antibacterial action, although not all are used for this purpose and the use may be off-licence: for example, erythromycin is unlicensed for this indication in the UK but authorised in the US. Erythromycin is the standard agent used for this purpose but is limited to short spells of treatment (less than 4 weeks), because with continual exposure, motilin receptors are down-regulated, and the drug becomes much less effective. In addition, the use of these important antibiotics for non-infective conditions may contribute to the increasing of multi-drug-resistant microbes. Novel motilin agonists are in development.

Serotonin Receptor Agonists

Examples: prucalopride, tegaserod

Serotonin stimulates peristalsis and secretion in the GI tract via an action on 5-HT$_4$ receptors. **Prucalopride** is a 5-HT$_4$-receptor agonist used to treat constipation that has not responded to other treatments. It accelerates gastric emptying, stimulates peristalsis, and decreases transit time. It has a long half-life, of around 20 hours, and is mainly excreted unchanged by the kidney. It is well tolerated, but it can cause GI disturbances including loss of appetite, abdominal pain, nausea, and vomiting. Rarely, prucalopride can cause cardiovascular problems, because although the main serotonin-receptor subtype in the heart is the 5-HT$_2$ receptor, 5-HT$_4$ receptors are also present. Care should be taken in patients with known cardiovascular conditions, including arrhythmias or ischaemic heart disease. Other 5-HT$_4$ agonists which reached the market included **tegaserod** and **cisapride,** now withdrawn from most health systems worldwide because of cardiovascular side-effects.

Guanylate Cyclase-C Receptor Agonists

Example: linaclotide

Linaclotide is converted to its active metabolite within the GI tract. It is taken orally, is not absorbed, and exerts its effect from the gut lumen. The enzyme guanylate cyclase converts guanosine triphosphate (GTP) to cyclic guanosine monophosphate (cGMP), an important second messenger responsible for a wide range of cell signalling functions. In intestinal epithelial cells, one of its actions is to activate cystic fibrosis transmembrane conductance regulator (CFTR) channels, which secrete Cl⁻ and HCO_3^- into the tract (dysfunction of these CFTR channels is the pathophysiological abnormality in cystic fibrosis). Linaclotide is a guanylate-cyclase agonist and increases cGMP levels, which in turn increases the activity of CFTR channels in the intestinal cells (Fig. 10.12). This efflux of ions creates an osmotic gradient, and water is pulled from the intestinal cells into the lumen, expanding and softening the faeces and promoting its easy passage. It also has an inhibitory action on sensory nerves in the intestines, reducing transmission of pain signals to the brain. Linaclotide is used to treat constipation and pain in IBS. Side-effects are mainly GI-related and include flatulence, bloating, and diarrhoea.

Future Possibilities

Ghrelin is a hormone released by the stomach, which stimulates appetite and GI secretion and motility. **Relamorelin** is a ghrelin analogue that increases gastric emptying and is currently in advanced clinical trials for the treatment of diabetic gastroparesis.

ANTIEMETICS

Vomiting (emesis) is an important protective reflex to rapidly expel actually or potentially toxic substances from the stomach. Although the muscular propulsion that forcibly ejects material comes mainly from the stomach and muscles that compress the stomach, intestinal smooth muscle can also generate peristaltic contractions to reverse the normal direction of tract flow and return contents back towards the stomach. Nausea is the unpleasant sensation that vomiting is imminent, may or may not precede vomiting, and may occur with autonomic symptoms such as pallor, sweating, and dizziness.

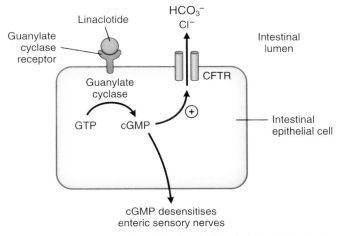

Fig. 10.12 The mechanism of action of linaclotide. CFTR, Cystic fibrosis transmembrane conductance regulator; cGMP, cyclic guanosine monophosphate; GTP, guanosine triphosphate.

THE PHYSIOLOGY OF VOMITING

The vomiting centre (VC) in the medulla oblongata is a loose collection of nerves which controls the vomiting reflex. It receives sensory impulses from a range of structures both within and outside of the CNS which can trigger emesis. Five main neurotransmitters are involved in the pathways feeding input to the VC, all of which offer potential targets for the action of anti-emetic drugs: **histamine**, acting on H_1 receptors; **ACh**, acting on muscarinic receptors; **dopamine**, acting on D_2 receptors; **serotonin** (5-HT), acting on $5-HT_3$ receptors; and **substance P,** acting on NK_1 receptors.

The key structures and their nerve pathways to the VC are shown on Fig. 10.13, which also shows the main neurotransmitters and the receptors involved with each pathway. The VC itself contains D_2, 5-HT, muscarinic, and H_1 receptors. Understanding the pathogenesis of vomiting is therefore essential for choosing the best anti-emetic in any given situation.

The Gastrointestinal Tract

Stretch receptors in the tract wall detect distension, like that caused by stasis in the tract or by obstruction, and send parasympathetic afferent impulses via the vagus nerve to the VC. Additionally, chemoreceptors in the tract respond to toxic or irritant substances: this releases 5-HT and substance P, which also activate vagal afferents to the VC. Vagal afferents from the GI tract also travel to the chemosensitive trigger zone (CTZ), which in turn sends input to the VC (Fig. 10.14). These pathways are at least in part responsible for vomiting caused by GI infection, obstruction, inflammation and radiotherapy. Drugs which irritate or inflame the GI tract, e.g. **NSAIDs** and some **cytotoxic agents,** can cause vomiting by this mechanism, as can drugs which inhibit GI motility and cause distension, e.g. **opioids**. The nausea, vomiting, and constipation associated with pregnancy is thought to be due to **progesterone**, which relaxes intestinal smooth muscle, delays gastric emptying, and reduces peristalsis.

Higher Centres

Unpleasant, frightening, or emotional situations may all trigger vomiting because the cortex, where these higher-order functions are housed, has input to the VC. Sights, smells, and memories may all induce vomiting. Pain can also be a powerful stimulant of vomiting. Raised intracranial pressure causes vomiting, although the reason for this is not clear.

The Chemosensitive Trigger Zone

This is a group of neurones in the floor of the fourth cerebral ventricle. They are exposed both to cerebrospinal fluid circulating within the ventricular system of the brain and to blood-borne substances, because the CTZ lies outwith the blood-brain barrier. This means that it detects potentially toxic substances both within the CNS and circulating in the bloodstream. There are receptors here for 5-HT, dopamine, substance P, and enkephalins. The CTZ may trigger vomiting in response to circulating toxins from GI and other infections, and to drugs including **digoxin**, **opioids**, **L-DOPA** (which is converted to dopamine, which acts directly on the D_2 receptors of the CTZ), the D_2 agonist **apomorphine,** and **cytotoxic agents**. In addition, disturbances of normal acid–base balance, electrolyte imbalances, and metabolic abnormalities, for example uraemia

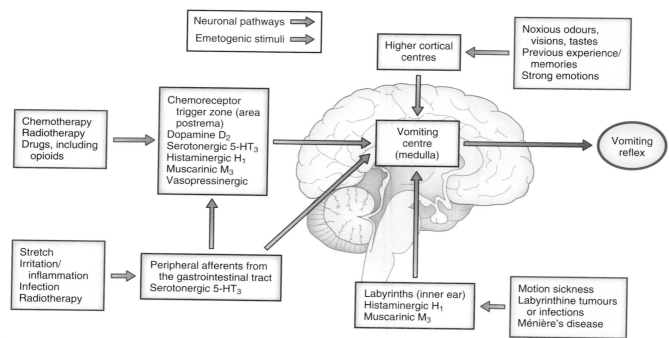

Fig. 10.13 The vomiting centre and key associated structures. (Modified from Quigley EM, Hasler WL, Parkman HP (2001) AGA technical review on nausea and vomiting. *Gastroenterology*, 120, 263–286.)

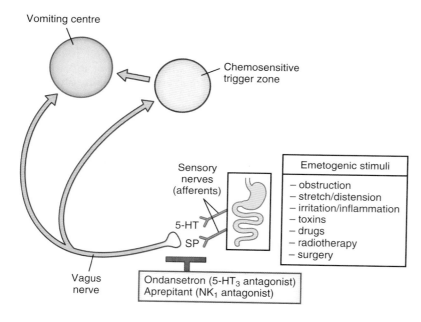

Fig. 10.14 Vomiting pathways between the gastro-intestinal tract, vomiting centre, and chemosensitive trigger zone. 5-HT, 5-hydroxytryptamine; NK, neurokinin; SP, substance P.

and diabetic ketoacidosis, directly stimulate the CTZ. Stimulation of the CTZ directly stimulates the VC (Fig. 10.14).

The Vestibular Nuclei

The four vestibular nuclei are collections of nerves in the brainstem which receive and integrate input from the balance mechanism of the middle ear, as well as from the eyes and proprioceptors in the musculoskeletal system. The two main neurotransmitters released here are histamine and ACh. Nausea and vomiting associated with motion sickness, vertigo, and middle ear infections are due to stimulation of the VC from the vestibular nuclei.

DOPAMINE ANTAGONISTS

Examples: domperidone, metoclopramide, phenothiazines

Dopamine, released in the VC and in the CTZ, is a powerful pro-emetic, and as described above has direct actions on the GI tract, decreasing motility and increasing transit time. Dopamine antagonists are therefore effective anti-emetics in a range of conditions including drug-, pregnancy-, and radiotherapy-induced vomiting and post-operative nausea and vomiting. However, because dopamine also has important functions in the nigrostriatal pathway and the regulation of voluntary muscle movement, dopamine antagonists that cross the blood-brain barrier can produce extrapyramidal movement disorders similar to those seen in Parkinson's disease (see also p. 53),

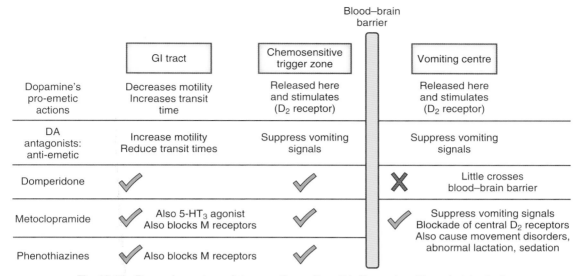

Fig. 10.15 Dopamine antagonists as anti-emetics. DA, Dopamine; GI, gastrointestinal.

and these drugs should be avoided in people with this disorder. Basal dopamine release in the tuberoinfundibular pathway suppresses prolactin production, and dopamine antagonists can therefore increase prolactin levels even in non-lactating people and cause galactorrhoea and gynaecomastia (Fig. 10.15).

Domperidone

Unlike other D_2 antagonists used to treat vomiting, domperidone does not readily cross the blood-brain barrier and so it is fairly free of central side-effects, including movement disorders and abnormal lactation, seen with the others in this group. It suppresses vomiting via its action on D_2 receptors in the CTZ; it also blocks D_2 receptors in the GI tract, which increases peristalsis and shortens gastric emptying times. For this reason, it is also used as a pro-kinetic agent in hypomotility disorders including GORD (see above). It is given orally and has a plasma half-life of around 7 hours.

Metoclopramide

Metoclopramide is related to the phenothiazines but is not used as an antipsychotic agent. It does, however, cross the blood-brain barrier, so extrapyramidal movement disorders and abnormal lactation are seen in its adverse effects profile. Its main action is via blockade of D_2 receptors, both in the CTZ and peripherally in the GI tract, but it also stimulates $5-HT_4$ receptors and blocks muscarinic receptors in the intestines, which aids motility and speeds up transit times. It is given orally or by injection, is well absorbed, and has a plasma half-life of around 5 hours, which is increased if kidney function is impaired. Intranasal preparations are available in some countries.

Phenothiazine Antipsychotic Drugs

Examples: chlorpromazine, droperidol, levomepromazine, prochlorperazine

Phenothiazines are used as D_2-receptor antagonists in the treatment of psychotic disorders (p. 64), but they are effective anti-emetics at much lower doses (around a third) of those used in psychiatry. They block D_2 receptors in the CTZ, but they also have antimuscarinic and antihistamine activity (antihistamines and phenothiazines are structurally

related). They are useful in controlling vomiting caused by most stimuli, including vestibular disorders because of their antihistamine activity. However, even at anti-emetic doses, adverse effects are common, including parkinsonian symptoms, sedation, abnormal lactation, and gynaecomastia.

5-HT₃ ANTAGONISTS

Examples: granisetron, ondansetron, palonosetron

$5-HT_3$ receptors are found in the GI tract and in the CTZ. $5-HT_3$ antagonists are used in post-operative nausea and vomiting, hyperemesis gravidarum, and drug-induced vomiting including with chemotherapy. The first $5-HT_3$-receptor antagonist developed as an anti-emetic, **ondansetron**, came on the market in the mid-1980s. It is given orally, rectally, or by intravenous or intramuscular injection and has a plasma half-life of 3 hours. **Palonosetron** has a longer half-life of up to 40 hours. Unlike antihistamines and phenothiazines, these drugs are non-sedating and are generally well tolerated; common side-effects include headache and constipation, the latter due to blockade of $5-HT_3$ receptors in the GI tract (Fig. 10.14). Rarely, they may cause arrhythmias including QT interval prolongation.

NEUROKININ-RECEPTOR ANTAGONISTS

Examples: aprepitant, fosaprepitant, netupitant (used in combination with palonosetron)

These drugs are anti-emetic because they block binding of substance P on NK_1 receptors in the GI tract (Fig. 10.14), VC, and CTZ, inhibiting input into and activation of the VC. They are used mainly to manage chemotherapy-induced vomiting and in some countries are also licensed for post-operative nausea and vomiting. **Fosaprepitant** is given intravenously and is converted to **aprepitant** in the liver; aprepitant has a half-life of 9–13 hours.

In addition to their anti-emetic action in blocking NK_1 receptors, neurokinin-receptor antagonists enhance the anti-emetic effect of $5-HT_3$ antagonists. **Netupitant** has a long half-life (around 90 hours) and is used in combination with the $5-HT_3$ antagonist **palonosetron** to treat chemotherapy-induced nausea and vomiting (CINV), particularly with regimens that include **cisplatin**, which is highly emetogenic. The acute phase of CINV in the hours immediately following administration of the cytotoxic drug is thought to be mainly due to 5-HT release in the GI tract, so both drugs contribute therapeutically at this time. The delayed phase of CINV, which manifests 25–120 hours after cytotoxic treatment, is thought to be mainly due to substance P acting on NK_1 receptors, and netupitant blocks this.

Adverse effects of these drugs include appetite suppression, constipation, and abdominal discomfort.

ANTIHISTAMINES

Examples: cinnarizine, cyclizine, doxylamine, promethazine

The most familiar use of antihistamines is in allergy (p. 122). The older antihistamines, the so-called first-generation agents, have significant antimuscarinic properties and cross the blood-brain barrier. They block H_1 and muscarinic receptors in the vestibular nuclei and muscarinic receptors in the VC itself. They relieve vomiting from most causes, although they are particularly helpful in preventing and treating nausea and vomiting associated with motion sickness and middle ear disorders such as Ménière's disease. The newer second- and third-generation antihistamines do not cross the blood-brain barrier and do not prevent or relieve motion sickness. When treating motion sickness, antihistamines are more effective as preventive treatment, taken in advance, than stopping established nausea and vomiting. **Cyclizine** is also used in palliative care, especially to counteract opioid-induced vomiting. It has a half-life of 20 hours.

Antihistamine anti-emetics block muscarinic receptors throughout the body and cause a range of antimuscarinic side-effects, including dry mouth, tachycardia, closed-angle glaucoma, and blurred vision. Sedation is a significant side-effect because histamine is also an important transmitter in central pathways that maintain daytime alertness (see also p. 124). Advice should always be given regarding likely drowsiness, e.g. avoiding driving and cycling; alcohol should be avoided because it enhances sedation.

ANTIMUSCARINIC AGENTS

Examples: hyoscine hydrobromide

Drugs with central antimuscarinic activity are anti-emetic because ACh stimulates vomiting via an action on muscarinic receptors in the VC and the vestibular nuclei. As discussed above, phenothiazines and first-generation antihistamines owe at least some of their anti-emetic activity to their ability to block muscarinic receptors in vomiting pathways. **Hyoscine** (scopolamine) and the closely related drug **atropine** are found in a range of poisonous plants including deadly nightshade and henbane. Hyoscine was first isolated in 1880; it is highly lipid-soluble, crosses the blood-brain barrier, and is a potent CNS depressant. Two formulations are currently in use, the main difference between them being their lipid solubility and therefore their ability to cross the BBB (see also **hyoscine butylbromide** above). **Hyoscine hydrobromide** is used as an anti-emetic because it crosses the blood-brain barrier and blocks muscarinic receptors in central vomiting pathways. Other central antimuscarinic side-effects include sedation, which may be beneficial in certain circumstances: for example, in the treatment of motion sickness in children,

in pre-medication, and in reducing respiratory secretions in palliative care. Peripheral antimuscarinic side-effects include dry mouth, urinary retention, and blurred vision. Its plasma half-life is around an hour, although this is extended if the drug is given subcutaneously or by transdermal patch.

NABILONE

Nabilone is a synthetic cannabinoid closely related to **tetrahydrocannabinol**, the main psychoactive substance in cannabis. Both the peripheral and central nervous systems possess cannabinoid receptors and several endogenous substances, collectively called the **endocannabinoids**, have been identified. This is a relatively new area of study, but the known functions of endocannabinoids relate to anti-inflammatory activity and modulation of pain. It is not certain why nabilone has anti-emetic activity, but it may inhibit 5-HT release in the VC. It is well absorbed orally and has a plasma half-life of around 2 hours. It is used to relieve CINV when standard anti-emetics have not been effective. Adverse effects include sedation, confusion, sleep disruption, psychotic symptoms, and GI upsets.

OTHER DRUGS WITH ANTI-EMETIC ACTIVITY

Dexamethasone is a synthetic glucocorticoid used mainly as an anti-inflammatory agent, but its anti-emetic properties are useful in a range of conditions including palliative care and cancer treatment, and when combined with other anti-emetics, it enhances their effectiveness. The glucocorticoids have such a wide range of physiological actions that their principal mechanism of action in preventing and alleviating nausea and vomiting has not been identified, although they may act through inhibiting the action of endogenous opioids or via inhibition of 5-HT. **Benzodiazepines** have no inherent anti-emetic activity of their own, but some drugs in this group, e.g. **lorazepam,** are sometimes used as adjuvants in chemotherapy-induced and post-operative nausea and vomiting, and in acute attacks of vertigo. They reduce the incidence and severity of nausea and vomiting and can reduce the requirement for anti-emetic treatment. Their beneficial action is believed to relate to their anxiolytic and calming effects. **Ginger** has been used for centuries in folk medicines for the relief of nausea and vomiting, including in pregnancy. There is evidence that, similar to the setron drugs such as **ondansetron**, ginger blocks $5-HT_3$ receptors, which would account for its anti-emetic action. Ginger and the setron drugs bind to different sites on the $5-HT_3$ receptor rather than competing for the same site, and there is evidence that ginger's action is additive when used with standard anti-emetic drugs in post-operative nausea and vomiting.

REFERENCES

Abrahami, D., McDonald, E.G., Schnitzer, M.E., et al., 2022. Proton pump inhibitors and risk of gastric cancer: population-based cohort study. Gut. 71 (1), 16–24.
Camilleri, M., Atieh, J., 2021. New developments in prokinetic therapy for gastric motility disorders. Front. Pharmacol. 12, 711500 art. no.
Denholm, D., Gallagher, G., 2021. Physiology and pharmacology of nausea and vomiting. Anaesth. Intensive Care Med. 22 (10), 663–666.
Ogawa, R., Echizen, H., 2011. Clinically significant drug interactions with antacids. Drugs 71 (14), 1839–1864.
Strand, D.S., Kim, D., Peura, D., 2017. 25 years of proton pump inhibitors: a comprehensive review. Gut. Liver. 11 (1), 27–37.

Antimicrobial Drugs

11

THE BIOLOGY OF MICROBES

The first living organisms on Earth were bacteria, appearing more than 3.8 billion years ago, and viruses probably evolved shortly afterwards. All life on Earth evolved from these ancient bacteria. The world in which the earliest human beings first appeared about 300,000 years ago already contained an enormous range of microbes, and throughout its existence, mankind has had to co-exist with, and defend itself against, these tiny organisms. Most microbes co-exist peacefully with humankind, and some are actively beneficial, including those used in producing wine, beer, or cheese and the bacteria in our digestive tract that synthesise vitamins, which we absorb and use. The industrial culture of microbes for the manufacture of biologically active substances, including drugs, is an expanding area of technology.

THE HISTORY OF MICROBIOLOGY

Infection, the growth and multiplication of micro-organisms within living cells and tissues of another organism, has been a major cause of death and disability throughout human history. Although the biology of micro-organisms could not begin to be understood until they were first viewed under the earliest microscopes in the mid-17th century, there is clear evidence dating back to earliest recorded human civilisation of people trying to prevent, treat, and control infection. With no basis in scientific fact, many practices were either useless or downright dangerous: bloodletting was recommended for pneumonia as late as the 1940s, and for hundreds of years from the 14th century on, syphilitic infections were treated with highly toxic mercury. Bubonic plague has caused regular epidemics globally over the past 1000 years and was much feared because of its sudden onset and very high death rate. Until the advent of antibiotics, doctors were powerless; common and entirely useless treatments included drinking vinegar or eating treacle, and topical application of onion or chopped-up snakes or pigeons. The causative organism of plague, *Yersinia pestis*, has been identified, and provided treatment is started early enough, the disease is usually curable.

Some practices could have been genuinely useful, although the practitioners did not understand why. The ancient Egyptians dressed wounds with mouldy bread; the idea that fungi and other micro-organisms protect themselves by releasing substances that kill other micro-organisms is very familiar to us today, and in fact the term 'antibiotic' in its original definition means an antimicrobial agent derived from another micro-organism. Honey was used in ancient Sumeria from 2000 BC to treat wounds. Honey contains antimicrobial substances, and its high sugar content gives it a very high osmolarity, which pulls water from microbial cells, dehydrating and killing them. Plant extracts were also used: cinchona bark was used as a treatment for malaria, even though **quinine,** its active principle, had not been identified.

The existence of invisible agents of infection was predicted in 1546 by an Italian doctor, Hieronymus Frascatorius, who correctly deduced that transmission of tiny particles between people accounted for the spread of infection. Proof of the presence of these agents did not come for more than a century, until people began to use magnifying lenses built into simple microscopes to examine objects from the natural world. Pioneers of early microscopy included Robert Hooke (1635–1703) and Antonie van Leeuwenhoek (1632–1723). Their lenses were crude but remarkably effective. Hooke made beautiful and detailed drawings of a range of biological specimens, including insects, plants, and fungi, and van Leeuwenhoek, working a few years later, extended and expanded the newly discovered microscopic world,

writing extensive and detailed descriptions of his own observations. Van Leeuwenhoek is credited with the discovery of bacteria; he put a drop of water mixed with pepper on his microscope stage because he was interested in what gave pepper its fiery taste and was amazed to see huge numbers of several different types of 'animalcules'. He examined a wide range of materials, including blood, sputum, and material scraped from his own teeth, finding these tiny creatures in huge numbers in almost every medium he studied; they were clearly alive because he could see them 'swimming' and 'playing'. By the middle of the 19th century, despite progressive development of the scientific process, rational and evidence-based thinking, and recognition of the importance of observation and accurate experimentation, the link between micro-organisms and human disease had not yet been proven. Additionally, many scientists believed that micro-organisms arose spontaneously in dead and dying tissues rather than having been transmitted in some way.

Several important reports that helped to establish the principles of transmissibility of infection appeared around this time. One key figure, Ignaz Semmelweiss (Fig. 11.1), saved countless newly delivered mothers from the dreaded childbed fever. The physical trauma associated with childbirth has always carried increased risk of infection, and in the mid-1840s, 1 in 10 women died of post-natal infection, also called childbed or puerperal fever. Semmelweiss, working in Vienna, noticed that women delivering in midwife-led units were 10 times less likely to die than women delivering in units led by obstetricians and medical students. He linked this to transmission of 'putrid matter' carried on their hands from autopsy rooms to the wards, and when he implemented a policy requiring handwashing before patient contact,

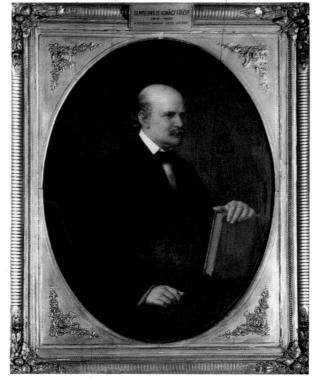

Fig. 11.1   Dr. Ignaz Philipp Semmelweiss (1818–1865), pioneer of antisepsis. (From Gloviczki P (2014) The best vascular care for every patient, every day. *Journal of Vascular Surgery*, 59 (3), pp. 843-856.)

death rates fell dramatically. Louis Pasteur (1822–1895) showed very clearly that microbial growth does not occur in sterilised materials sealed inside sterilised containers, convincingly disproving the theory of spontaneous generation; pasteurisation of foodstuffs is now used worldwide to minimise microbial contamination and extend their shelf-life. The science of microbiology, by now on a firm footing, expanded rapidly from the 1850s onwards, driven by work done by notable scientists such as Robert Koch, whose significant contributions included identification in 1822 of *Mycobacterium tuberculosis* as the organism responsible for tuberculosis (TB), and isolating and growing it in pure cultures. Joseph Lister, an Edinburgh surgeon, began to use antiseptics in handwashing and in the cleaning of surgical instruments and materials, resulting in significant reduction in the rates of post-operative infection in his patients.

Isolation, visualisation (with microscopes), and study of bacteria, protozoa, and fungi formed the basis of early microbiological knowledge, but viruses, being much smaller, were impossible to detect directly using technology available at the end of the 19th century. However, their existence was deduced indirectly when it was shown in 1892 that extracts of diseased leaves from tobacco plants caused the same disease in healthy plants, even after being passed through filters known to stop the passage of bacteria. Direct viewing of viral particles had to wait until the development of the electron microscope in 1931, which gave significantly higher magnification than the standard light microscope. Fittingly, the first virus to be seen under the electron microscope was the tobacco mosaic virus, the same virus whose existence was indirectly demonstrated in the 1892 filter experiments (Fig. 11.2).

MICROBIAL ADAPTABILITY

Microbes are the most varied and adaptable forms of life on Earth. Underlying their evolutionary success throughout their billions of years of existence is their seemingly inexhaustible ability to constantly adapt to changing environments. They survive and flourish in the face of a wide range of intensely hostile conditions: in ice, around volcanic craters, deep in the ocean, and in deserts. Some bacteria are even resistant to radiation and survive for years in the inhospitable environment

of space. Despite reproducing asexually, i.e. each new daughter cell in theory should be an exact copy of the parent cell, microbes constantly mutate and evolve, sometimes through random genetic mutations, sometimes through errors in copying genetic material during cell division, and sometimes in response to changing environmental conditions. The ability of microbes to produce and survive quite significant degrees of genetic mutation means that often not all microbes in a colony of apparently identical microbes are genetically identical. This gives the colony, as a whole, a survival advantage. If a mutation in a microbe's genetic material improves its ability to survive and reproduce in its current environment or in changing environmental conditions, it is more likely than its less well-equipped neighbours to divide and proliferate, passing its beneficial mutation to its daughter cells. In this way, if a colony is exposed to a toxin or other stressor, susceptible microbes will perish, but better adapted ones survive to generate a new colony capable of thriving in their new environment (Fig. 11.3). This adaptability is the basis for the development of antimicrobial drug resistance.

Antimicrobial Drug Resistance

The ability of microbes to rapidly adapt to changing environmental conditions presents major problems in treatment of infections. In response to exposure to an antimicrobial agent, microbes can quickly develop mechanisms to protect themselves from the drug. A microbe not killed or not prevented from dividing by an antimicrobial drug is said to be resistant to that drug. Strains of microbes, particularly bacteria, that have developed multi-drug resistance cause infections that cannot be effectively treated, a problem of global proportions identified in 2019 by the World Health Organisation as one of the top 10 public health threats facing humanity. Without effective antimicrobial drugs, common infections cannot be treated, a potential problem for even healthy individuals but particularly for the vulnerable, e.g. the very young or older people. The risks associated with post-operative infections are significantly magnified, and even trivial procedures can become life-threatening. The dangers of childbirth increase, and prevention and treatment of infection in immunocompromised people, i.e. in cancer patients and in those receiving organ transplant, may become almost impossible. Although the challenge presented by antimicrobial resistance threatens all populations on Earth, impoverished countries with underfunded healthcare systems, poor sanitation, lack of access to clean water, and unhygienic living conditions are particularly vulnerable. Specific mechanisms by which each type of microbe develops drug resistance are explained below.

Antimicrobial Stewardship

From the first half of the 20th century, clinical medicine has had access to an expanding range of effective antimicrobial drugs, leading to a steady increase in global use. The bulk of antimicrobial use, however, is not in human medicine, but in plant agriculture, animal husbandry, food production, veterinary medicine, and a range of industrial applications, and significant quantities of these drugs are washed into the natural environment, including soil and water. This has led to widespread microbial exposure to antimicrobial drugs, contributing to the consequent widespread emergence of multiple resistant strains. This phenomenon was recognised relatively quickly in the antimicrobial era, with warnings in the literature as early as the 1950s that antibiotic efficacy

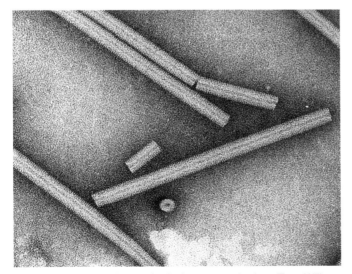

Fig. 11.2 Electron micrograph of tobacco mosaic virus. (From Williams RC and Fisher HW (1974) An electron micrographic atlas of viruses. Charles C. Thomas, Springfield, Il, with permission.)

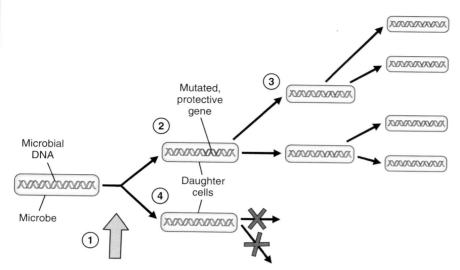

Fig. 11.3   Genetic mutations can give microbes a survival advantage in changing environmental conditions. 1. A microbe is exposed to an environmental stressor, e.g. a natural toxin or an antimicrobial drug. 2. One daughter cell develops or acquires a mutated gene that protects against the stressor. 3. Daughter cells produced from this line inherit the protective gene and are more likely to survive and proliferate, producing a colony with a selective survival advantage. 4. Daughter cells lacking the mutated protective gene are much less likely to survive.

was at serious risk. However, optimism that the continual production of new drugs would offset the issue, as well as resistance from agriculture and industry to any regulation of antibiotic use, has meant that the worldwide approach required to tackle the issue has been slow and piecemeal.

Much antimicrobial use, including prescribing in human medicine, is generally accepted as inappropriate, unnecessary, and indiscriminate, and global agreements and targets for limiting it have been put in place. Rational and directed use of antimicrobials is called antimicrobial stewardship, which at the most fundamental level means that every dose of an antimicrobial drug should be justified: the right antimicrobial at the right dose by the correct route for the shortest time necessary. This approach, provided it is followed across an entire organisation or healthcare system, should reduce overall antimicrobial consumption, ensure that those antimicrobials that are used are likely to be effective, and reduce the emergence of resistant strains.

ANTIMICROBIAL DRUGS AND SELECTIVE TOXICITY

Antimicrobial drugs are inherently cytotoxic: they are used with the intention of killing or fatally disabling the target microbe. The potential for host cell damage is high, and avoiding or minimising damage to healthy cells is an integral consideration when developing and using antimicrobials. The principle of selective toxicity depends on identifying a biochemical process or structural feature present in the microbe but not in human cells and finding or designing a drug that targets it. This should maximise microbial toxicity while limiting damage to host cells. It is a significant challenge, however, reflected in the limited number of new antimicrobials that have come to market in the past 30 years.

ANTIBACTERIAL DRUGS

There are more antibacterial drugs in clinical use than any other category of antimicrobial agents, because bacterial cells are sufficiently different in structure and function to human cells to offer a range of potential drug targets. The term 'antibiotic' is used throughout this section to mean any antibacterial drug, natural or synthetic, used to treat bacterial infections.

Although the definitions above are straightforward, the action of individual drugs can be either bactericidal or bacteriostatic depending on drug dose, bacterial numbers, and how favourable the growth medium is; most antibiotics can be either, depending on the conditions. Clearing an infection is the result of a combined action of effective antibacterial treatment and the efforts of the host's own immune system; therefore, treating infections in immunocompromised people is often harder than in individuals with functional immunity. For this reason, bactericidal antibiotics may be preferred if the patient has weakened immunity.

The Biology of Bacteria

Fig. 11.4 illustrates the key features of bacterial cells targeted by some important antibiotics.

The Cell Wall and Cell Membrane

Bacteria possess a phospholipid cell membrane, similar in many respects to the human cell membrane, and which is too fragile to protect the cell from its external environment. Overlying the membrane and forming the outer coating of the cell is a rigid and robust cell wall. An intact cell wall is essential for bacterial survival. Cell walls are not found in human cells, and because they are made largely of peptidoglycans, molecules not found in human biology, they offer an excellent selective target for antimicrobial drugs: the **penicillins** and **cephalosporins**, among others, are lethal to bacteria because they disrupt the cell wall. Peptidoglycan is formed of long, chain-like molecules which extensively cross-link, giving the cell wall its strength. The cell wall varies in thickness and composition between types of bacteria, which in turn alters the stains they take up in the laboratory. Thick, peptidoglycan-rich cell walls take up crystal violet dye, staining the bacterium deep

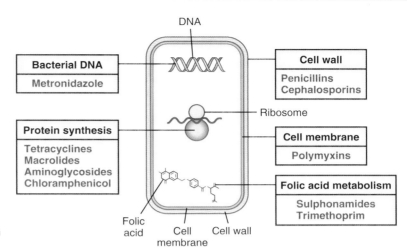

Fig. 11.4 The main antibacterial drug targets, with examples of drugs that attack each.

blue when seen under the microscope. These organisms are said to be Gram-positive, after the scientist who first made the observation (Fig. 11.5A). The Gram stain is one of the most important laboratory techniques used to identify the causative bacteria in infections. Gram-positive organisms include all staphylococci and all streptococci. Gram-negative organisms do not retain the stain because they have much less peptidoglycan and much thinner cell walls. However, because their cell wall is so thin, they also have a complex lipid-rich outer membrane lying over it to protect it. This outer membrane contains several pathologically important molecules, including endotoxin (lipopolysaccharide, LPS) which stimulates host cell defence responses (Fig. 11.5B). **Polymyxins** bind to the LPS component of Gram-negative outer cell membranes, disrupting membrane structure and increasing permeability. Antibiotic resistance is more widespread in Gram-negative organisms because the complex outer membrane contains a range of pumps, pores, and enzymes which can rapidly adapt to exclude or destroy drugs in its local environment.

KEY DEFINITIONS

- Broad-spectrum antibiotics are effective against a range of both Gram-positive and Gram-negative bacteria. Narrow-spectrum antibiotics are effective only against one type or the other.

Bacterial DNA and Protein Synthesis

The cytoplasm contains a range of specialised structures, including ribosomes for protein synthesis. Human cells also synthesise proteins on ribosomes, but bacterial ribosomes are smaller, providing a target for protein synthesis inhibitors including the **tetracyclines** and **chloramphenicol**. Bacterial cells do not contain a nucleus, i.e. they are prokaryotic, and their DNA is present as a single long strand rather than separate chromosomes. Bacterial enzymes involved in DNA replication or in transcription may be sufficiently different from their human equivalent to be drug targets: for example, **metronidazole** inhibits replication of bacterial DNA.

Bacterial Metabolism

Like human cells, bacteria contain thousands of different enzymes to catalyse the wide range of biochemical reactions required for life. Although microbial and human biochemistry share similar pathways, it is possible to find metabolic processes present in bacterial cells but not in human cells, including their handling of folic acid. **Trimethoprim** and the **sulphonamides** are examples of antibiotics that interfere with folic acid metabolism.

ANTIBACTERIAL RESISTANCE

If a population of bacteria is exposed to an antibiotic, all susceptible cells will die, but resistant cells will proliferate, so that eventually all bacteria in the population will be resistant to that drug. Broad-spectrum antibiotic use induces the development of resistance more effectively than narrow-spectrum antibiotics because it affects a wider range of bacteria. Some bacteria develop resistance more readily than others: for example, *Staphylococcus aureus*, a common bacterium often found living harmlessly on skin and mucous membranes, but which causes a range of skin, wound, and other tissue infections, rapidly develops resistance to nearly all known families of antibiotics. Methicillin-resistant *S. aureus* (MRSA) infections are a major global problem, particularly in healthcare settings and in vulnerable people, e.g. the very old and the very young. Bacteria can develop or acquire protective genes against a drug, i.e. develop resistance to that drug, in a range of ways. Once the bacterium possesses one or more genes that protect it against a drug, it copies them, and in the ways described below, the gene(s) can be spread through a rapidly dividing bacterial population in a matter of hours (Fig. 11.6).

Transfer of Protective Genes From One Bacterium to Another

Bacteria can pass protective genes between themselves in a process called conjugation (Fig. 11.7A). These genes are usually found on DNA fragments called plasmids, which the bacteria copy and transfer into adjacent bacteria through a connecting tube called a pilus (Fig. 11.7B). Plasmids can carry multiple resistance genes, giving resistance to more than one drug, and are therefore a very important mechanism for spreading drug resistance in a colony. In addition, bacteria can pick up plasmids released when bacteria die and lyse.

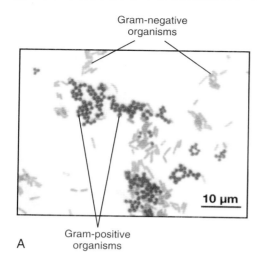

A

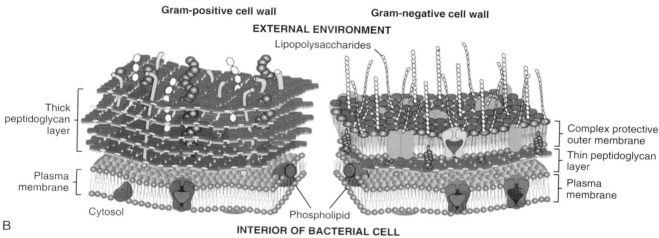

B

Fig. 11.5   Gram-positive and Gram-negative organisms. A. Mixed bacterial culture showing both Gram-positive and Gram-negative bacteria. B. The structure of the cell wall and associated membranes in Gram-positive and Gram-negative bacteria. (Modified from (A) Lo KK-W (2017) Inorganic and organometallic transition metal complexes with biological molecules and living cells, Fig. 7.2. St. Louis: Academic Press and (B) Tripathi P, Beaussart A, Andre G, et al. (2012) Towards a nanoscale view of lactic acid bacteria. *Micron*, 48, (12), pp. 1323–1330.)

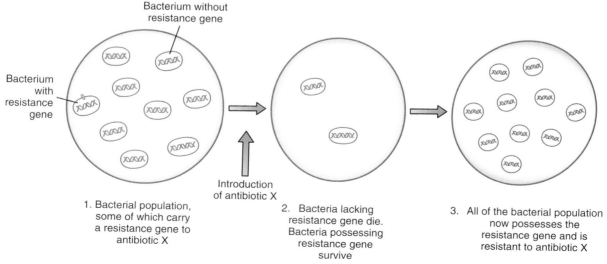

Fig. 11.6   Emergence of drug-resistant bacterial populations.

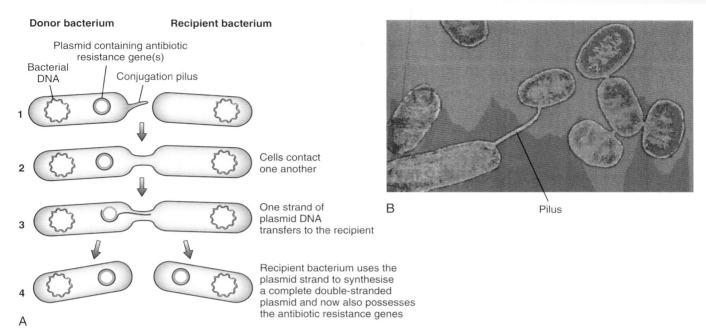

Donor bacterium   **Recipient bacterium**

Plasmid containing antibiotic
resistance gene(s)

Bacterial
DNA
Conjugation pilus

1

2   Cells contact
one another

3   One strand of
plasmid DNA
transfers to the recipient

B   Pilus

4   Recipient bacterium uses the
plasmid strand to synthesise
a complete double-stranded
plasmid and now also possesses
the antibiotic resistance genes

A

Fig. 11.7   Bacterial conjugation. A. Bacteria can pass genes that give antibiotic resistance to each other, spreading resistance in a population. B. False-coloured micrograph of bacteria, showing pilus bridges between the large bacterium (bottom left) and its neighbour, and the bacterium (middle right) and three of its neighbours. (Modified from (A) VanMeter KC, Hubert RJ, and VanMeter WG (2010) Microbiology for the healthcare professional, Fig. 25.2. St. Louis: Mosby and (B) Fitzgerald-Hayes M and Reichsman F (2010) DNA and biotechnology, 3rd ed, Fig. 4.6. San Diego: Academic Press.)

Spontaneous Mutation

As mentioned before, bacteria are genetically unstable: that is, unlike human cells, which have rapid and robust mechanisms for eliminating errors from their genetic material, they tolerate significant mutations in their DNA. The mutations are random, but because bacteria replicate so fast, they occur very frequently. Some will be beneficial and will appear in all cells descending from the original (Fig. 11.3).

Mechanisms of Drug Resistance

Resistance genes can protect the bacterium against the drug in one of four main ways.

The Gene May Code for an Enzyme That Breaks Down the Drug

For example, when exposed to **penicillin**, bacteria with the gene that produces β-lactamase survive because β-lactamase destroys the penicillin molecule.

The Gene May Change the Cell-Surface Receptor That Allows the Drug to Bind to the Bacterium

For example, when exposed to **penicillin**, bacteria that do not make penicillin-binding receptors survive, because penicillin cannot latch onto the bacterial cell surface and penetrate it.

The Gene May Increase the Bacterium's Ability to Excrete the Drug

For example, bacteria that produce pumps to excrete a drug survive, because they can keep the drug levels in their cytoplasm too low to cause damage. *Pseudomonas aeruginosa*, a microbe responsible for a wide range of clinically important infections and which readily evolves into multi-drug resistance strains, quickly generates efflux pumps to clear antibiotics from their internal environment.

The Gene May Change the Permeability of the Bacterial Cell Wall, Blocking Drug Entry

For example, structural changes to pores in the bacterial cell membrane can allow the bacterium to exclude particular drugs: this is a common mechanism and accounts for resistance to a wide range of bacteria.

COMBINATION THERAPY

Using more than one antibiotic simultaneously (combination therapy) can be advantageous in two main ways (Fig. 11.8).

Prevention of the Emergence of Drug-Resistant Bacteria

Combination therapy is used in hard-to-treat, serious, and chronic infections such as TB, or to eradicate gastric *Helicobacter pylori* infection, which is strongly associated with peptic ulcer disease (p. 188). It is also used in immunocompromised or vulnerable individuals, whose own defence mechanisms are unable to contribute significantly to clearing the infection. The principle is that by using more than one drug, a larger proportion of bacteria are cleared as fast as possible at the beginning of treatment, increasing the chances that the host immune system can eradicate the remainder (Fig. 11.8A). There are however risks to this approach, including the increased incidence of side-effects from multiple drugs, and the likelihood that if treatment is not successful and the infection is not cleared, surviving organisms will be multi-drug resistant.

Antibiotic Synergism

In some situations, antibiotics work synergistically, and their combined antibacterial effect is greater than the sum of their individual action. Fig. 11.8B shows a hypothetical

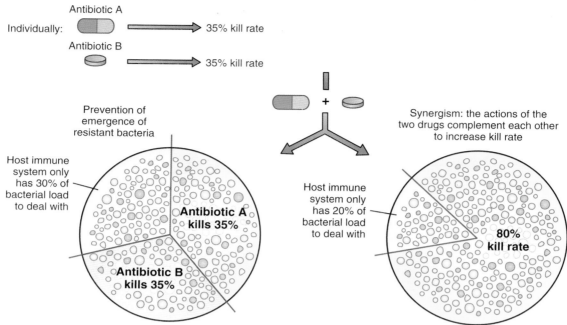

Fig. 11.8   The value of combination therapy in treatment of complex or chronic infections.

example, where antibiotics A and B individually have a 35% kill rate for a particular infection, but because of synergism, when combined, their total kill rate is 80%. For example, **trimethoprim** and the **sulphonamides** work synergistically because although they both interfere with bacterial folate use, they inhibit different steps in the biochemical pathway. **Ampicillin** and **gentamicin** work synergistically when treating enterococcal infections, e.g. infective endocarditis, because ampicillin increases bacterial uptake of gentamicin (although this synergy does not work for all aminoglycosides, such as **amikacin**).

GENERAL ADVERSE EFFECTS OF ANTIBIOTIC TREATMENT

Some adverse effects of antibiotic treatment are common to many antibiotics.

Superinfection

There are about the same number of bacteria living in or on the healthy individual as there are cells in the body: a huge number, running into the tens of trillions. The umbrella term given to these organisms is the human microbiome, and the importance to human health of this symbiotic relationship is becoming increasingly clear. One benefit of the healthy microbiome is that by colonising both internal and external body surfaces, they prevent other, potentially pathogenic organisms from establishing themselves. Introducing an antibiotic into the body, especially if broad-spectrum, kills not only the target pathogen, but also normal body flora, and can allow pathogens to colonise and proliferate. This is called super-infection. A common example is candidiasis (thrush), caused by the yeast *Candida albicans*.

Gastrointestinal Adverse Effects

These are common, affecting about 10% of people, and are more common in broad-spectrum therapy. They include diarrhoea, nausea, vomiting, abdominal bloating, and discomfort, and are believed to be due to loss of normal gut flora. There is probably more than one reason why eliminating

normal gut flora disturbs gastrointestinal (GI) function. Some superinfecting organisms (see above) probably have direct pathogenic activity in the tract. Antibiotic-associated colitis, sometimes called pseudomembranous colitis or *Clostridium difficile* colitis, is caused by overgrowth of *C. difficile*. The toxin produced by this organism causes severe inflammation and bleeding of the colon, with watery, profuse diarrhoea; bloody stool; and possible dehydration and electrolyte imbalance. In addition, the normal gut flora helps to digest large-molecular-weight carbohydrates, and if this is impaired because the normal gut organisms have been killed, the undigested carbohydrates have an osmotic effect, retaining water in the gut contents and contributing to watery diarrhoea. In addition, the normal microbiome helps to regulate GI motility: when it is lost, motility is increased.

Allergy

Allergies, often manifested as skin reactions, are common, especially with certain groups of drugs including the **penicillins** and **cephalosporins**. Many antibiotic-triggered allergies are due to a type I hypersensitivity reaction, with histamine release and rapid onset of symptoms, including itchy, raised blisters (urticaria). Other antibiotic-related allergies are due to a type IV (delayed type) hypersensitivity reaction and may not appear until up to 2 weeks after the antibiotic has been started, often after the course is finished. This is sometimes called post-antibiotic rash and is more common in children. The immunology of drug-related allergy is described in more detail on p. 37.

ANTIBIOTICS THAT INHIBIT PROTEIN SYNTHESIS

Proteins are composed of amino acids and are the fundamental building blocks of living cells. As in human biology, microbial DNA codes for the production of proteins needed for the bacterial cell to carry out all functions essential to life. The sections of functional code within the DNA—the genes—are used as templates to make molecules of messenger RNA (mRNA) in a process called transcription. Each mRNA molecule therefore carries the code for a specific protein, and travels into the cytoplasm and attaches to ribosomes within the bacterial cell, where its code is translated into the final protein. This is a complex, multi-stage process, and many protein synthesis inhibitors are currently used as antibacterials, each of which blocks the process at different steps (Fig. 11.9).

The Stages of Bacterial Protein Synthesis

The bacterial ribosome is composed of two protein units, a larger one (the 50S subunit) and the smaller one (the 30S subunit). The actual process of protein synthesis, by adding new amino acids to the growing protein chain, takes place on the 30S unit because this is where the mRNA and amino acid binding sites are. Protein synthesis is described in four stages (Fig. 11.9).

Initiation

In initiation (Fig. 11.9A), an mRNA molecule, containing the code for the new protein, binds to the 30S subunit so that its code can be read and a new protein molecule assembled. The first amino acid to be added is usually an N-formylmethionine residue and is called the initiating amino acid. This amino acid is not found in human proteins. It binds to what is called the P site. The next amino acid slots into an adjacent binding site, called the A site, and the two amino acids are joined together with a peptide bond (Fig. 11.9B and C).

Elongation

As soon as the two amino acids in the A and P sites are linked with a peptide bond, the ribosome slides along the mRNA molecule to the next coding section. The A site is now free for the next amino acid; a third amino acid is therefore added according to the mRNA code, joined to the second with a peptide bond, and the ribosome shifts along again. This is called elongation (Fig. 11.9D). The new protein emerges from the ribosome through an exit tunnel, pushed out as new amino acids are added via the A site. This proceeds until the ribosome has read the entire code along the mRNA molecule and the new protein is complete.

Termination

Once the ribosome has finished reading the mRNA code, the new protein is released. The mRNA itself, its job done, is degraded by enzymes in the cytoplasm.

KEY POINT: SELECTIVE TOXICITY OF PROTEIN SYNTHESIS INHIBITORS

Although the basic process of protein synthesis is the same in both human and bacterial cells and both have ribosomes for protein synthesis, bacterial ribosomes are smaller than human ones. This structural difference offers a selective target for the action of protein-inhibitor antibacterial drugs.

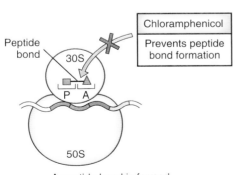

Initiation. Amino acid binds to the
A   P site, according to the mRNA code

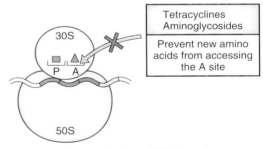

A second amino acid binds to the
B   adjacent A site, again according to the mRNA code

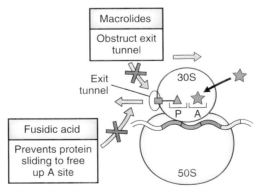

A peptide bond is formed
C   between the two amino acids

Elongation. The ribosome slides along the mRNA
to the next part of the code. The protein slides along
D   one slot, freeing up the A site for the next amino acid

Fig. 11.9   The stages of protein synthesis and examples of drugs that inhibit different steps.

AMINOGLYCOSIDES

Examples: streptomycin (the first), gentamicin, tobramycin, neomycin, amikacin

Streptomycin was isolated in 1944 from the soil bacterium *Actinomyces griseus*. Its use now is almost exclusively in TB treatment, and **gentamicin** is the most frequently used aminoglycoside. Aminoglycosides bind irreversibly to the 30S ribosomal subunit, preventing new amino acids from accessing the A binding site (Fig. 11.9B). The new protein is forced to terminate while only partially complete and is therefore non-functional. Anaerobic organisms are not susceptible to aminoglycoside action because the uptake mechanism needed to absorb the drug into the microbe is oxygen-dependent and not present in anaerobes. They are broad-spectrum agents, with higher activity against Gram-positive than Gram-negative organisms, and are usually reserved for serious infections such as sepsis because they have highly unpleasant side-effects.

Pharmacokinetics

Aminoglycosides are large, highly charged molecules and so are not absorbed across the wall of the GI tract; they are usually given by intravenous or intramuscular injection. **Tobramycin** is also available for nebulisation in respiratory infections. **Neomycin** is too toxic for systemic use, but it is used for topical infections; because it is not absorbed, it is given orally to sterilise the GI tract before surgery. Aminoglycosides have relatively short half-lives of 2–3 hours and cross the placenta but not the blood–brain barrier. They are not metabolised, mainly because they are too large and electrically charged to enter liver cells, so their clearance depends largely upon renal excretion. Active drug can accumulate very quickly in the renal tubules if kidney function is impaired, and renotoxicity is one of these drugs' most dangerous side-effects.

Adverse Effects

Aminoglycosides have significant side-effects, which are generally dose-related, and therapeutic drug monitoring is recommended to guide dosing. Renal toxicity is described above, and kidney function must be monitored and the drug stopped at the first sign of impairment. Ototoxicity, leading to permanent hearing loss, occurs in up to one-third of patients. The drugs accumulate in the fluids in the cochlea of the inner ear, where they may persist for extended periods of time and permanently damage the sensitive hair cells responsible for hearing. High-pitched sounds are lost first, and progressive hearing impairment can occur over several months following drug administration because of the slow clearance from inner ear fluids. **Neomycin** is particularly toxic to the hearing apparatus of the inner ear and so is not used systemically. There may also be toxicity to the vestibular system, causing dizziness and problems with balance. **Gentamicin** and **streptomycin** are more vestibulotoxic than cochleotoxic. Aminoglycosides should not be used in myasthenia gravis, and care should be taken with neuromuscular blockade in surgery, because they block acetylcholine release at the neuromuscular junction and can cause paralysis, including of the respiratory muscles.

CHLORAMPHENICOL

Chloramphenicol was isolated in 1947 from the bacterium *Streptomyces venezuelae*. It binds to the 50S subunit of the ribosome and prevents peptide bond formation between amino acids in the growing protein (Fig. 11.9C). Microbial resistance is usually due to the acquisition of a gene that codes for an enzyme that breaks down the drug.

Pharmacokinetics

The plasma half-life of chloramphenicol is 2–3 hours. It is broad-spectrum and active against a wide range of Gram-positive and Gram-negative bacteria. It is well absorbed orally, but because of its significant toxicity, systemic use is limited to life-threatening infections that do not respond to other, safer agents. Topically, it is widely and safely used to treat bacterial conjunctivitis. Chloramphenicol is an enzyme inhibitor and reduces metabolism of a range of other drugs, including **phenytoin** (p. 73) and the **coumarin anticoagulants** (p. 150).

Adverse Effects

The most dangerous side-effect of chloramphenicol is irreversible bone-marrow suppression, which occurs in 1 in 10,000 people and is always fatal. In newborn babies, it can cause 'grey baby syndrome', which carries a 40% fatality rate. The characteristic ashen colour of affected babies is due to progressive circulatory collapse caused by chloramphenicol interfering with the ability of myocardial cells to use oxygen to produce energy. The younger the baby, the greater the risk, probably due to liver immaturity and a reduced capacity to metabolise the drug.

FUSIDIC ACID

Fusidic acid was first isolated from the fungus *Fusidium coccineum* and prevents the new protein from sliding along the ribosome to free up the A site for an incoming amino acid (Fig. 11.9D). It is bacteriostatic and narrow-spectrum, effective only in staphylococcal infections. Because resistance develops rapidly, it is used in combination with other agents when treating systemic infections. It is chemically related to steroids, so is very fat-soluble and distributes very well through all body tissues (including bone and joints), crosses the placenta, and appears in breast milk.

Pharmacokinetics

It is narrow-spectrum, and its plasma half-life is 10–14 hours. It is well but unpredictably absorbed from the GI tract and is better absorbed from tablet formulations than from suspensions. It is used topically for a range of staphylococcal skin and eye infections and can be given intravenously if required.

Adverse Effects

Topical preparations can cause local irritation, including skin rashes and eye dryness and discomfort. Side-effects from oral administration include GI upset, dizziness and drowsiness, and impaired liver function.

MACROLIDES

Examples: erythromycin, clarithromycin, azithromycin

Erythromycin was first isolated from the soil bacterium *Streptomyces erythraeus* in 1950. It is a first-generation macrolide, and a range of second-generation agents including clarithromycin and **azithromycin** were developed from erythromycin to produce drugs more stable in stomach acid. They have broad-spectrum activity and are effective in a wide range of important infections, but widespread use led to widespread bacterial resistance, and in recent decades research effort has focussed on development of novel macrolides. Third-generation agents entered the market in the 1990s but have largely been withdrawn because of serious side-effects; fourth-generation agents are currently in clinical trials. Macrolides block the exit tunnel in the ribosome through which the new protein emerges (Fig. 11.9D). As a group, they are more active against Gram-positive bacteria than Gram-negative because they are bulky molecules which do not easily penetrate the complex outer cell membrane of Gram-negative bacteria (Fig. 11.5). Different members of the group have different activity profiles; for instance, **azithromycin** is more active than **erythromycin** against *Haemophilus influenzae.*

Pharmacokinetics
Erythromycin is degraded by stomach acid, poorly absorbed across the gut wall especially in the presence of food, and normally almost completely metabolised in the liver. **Azithromycin** and **clarithromycin** are acid-stable and better absorbed. **Erythromycin** and **clarithromycin** are both enzyme inhibitors, and so decrease the activity of metabolising enzymes in the liver; this interaction can increase the plasma concentrations of a wide range of other drugs.

Adverse Effects
Erythromycin can interfere with liver function, giving abnormal liver enzyme levels and sometimes cholestatic jaundice. Both **erythromycin** and **clarithromycin** block potassium channels in cardiac muscle, and high doses can cause arrhythmias, including QT prolongation.

OXAZOLIDINONES

The two antibiotics in this group, **linezolid** and **tedizolid**, released in 2000 and 2014, respectively, are synthetic drugs most active against Gram-positive bacteria, including MRSA. **Tedizolid** is more potent with a wider range of activity than **linezolid** and has a longer half-life, meaning that it needs to be given only once daily. These drugs bind to the P binding site on the ribosome (Fig. 11.9A) and prevent initiation of protein synthesis. Currently, microbial resistance is not a major problem but is increasing, mainly due to bacterial alterations in ribosome structure, preventing the drugs from binding. They are well absorbed orally and can be given intravenously. Both agents can cause GI upsets, headache, and rash. **Linezolid** can cause irreversible optic neuritis and potentially dangerous blood disorders, including low blood platelet levels; patients should be advised to report any visual symptoms, and full blood counts performed regularly.

TETRACYCLINES

Examples: tetracycline, doxycycline, minocycline, oxytetracycline
Tetracyclines are produced by soil-dwelling bacteria of the *Actinomycetes* species.

They were first discovered in 1948 and widely used in the years following their introduction because they are broad-spectrum agents effective in a very wide range of infections. However, although development of second- and third-generation tetracyclines produced newer and more effective drugs, widespread resistance has limited their usefulness. Resistance is spread mainly by plasmids (Fig. 11.7), which often carry genes for resistance to other antibiotics as well as tetracyclines, increasing multi-drug resistance. These drugs work by blocking access of new amino acids to the A site on the ribosome, preventing elongation of the new protein (Fig. 11.9A).

Pharmacokinetics
Following oral administration, many tetracyclines are irregularly and unpredictably absorbed, although **doxycycline** and **minocycline** are slowly but completely absorbed. All tetracyclines form insoluble complexes with iron, calcium, magnesium, and aluminium, significantly inhibiting absorption. Dairy products, **iron** supplements, and **antacids**, which frequently contain aluminium, calcium, or magnesium salts, should therefore be avoided.

Adverse Effects
Tetracyclines can cause photosensitivity, super-infections, and GI disturbances. They bind to calcium, are taken up into bones and teeth, and can permanently stain growing teeth. The presence of the drug in developing bone and tooth tissue can also interfere with its normal structure, leading to weakening or deformity. Tetracyclines are therefore contra-indicated in pregnancy or breast-feeding women and not given to children. In common with several other drugs, tetracyclines can cause drug-induced autoimmunity. The drug binds to specific proteins, including collagen, in any of a range of tissues, including skin and liver, and triggers an immune response against that tissue. **Minocycline** is the most strongly implicated, with clear causative links to systemic lupus erythematosus-like syndromes and autoimmune hepatitis.

ANTIBIOTICS THAT INTERFERE WITH CELL WALL INTEGRITY

KEY POINT: SELECTIVE TOXICITY OF ANTIBIOTICS TARGETING BACTERIAL CELL WALLS

Cell wall synthesis and/or structure is an excellent selective target for antibiotics because human cells do not use the peptidoglycans needed by bacteria for cell wall synthesis.

Cell Wall Structure
Individual peptidoglycan chains are cross-linked firmly together with peptide bonds, giving the cell wall a rigid mesh-like structure, enclosing the bacterium in a robust protective wrapping (Fig. 11.10). Without these stabilising

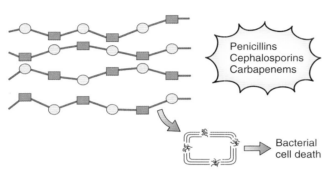

Peptide bonds
formed by transamidase

Peptidoglycan chains

A   Normal cell wall peptidoglycan structure, showing
peptide bonds holding the peptidoglycan chains together

Penicillins
Cephalosporins
Carbapenems

Bacterial
cell death

B   If peptide bond formation is prevented, the
peptidoglycan structure is weakened and the cell wall loses its
integrity. β-lactam antibiotics inhibit the transpeptidase
enzyme that produces the peptide bond links

Fig. 11.10 The mechanism of action of the β-lactam antibiotics. A. Normal cell wall peptidoglycan structure, showing peptide bonds holding the peptidoglycan chains together. B. If peptide bond formation is prevented, the peptidoglycan structure is weakened and the cell wall loses its integrity. β-lactam antibiotics inhibit the transpeptidase enzyme that produces peptide bond links.

bonds, the peptidoglycan layers lose strength and structure, and the cell wall is disrupted, losing its ability to protect the bacterium from its external environment. The enzyme responsible for synthesising the peptide bonds is called transpeptidase.

THE β-LACTAM ANTIBIOTICS

The β-lactam antibiotics include the penicillins, the cephalosporins, and the carbapenems.

The β-lactam ring is a simple four-membered ring built from three carbon atoms and a nitrogen atom, and antibiotics containing this structure are called β-lactam antibiotics. Fig. 11.11A shows the core chemical structure of penicillin, containing its β-lactam ring. The β-lactam ring inhibits transpeptidase and so is essential for drug activity. In the presence of a β-lactam antibiotic, the cell wall structure is disrupted and loses its integrity, leading to bacterial cell death (Fig. 11.10).

Resistance to β-Lactam Antibiotics

The main mechanism by which bacteria develop resistance to β-lactam antibiotics is by producing an enzyme called β-lactamase that destroys the β-lactam ring (Fig. 11.11B). With the ring destroyed, the antibiotic loses its ability to inhibit cell wall synthesis. β-lactamase inhibitors in clinical use are designed to bind to and inhibit the activity of bacterial β-lactamase, thus preserving the antibiotic and prolonging its activity (Fig. 11.11C). **Clavulanic acid** is used with **amoxycillin** (co-amoxiclav) and **avibactam** and **tazobactam** with some cephalosporins.

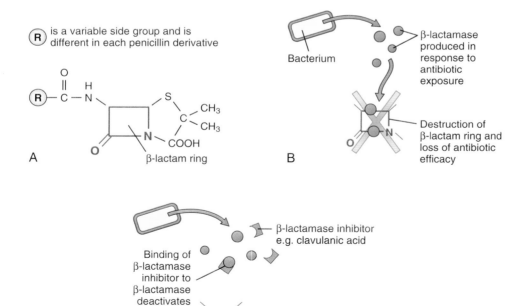

R is a variable side group and is different in each penicillin derivative

A   β-lactam ring

Bacterium

β-lactamase produced in response to antibiotic exposure

Destruction of β-lactam ring and loss of antibiotic efficacy

B

Binding of β-lactamase inhibitor to β-lactamase deactivates the enzyme

β-lactamase inhibitor e.g. clavulanic acid

β-lactam ring remains intact and the antibiotic remains active

C

Fig. 11.11 A. The core chemical structure of the penicillins, showing the β-lactam ring. R is a variable side group and is different in each penicillin derivative. B. Bacteria produce β-lactamase to destroy the β-lactam ring. C. β-lactamase inhibitors are given with β-lactam antibiotics to protect the drug from destruction by β-lactamase.

Focus on: The Penicillins

Examples: benzyl penicillin, amoxicillin, ampicillin, flucloxacillin

The discoverer of penicillin, the Scotsman Alexander Fleming, made his historically famous observations in 1928. On returning from holiday, he noticed that some of his staphylococcus culture plates had become contaminated with a fungus called *Penicillium notatum*, and that surrounding the fungal colonies were large, clear areas where bacteria were unable to grow. He reasoned that the fungus was producing a substance toxic to the bacteria. His findings were published and picked up by a team of scientists led by Howard Florey and Ernst Chain working in Oxford, who diverted their research efforts into identifying and purifying the fungal antibacterial agent. At the beginning of World War II, realising the impact an effective antibiotic would have in treating the infections caused by battlefield injuries, the team relocated to the United States where penicillin production was refined and begun on an industrial scale. Over the remaining years of the war, it saved thousands of lives (Fig. 11.12). Fleming, Florey, and Chain were jointly awarded the Nobel Prize for Medicine in 1945, recognising the massive impact of their work in human health. Today's penicillin family of antibiotics include the original, **benzyl penicillin** (**penicillin G**), and about 15 further agents produced by chemically modifying the core penicillin molecule.

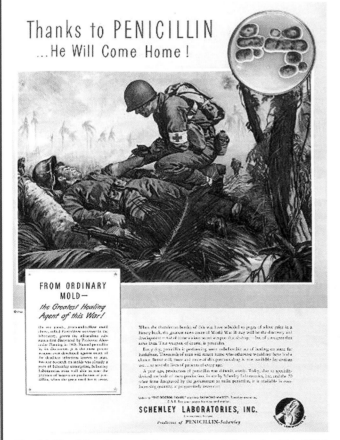

Fig. 11.12 Advertisement for penicillin, Life magazine, 1944.
(From Science Museum London, CC BY 4.0)

Modifications and Altered Activity

Modifying the chemical structure of the basic penicillin core by adding different side chains (position R in Fig. 11.11A) has produced different classes of penicillins with different spectra of activity. This has yielded broad-spectrum drugs effective against Gram-negative and Gram-positive organisms. They include the aminopenicillins (e.g. **amoxicillin** and **ampicillin**, developed in the 1960s) and the newer carboxypenicillins (e.g. **carbenicillin**) and piperazine penicillins (e.g. **piperacillin**).

β-lactamase-Resistant Penicillins. These are prepared by adding additional chemical groups to the β-lactam ring, which shield it from bacterial β-lactamase and allow the drug to remain active even in the presence of bacteria producing this enzyme. There is a trade-off, however, in terms of antibacterial activity: by tucking the β-lactam ring deeper into the drug molecule, its ability to inhibit cell wall synthesis is also reduced, so penicillins modified in this way lose efficacy. Examples of β-lactamase-resistant penicillins include **methicillin, flucloxacillin, and temocillin**.

Pharmacokinetics

Although **benzyl penicillin** is highly potent, it is almost completely destroyed in the acidic juices of the stomach and so must be given parenterally. It is also narrow-spectrum, with little activity against Gram-negative bacteria, and bacteria quickly develop resistance via β-lactamase production. **Phenoxymethylpenicillin (penicillin V)** was developed in 1948, and although it is less active than benzyl penicillin and is narrow-spectrum, it survives the acid environment of the stomach and can be given orally. Most penicillins can be given orally, although absorption varies from drug to drug: **ampicillin** is poorly absorbed whereas **amoxycillin** and **flucloxacillin** are well absorbed. Most penicillins do not enter liver cells and so liver metabolism is limited, and the drugs are largely excreted unchanged by the kidney. The kidney clears penicillin rapidly from the bloodstream, so plasma half-lives are generally short; the half-life of **benzyl penicillin** is only about 30 minutes, and the half-life of **amoxycillin** is 1 hour. Renal impairment can therefore significantly extend plasma half-lives. In general, penicillins are well distributed, although they do not cross the blood–brain barrier in appreciable quantities unless the meninges are inflamed. Penicillin must not be given intrathecally because of the risk of convulsions.

Adverse Effects

Penicillins can cause any of the range of antibiotic-related adverse effects (see above), including GI upsets, superinfection, and allergy. Penicillin allergy can be severe. About 10% of people report a reaction to penicillin, although it is estimated that fewer than 1% of these people have a true allergy. The most severe form of allergy, anaphylaxis, is a type I hypersensitivity reaction, with massive release of histamine and other inflammatory mediators into the bloodstream. This causes urticaria and GI changes, and potentially life-threatening bronchoconstriction, vasodilation, hypotension, and cardiovascular collapse.

Cephalosporins

Examples: cephalexin, cefuroxime, cefotaxime

The first cephalosporin, cephalosporin C, was identified in 1953 from the fungus *Cephalosporium*, grown from sewage. It contained a β-lactam ring, but unlike the penicillins, which by this time were in widespread use and had caused widespread resistance, it was less susceptible to β-lactamase. Thousands of semi-synthetic derivatives have been produced, leading to the introduction of several generations of cephalosporin antibiotics, each giving improved activity against Gram-negative infections and increased stability to β-lactamase. The newest agents have good activity against both Gram-negative and Gram-positive organisms and do not lose activity when exposed to bacterial β-lactamase.

Pharmacokinetics

Absorption in this group is variable: some can only be given intramuscularly or intravenously because they are not absorbed across the wall of the GI tract (e.g. **ceftriaxone**), whereas some, e.g. **cephalexin**, can be given orally. They distribute well, including into the cerebrospinal fluid, especially the newer agents. As with the penicillins, they are not significantly metabolised in the liver and rely on renal excretion for clearance from the body.

Adverse Effects

Like their close cousins the penicillins, the cephalosporins are generally well tolerated. There is penicillin cross-allergy, so a penicillin-allergic individual has an increased risk of cephalosporin allergy too. Antibiotic-associated colitis (see above) is more common with the cephalosporins than most other antibiotics.

Carbapenems

Examples: imipenem, meropenem

These β-lactam antibiotics were developed in the 1980s from **thienamycin**, produced by a bacterium of the *Streptomyces* family.

Pharmacokinetics

Carbapenems are not absorbed across the wall of the GI tract and so must be given intravenously. **Imipenem**, the original, is an effective broad-spectrum drug resistant to β-lactamase but is rapidly deactivated by enzymes in the kidney. It is therefore given with an inhibitor of these enzymes, **cilastatin**, to preserve it from renal metabolism and prolong its activity. Carbapenem half-lives range from 1–5 hours. They are not metabolised significantly in the liver and are therefore cleared from the body mainly by the kidneys.

Adverse Effects

GI side-effects are very common. These drugs can also cause neurotoxicity (especially **imipenem**) and renal toxicity.

BACITRACIN

Bacitracin is produced by the bacterium *Bacillus subtilis*. It interferes with cell wall synthesis by blocking the biochemical pathway that transports peptidoglycan molecules into the growing cell wall structure. It is toxic in systemic use, including nephrotoxicity and allergy, and is not licensed for use in all countries. Topical preparations are available in some countries to treat eye and skin infections.

TEICOPLANIN AND VANCOMYCIN

These two glycopeptide drugs are structurally similar and possess similar activity spectra. They are both more active against Gram-positive than Gram-negative bacteria because they cannot penetrate the complex outer membrane of Gram-negative organisms and are particularly active against staphylococcal species including MRSA. Generally, they are reserved for serious infections that do not respond to other antibiotics. Both drugs work by inhibiting the linking of peptidoglycans in cell wall synthesis: the cell wall is therefore weakened and loses its protective function. They are not absorbed after oral administration, so are given by intramuscular or intravenous injection for systemic infection; however, given orally they clear GI infection, including *C. difficile*. **Teicoplanin** has a long half-life of up to 100 hours while **vancomycin's** is much shorter (4–11 hours), and renal impairment significantly increases both. This is compounded by the fact that both can cause nephrotoxicity, vancomycin more so than teicoplanin. Both drugs cause a range of side-effects including blood abnormalities, nausea, and allergy (there is cross-allergy between the two drugs).

ANTIBIOTICS ACTING ON THE BACTERIAL CELL MEMBRANE

POLYMYXINS

Examples: colistimethate sodium

Polymyxins are highly active against Gram-negative organisms because they bind avidly to LPS on their protective outer cell membrane (Fig. 11.5). This disrupts the membrane integrity, and it loses its barrier function. It also allows the polymyxin molecules to travel through the bacterial cell wall to deeper structures, where they cause further damage, increase membrane permeability and lead to lysis of the cell. They are not active against Gram-positive bacteria.

Pharmacokinetics

Colistimethate is not absorbed across the wall of the GI tract because it is highly charged and is given intravenously for systemic infections. It is also used by nebuliser for respiratory tract infection, usually in cystic fibrosis in children, and can be given orally to clear the bowel of Gram-negative organisms prior to surgery. It is not significantly metabolised and is excreted unchanged by the kidney. Care is therefore needed in reduced renal function, which may significantly extend the normal half-life of 2–3 hours.

Adverse Effects

Polymyxins can cause a range of unpleasant side-effects, including neurological and renal toxicity.

ANTIBIOTICS ACTING ON BACTERIAL DNA

KEY POINT: SELECTIVE TOXICITY OF ANTIBIOTICS TARGETING DNA SYNTHESIS

This group of drugs has no one target in common because DNA synthesis is common to both mammalian and bacterial cells. Individual selective targets are described for individual drugs below.

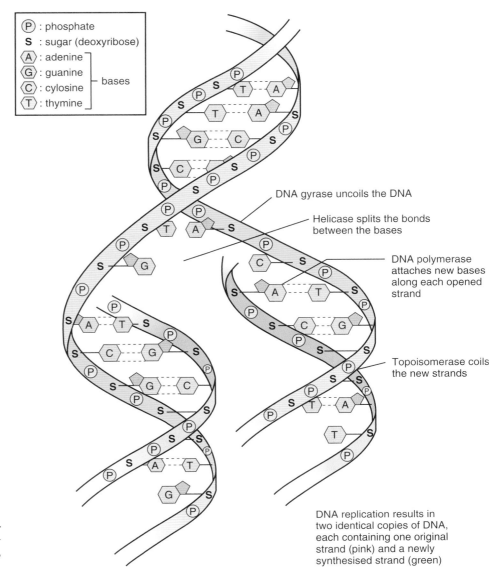

P : phosphate
S : sugar (deoxyribose)
Ⓐ : adenine ⎤
Ⓖ : guanine ⎥
Ⓒ : cylosine ⎥ bases
Ⓣ : thymine ⎦

DNA gyrase uncoils the DNA

Helicase splits the bonds between the bases

DNA polymerase attaches new bases along each opened strand

Topoisomerase coils the new strands

DNA replication results in two identical copies of DNA, each containing one original strand (pink) and a newly synthesised strand (green)

Fig. 11.13 The steps in DNA replication. (Modified from HESI (2021) Admission assessment exam review, 5th ed, Fig. 5.11. St. Louis: Elsevier.)

Several important antibiotics interfere with DNA structure, replication, or transcription. Because the basic structure of DNA is the same in human and bacterial cells, identifying a selective target that damages the infecting microbe and not host cells is challenging.

DNA Replication

To divide and produce two daughter cells, bacteria first replicate their DNA, a copy for each daughter cell. Fig. 11.13 shows the main steps, the enzymes responsible for catalysing each step, and the antibiotics that target the process. The molecule must first be uncoiled, an action facilitated by an enzyme called DNA gyrase, and the two bases forming each rung separated, performed by an enzyme called DNA helicase. Using the two halves of the original molecule as templates, an enzyme called DNA polymerase attaches new bases in sequence to each half-ladder unit and links them together, restoring the original ladder structure, and then an enzyme called topoisomerase coils the DNA back up. The

process ends up with two identical DNA molecules, one for each daughter cell.

Metronidazole

Metronidazole is a pro-drug. It diffuses passively into cells, including host cells and microbes. Some protozoa and some anaerobic bacteria, e.g. *C. difficile* and *H. pylori*, possess an enzyme that converts metronidazole to a very reactive and toxic metabolite. This metabolite binds to DNA and breaks it up (Fig. 11.14). This is a bactericidal action, because the damaged DNA can neither be used to make new proteins nor can it be copied to allow the microbe to divide. Aerobic cells, including human cells, lack this enzyme and so do not produce the toxic metabolite. It also means, of course, that aerobic microbes are resistant to metronidazole. Metronidazole is broad-spectrum and used to treat a range of anaerobic infections, including vaginal, pelvic, and intestinal infections, but formerly susceptible organisms are steadily developing resistance, mainly due to reducing their uptake

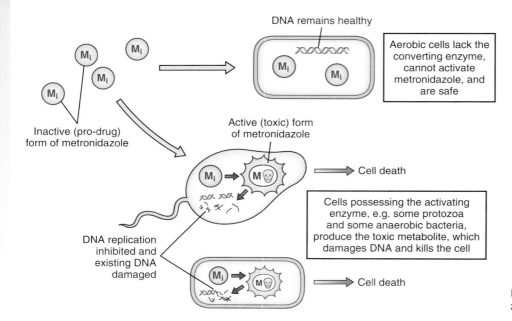

Fig. 11.14 Activation of metronidazole in anaerobic organisms.

of the drug. **Tinidazole** is in the same class and has a similar spectrum of action to metronidazole.

Pharmacokinetics

Metronidazole is available in a range of formulations and is usually given orally, intravenously, rectally, or vaginally. It is well absorbed when given orally, with a bioavailability of over 90%. It distributes into the CSF, crosses the placenta, and appears in breast milk. It is not highly plasma protein-bound and has a half-life of 6–9 hours. Most is metabolised in the liver and the metabolites excreted in the urine, so doses may need to be reduced in reduced liver function.

Adverse Effects

Metronidazole can give an unpleasant metallic taste in the mouth, muscle pain, and GI upsets. Current advice is to avoid alcohol while taking this drug because a disulfiram-like reaction has been reported, although the validity of this is increasingly being questioned because the evidence is weak.

Nitrofurantoin

Nitrofurantoin is a synthetic agent and a pro-drug. Susceptible bacteria possess enzymes that convert it to toxic metabolites that interfere with certain key biochemical processes, including synthesis of DNA, RNA, and protein. Cells lacking these enzymes, including animal cells, do not produce the toxic metabolites. The drug can cause serious side-effects and so is not used as a first-line agent. Nitrofurantoin is concentrated in the urine in its active form because it is actively secreted into renal tubules, and so is used in urinary tract infection. It is highly effective against *Escherichia coli*, which is responsible for 80% of uncomplicated urinary tract infections, and resistance rarely develops. It must, however, be used with caution or avoided altogether, in renal impairment, because the drug can quickly accumulate and cause toxicity, including peripheral neuropathy.

Pharmacokinetics

The half-life is short, less than 1 hour, and nitrofurantoin is very heavily plasma protein-bound (up to 90%). Up to half of a dose is excreted unchanged in the urine. It is well absorbed orally, especially if taken with food.

Adverse Effects

Mild GI side-effects are common, but nitrofurantoin can cause a range of serious adverse effects, including acute pulmonary disease and bone marrow failure.

Quinolones (Fluoroquinolones)

Examples: ciprofloxacin, levofloxacin, ofloxacin

These broad-spectrum synthetic antibiotics are used in a wide range of infections, including serious respiratory and enteric infections. They inhibit DNA gyrase and topoisomerase (Fig. 11.13) and so prevent correct coiling and uncoiling of bacterial DNA, in turn preventing DNA replication and bacterial cell division. Resistance is usually due to the bacteria altering their binding site for the drug, or due to production of efflux pumps which pump the drug out of the bacterial cell. The original drugs in this group, including **nalidixic acid**, are narrow-spectrum, but incorporation of a fluoride atom into the quinolone molecule produced fluoroquinolones, which are more potent and broad-spectrum.

Pharmacokinetics

The quinolones are usually given orally or intravenously and distribute well throughout body tissues. **Levofloxacin** is available for nebulisation, e.g. to treat chronic respiratory infection in cystic fibrosis. Foodstuffs, **iron** preparations, and **antacids** in the GI tract reduce absorption. Some of the drugs in this class, e.g. **ciprofloxacin**, are enzyme inhibitors, decreasing the metabolising activity of cytochrome P450 in the liver and inhibiting the metabolism of some other drugs, including **warfarin**.

Adverse Effects

Fluoroquinolones are generally well tolerated, but their more severe side-effects include tendinitis, with possible rupture, especially in older people and most often affecting the Achilles tendon. Central nervous system effects include headache, dizziness, and, rarely, convulsions. They can also cause GI upsets, skin rashes, and cardiac arrhythmias.

ANTIBIOTICS INTERFERING WITH FOLIC ACID METABOLISM

THE SULPHONAMIDES AND TRIMETHOPRIM

These antibiotics interfere with folic acid metabolism. Folic acid (dihydrofolic acid) is an essential precursor in protein and DNA synthesis in both human and bacterial cells; however, there are important differences in the folic acid pathway between them, generating selective targets for antimicrobial action. Sulphonamides, the first antimicrobial drugs, were developed in the 1930s by the German doctor Gerhard Domagk, who won the Nobel Prize for this ground-breaking work. The original agent, **prontosil**, is no longer used because of toxicity, and sulphonamide use in general has declined because of widespread bacterial resistance. It is interesting that the sulphonamides are chemically closely related to a range of other clinically important drugs, including the diuretic **acetazolamide**, the antidiabetic **sulphonylureas**, the anti-inflammatory **sulfasalazine**, and **loop and thiazide diuretics**, because they are all derived from the same family of sulphur-containing dyes. Cases of cross-allergy between these groups of drugs have been reported.

The Folic Acid Pathway

A simplified representation of the folic acid pathway, and the sites of sulphonamide and trimethoprim action, are shown in Fig. 11.15. Bacteria must synthesise their own dihydrofolic acid because they have no way of absorbing it from their environment. They use the enzyme dihydropteroate synthase to produce dihydrofolic acid from the precursor molecule para-aminobenzoic acid (PABA). Human cells do not possess this enzyme because mammalian biology has evolved to absorb pre-formed dihydrofolic acid from the diet and cells do not need to make their own. Dihydropteroate synthase is therefore an ideal selective target and is inhibited by **sulphonamides**. In both human and bacterial cells, folic acid is converted to its active form, tetrahydrofolic acid, by the enzyme dihydrofolate reductase, but the enzyme takes slightly different forms in the two different cells. **Trimethoprim** inhibits bacterial dihydrofolate reductase far more effectively than the human enzyme, and therefore prevents bacterial synthesis of amino acids and nucleic acids. Because they block sequential steps in folic acid metabolism, trimethoprim and sulphonamides act synergistically and are often used together; the sulphonamide usually used is **sulphamethoxazole** and the combination drug is called **co-trimoxazole**.

Methotrexate (p. 237) inhibits the human form of dihydrofolate reductase.

Sulphonamides

Examples: sulphamethoxazole, sulfadiazine

Sulphonamides exert their antibacterial action because they are very closely related to PABA (Fig. 11.15). This means that the enzyme dihydropteroate synthase mistakenly binds to the drug instead of PABA, significantly reducing folic acid production. They are broad-spectrum agents, used mainly in GI, respiratory, and urinary tract infections. Microbial resistance is now very common amongst all groups of previously susceptible bacteria, mainly because the bacteria begin producing variants of dihydropteroate synthase. These enzyme variants are still capable of generating folic acid for the bacterium, but their binding sites for the sulphonamide drugs are subtly changed to prevent the drug from latching on.

Pharmacokinetics

The most common sulphonamide, **sulphamethoxazole**, has a plasma half-life of 10 hours and is mainly excreted in its unchanged form by the kidney. Care is therefore needed in reduced renal function. It is well absorbed after oral administration and distributes well, crossing the blood–brain barrier and the placenta.

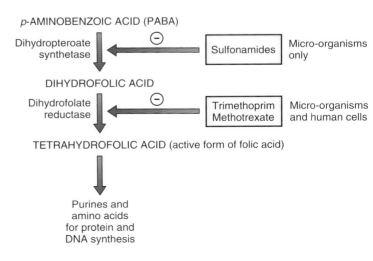

Fig. 11.15 The mechanism of action of sulphonamides and trimethoprim. (Modified from Waller DG, Sampson A, and Hitchings A (2022) Medical pharmacology and therapeutics, 6th ed, Fig. 51.4. Oxford: Elsevier.)

Adverse Effects

Sulphonamides commonly cause allergic reactions, including potentially fatal anaphylactic events. Serious hypersensitivity reactions include Stevens–Johnson syndrome (see Fig. 3.13) and other serious skin reactions and can trigger or worsen systemic lupus erythematosus. They can cause folic acid deficiency and so should be used with caution in people predisposed to this, e.g. in alcohol dependency, pregnancy, or malabsorption syndromes. Use is contra-indicated in the first trimester of pregnancy because its antifolate action can cause developmental abnormalities in the fetus. Other significant side-effects include bone marrow suppression, blood abnormalities, and renal toxicity.

Trimethoprim

The clinical pharmacology of trimethoprim is very similar to that of the sulphonamides, unsurprisingly so because of their closely related activities. Trimethoprim is also broad-spectrum and is more frequently used as monotherapy than the sulphonamides. Rarely, it can precipitate serious blood disorders, and patients on long-term therapy should be monitored. Its half-life is between 8 and 10 hours, which can be prolonged in renal impairment because a significant proportion of the drug is excreted in its unchanged form.

Focus on: Mycobacteria and Anti-Tuberculosis Drugs

Mycobacteria are slow-growing microbes characterised by a thick cell wall rich in lipids called mycolic acids. Mycolic acids make the cell wall much less permeable to laboratory stains, more resistant to damage by detergents and antiseptics, and more resistant to most of the main families of antibiotics and to the body's immune defences. Effective treatment of mycobacterial infections is therefore restricted to a small number of drugs, to which microbial resistance is an increasing problem. Important diseases caused by mycobacteria include leprosy (*Mycobacterium leprae*) and tuberculosis (TB) (*Mycobacterium tuberculosis*).

Tuberculosis

Globally, TB is the leading cause of death from a single infectious agent and World Health Organisation data estimates that one-quarter of the world's population in 2020 was infected with *M. tuberculosis*. Although infection rates are slowly declining, the TB epidemic remains a massive worldwide healthcare challenge. *M. tuberculosis* is an intracellular pathogen, spread by inhalation, and once in the airways is phagocytosed by alveolar macrophages. Normally, macrophages destroy phagocytosed microbes using their range of digestive enzymes and toxins, but *M. tuberculosis* deactivates these mechanisms and survives and replicates within the macrophage. Although initial infection involves the lungs (pulmonary TB), untreated disease frequently becomes latent, walled-off but protected within lesions (granulomas) formed in the lungs as the immune system, unable to eradicate the infection, tries to contain it. Latent disease can be re-activated and spread to involve most oth-

er body tissues, including the brain, skin, heart, and bone. TB treatment regimens vary from country to country, but an extended period of treatment, usually between 6 and 9 months, with multiple antimycobacterial agents is the norm. First-line drugs include **isoniazid**, **rifampicin**, **ethambutol**, and **pyrazinamide**, used in varying combinations because monotherapy with any one alone rapidly produces resistant strains. Despite this, multi-drug resistance is becoming an increasing problem. Fig. 11.16 shows the targets exploited by the main anti-tuberculous agents.

Isoniazid

This antibiotic is highly effective against *M. tuberculosis* and is an important first-line drug in TB treatment. It is a pro-drug, activated inside mycobacteria to an inhibitor of an enzyme that catalyses the production of mycolic acids in the mycobacterial cell wall. This prevents normal cell wall synthesis, and without an intact cell wall, the mycobacterium cannot survive or replicate.

Pharmacokinetics. Isoniazid is well absorbed from the gastrointestinal tract and has a half-life of 0.5–5 hours, depending on the individual's ability to metabolise it. Most of a dose is metabolised in the liver to a range of metabolites, including highly reactive free radicals which can cause significant liver injury. Particular care is therefore needed in liver impairment, including regular monitoring of hepatic function. Isoniazid is a potent inhibitor of the cytochrome P450 family of hepatic metabolising enzymes and increases circulating levels of a number of other drugs, including **anticonvulsants**.

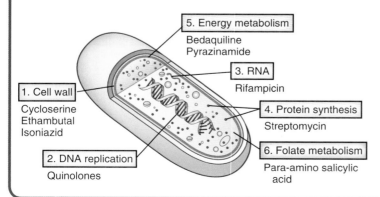

Fig. 11.16 *Mycobacterium tuberculosis:* **targets for drug action.** (Modified from Bhat ZS, Rather MA, Maqbool M, et al. (2018) Drug targets exploited in *Mycobacterium tuberculosis*: pitfalls and promises on the horizon. *Biomedicine & Pharmacotherapy*, 103, pp. 1733-1747.)

Adverse Effects. Isoniazid is generally well tolerated. Liver impairment, renal impairment, and ototoxicity are among the most serious side-effects. It can cause peripheral neuropathy because it inhibits cellular use of vitamin B_6 (pyridoxine), essential for a wide range of important metabolic pathways including myelin synthesis. Co-administration of vitamin B_6 supplements prevents this and is important in people at particular risk of nutritional deficiency, including in those who are alcohol-dependent, in malnutrition, and in older people. It reduces the efficacy of **L-DOPA** in the treatment of Parkinson's disease because it inhibits the enzyme dopa decarboxylase, which converts L-DOPA to dopamine (p. 54).

Rifamycins

This group of drugs includes **rifampicin** and **rifabutin**; rifampicin (rifampin) is the main one used in TB. It is broad-spectrum, bactericidal, and particularly useful in mycobacterial infections, including leprosy. It inactivates the bacterial enzyme RNA polymerase so that the bacteria are unable to make RNA, including mRNA. Because mRNA is the molecule used to transfer the genetic code from DNA to the ribosome for protein synthesis, this prevents the microbe from producing essential proteins, and it dies. It is used in short courses for a range of infections, including meningococcal meningitis, but in TB it is given for up to 6 months.

Pharmacokinetics. Rifampicin is well absorbed when given orally and is taken up and concentrated within macrophages and other immune cells, explaining its ability to target the intracellular pathogen *M. tuberculosis*. It is a strong inducer of a range of liver enzymes, and so it increases the rate at which a range of other drugs are cleared from the plasma. Drugs affected include **oestrogen** (so rifampicin can cause contraceptive failure), **warfarin**, **phenytoin**, and **sulphonylureas**. It is metabolised in the liver and has a plasma half-life of around 3.5 hours. Care is needed in patients with reduced liver function, in whom the drug can accumulate.

Adverse Effects. Rifampicin commonly causes nausea and vomiting. It distributes well, including into the CSF, and can cause an orange discolouration of body fluids, including urine and tears, which can stain soft contact lenses. It can cause blood disorders, and blood counts should be monitored regularly in long-term therapy.

Ethambutol

Although the mechanism of action of this bacteriostatic agent is not known, it is believed to block production of a substance called arabinogalactan, which mycobacteria use in their cell wall. Because other types of microbes do not use these pathways, the drug is only effective in mycobacteria. In the presence of ethambutol, dividing bacteria cannot produce an intact cell wall and do not survive. It is given orally and work is currently under way to develop a dry powder formulation for inhalation. This would reduce the drug dose required and therefore limit systemic toxicity. Some of the drug is metabolised in the liver, but about 50% is excreted unchanged by the kidney. In people with normal renal function, its half-life is 3–4 hours, but because of the large contribution made by the kidney to clearing

unchanged drug from the plasma, renal impairment can significantly extend this. It enters the CSF, so is effective in tuberculous meningitis. Its most significant side-effect is a dose-dependent neuropathy of the optic nerve, leading to reduced visual acuity and red–green colour blindness. Although some restoration of vision can occur if the drug is stopped as soon as vision problems are detected, there is often residual and permanent vision loss.

Pyrazinamide

Pyrazinamide is bacteriostatic and a pro-drug. It is taken up into infected macrophages and enters the cell's lysosomes, where the macrophage has enclosed the mycobacteria in an effort to destroy them. The environment in these lysosomes is acidic, which activates the drug. Once activated, the drug inhibits microbial synthesis of important fatty acids, disrupting membranes within the cell. Energy production takes place on internal membranes, so interfering with membrane structure interferes with energy production and depletes the mycobacterium's energy stores, without which it cannot survive. Pyrazinamide is given orally and has a long half-life of 10 hours. It distributes well, including across the blood–brain barrier, so is effective in treating tuberculous meningitis. About 70% of a dose of the drug is excreted unchanged in the urine, so care must be taken in reduced renal function. It can cause liver impairment, and liver function should be checked before commencing treatment. Other side-effects include reduced appetite, skin reactions, and development or worsening of gout.

Other Antimycobacterial Drugs

Several other antibiotics are used as second-line agents or in multi-drug-resistant TB. Macrolides including **azithromycin** can be useful. Other agents include **cycloserine**, **amikacin,** and **streptomycin** and some **quinolones**

Aminosalicylic Acid. This is a pro-drug converted to its active form after uptake by the mycobacterium. In its active form, it closely resembles para-aminobenzoic acid, which is the precursor converted to folate in the folic acid pathway (Fig. 11.15). It is therefore used in the pathway instead of PABA and so reduces microbial production of folate. It is given orally and can cause gastrointestinal disturbances and hypersensitivity reactions.

Bedaquiline. Bedaquiline is a synthetic antibiotic used in the treatment of multi-drug-resistant TB. It is bactericidal because it inhibits mycobacterial ATP synthase, an enzyme essential for ATP production. Inability to produce ATP leads to bacterial death. It is well absorbed when given orally and is over 99% bound to plasma proteins. It distributes widely through body tissues, including into respiratory secretions. It has a very long half-life, averaging 5.5 months, probably because it binds to proteins in peripheral tissues and is released very slowly from these sites. It is only partly metabolised in the liver, and most of the drug is excreted unchanged in the faeces, with very little excreted in the urine. Bedaquiline causes nausea, headache, myalgia, and changed liver function and should be used with care in certain cardiac disorders including heart failure and arrhythmias because it extends the QT interval.

ANTIVIRAL DRUGS

Compared to antibiotics, there are relatively few antiviral drugs because viruses are obligate intracellular parasites: that is, they enter host cells and insert viral DNA into the host cell DNA. Directed by viral genes, host cell organelles and biochemical pathways produce new viral proteins and nucleic acids, which the host cell then assembles into new viral particles. Because each step in viral replication is performed by host cell machinery, finding a selective drug target and avoiding poisoning the host cell is a challenge. Many antiviral agents are significantly toxic and cause serious adverse effects, especially in systemic use.

The Biology of Viruses

Viruses are much smaller than human cells and most bacterial cells. Because they are not capable of independent life, viruses are not categorised as living cells: instead, they are referred to as viral particles, and infect a wide range of host cells including animals, plants, and even bacteria. Structurally, they are much simpler than living cells, and comprise an outer shell, called a capsid, which contains only their genetic material and a few essential viral enzymes: there are no organelles or other internal metabolic structures. Some viruses carry their genetic material in the form of DNA (DNA viruses) but others (RNA viruses) have only RNA. Clinically important DNA viruses include herpesviruses, human papilloma virus, and hepatitis B virus. DNA viruses may increase the risk of cancer in infected tissues because the act of inserting their viral DNA into the host cell genome generates a mutation, the key event in carcinogenesis. Clinically important RNA viruses include influenza virus, coronaviruses, rhinoviruses, and most hepatitis viruses.

Replication of DNA Viruses

The main stages of the viral replication cycle for DNA viruses are shown in Fig. 11.17. The virus latches on to the target cell membrane and enters the cytosol. Here, it uncoats: its capsid breaks apart and releases the viral DNA, which enters the host cell nucleus and is integrated into the host cell's own genome. The host cell then transcribes the viral DNA into viral RNA, which carries the code for viral proteins. Viral RNA travels out of the nucleus to the host cell ribosomes, which translate the viral protein code into new viral proteins. At the same time, host cell enzymes make copies of the viral DNA. As new viral proteins and DNA are synthesised, they are assembled into new viral particles, which are released from the host cell and infect adjacent cells.

RNA viruses cannot insert their RNA directly into the host cell genome because RNA is single-stranded and DNA is double-stranded. Their RNA is used directly by host ribosomes to produce new viral proteins.

Replication of Retroviruses

Retroviruses are a type of RNA virus and contain RNA, which they convert to DNA using an enzyme called reverse transcriptase which they carry with them in their capsid. This DNA can then be inserted into the host cell DNA. Because reverse transcriptase is a uniquely viral enzyme, it is an ideal selective target for drug action. Clinically important retroviruses include HIV, and their biology is discussed in the section on HIV treatment.

ANTIVIRAL RESISTANCE

As with antibacterial agents, viral resistance to antiviral drugs is spreading, compromising the treatment of a range of infections. Viruses mutate readily and, unlike animal cells, can remain viable even following significant alterations in their genetic material. This further complicates efforts to

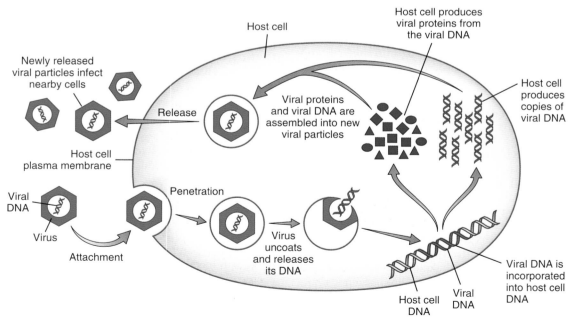

Fig. 11.17 The replication cycle of a DNA virus. (Modified from Ryu W-S (2017) Molecular virology of human pathogenic viruses, Fig. 3.1. Boston: Academy Press.)

find effective antiviral drugs, as well as effective vaccines: if the virus constantly mutates, it presents the equivalent of a moving target. Some clinically important viruses, such as rhinoviruses, responsible for the common cold, exist as many serotypes, i.e. variants of the virus, all possessing slightly different surface proteins. This means that even if a drug (or a vaccine) is developed against one serotype, it is not necessarily effective against others. It also explains why it is possible to catch the common cold on multiple occasions: antibodies produced against the serotype causing this week's cold will not protect against a different serotype prevalent in 2 weeks' time.

Latency

Latency is associated mainly with viruses of the herpes family, which have evolved this strategy to resist elimination from their host organism and presents a significant challenge to effective antiviral therapy. Herpes viruses are DNA viruses that include herpes simplex (cold sores, genital sores, eye and central nervous system infections), varicella zoster (chickenpox and shingles), Epstein–Barr virus (infectious mononucleosis and a range of malignancies including Hodgkin's disease), and cytomegalovirus (a range of infections including hepatitis, and stillbirth and congenital abnormalities). In latency, the virus scales all metabolic activity down to a very low level but retains all its genetic material and is capable of rapid re-activation. Concealed within its host cell, the virus effectively evades immune mechanisms, and because it is metabolically inactive, is unaffected by antiviral drugs.

ANTIVIRAL DRUGS

Most antiviral drugs are only effective when the virus is replicating because they inhibit the synthesis of viral nucleic acids. Other mechanisms of action include prevention of the uncoating step and inhibition of viral protein synthesis. Because of the pared-down, relatively simple nature of viral biology, there is a limited range of viral-specific enzymes available as drug targets.

INHIBITORS OF VIRAL NUCLEIC ACID SYNTHESIS

These drugs inhibit the production of viral nucleic acids: DNA and RNA. Nucleic acids are built of units called nucleotides, which contain a base (adenine, cytosine, guanine, or thymine) linked to a sugar unit (ribose in RNA and deoxyribose in DNA) which in turn is linked to a phosphate group. A nucleoside refers to the base and sugar only (Fig. 11.18A). RNA is a single chain of nucleotides, and DNA is a double chain, linked by the bases (Figure 11.18B). Nucleic acids are built by enzymes called polymerases: RNA polymerase builds single-stranded RNA and DNA polymerase builds double-stranded DNA.

Nucleoside Analogues

Examples: acyclovir, famciclovir, ganciclovir, ribavirin

These are sometimes called false nucleosides and are structurally very similar to the nucleoside units assembled into new viral DNA. **Acyclovir, famciclovir, ganciclovir,** and **ribavirin** all contain the normal base guanine (and so are sometimes referred to as guanosine nucleosides), but instead of a normal sugar, they are attached to a different chemical group which does not bind to incoming nucleotides. DNA polymerase mistakes the drug molecule for the true nucleoside and inserts it into the growing nucleotide chain. However, once the drug molecule is incorporated into a new nucleotide chain, no further nucleotides can be added, and synthesis is terminated (Fig. 11.18C). Viral DNA synthesis cannot be completed and so the production of new viral particles stops. These drugs are most useful against herpesviruses, including cytomegalovirus. **Ribavirin** is also used in hepatitis C and a range of respiratory infections.

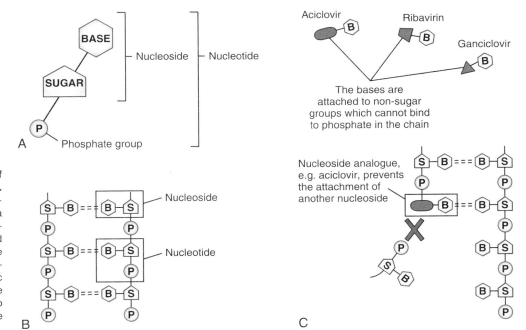

Fig. 11.18 The mechanism of action of nucleoside inhibitors. A. Nucleoside and nucleotide structure. B. Nucleotides linked in a section of DNA. C. Nucleoside analogues, e.g. acyclovir, ribavirin, and ganciclovir, are so similar in structure to the true analogue that the polymerase enzyme builds new nucleic acid using them instead of the true nucleosides. They cannot attach to incoming nucleosides, and so the chain synthesis is terminated.

Acyclovir (Aciclovir)

This was the first drug in this class to be developed and entered the market in the mid-1970s. When used topically, it is remarkably free of side-effects even though it blocks DNA synthesis. Its selective toxicity is based on the fact that it is thirty times more active against viral DNA polymerase than human DNA polymerase. In addition, it is a pro-drug: it is only activated in host cells that have been infected with a virus. The result is that it has very little effect on healthy host cell DNA production but is highly effective against viral DNA synthesis in infected cells. However, viral resistance is an increasing problem, usually because the virus produces slight variants of its DNA polymerase not affected by the drug. Acyclovir is used topically, e.g. to treat cold sores, but needs to be applied early to achieve effect. It is also given intravenously and orally to treat systemic infections, and distributes well throughout body fluids, including crossing the blood–brain barrier. Its very high selectivity for viral DNA polymerase means that even with systemic use, it is usually well tolerated and does not cause significant adverse effects, although encephalopathy has been reported. In systemic use, a good fluid intake is important, because the drug can crystallise out in renal tubules, leading to inflammation and renal impairment.

Foscarnet

Foscarnet binds to the active site on viral DNA polymerase and blocks its ability to add nucleotides to a growing nucleotide chain. It is 100 times more selective for the viral enzyme than the human enzyme, and so effectively blocks viral DNA production at concentrations much lower than are needed to affect the host cell. It is most effective in herpesvirus infections and is usually used in cytomegalovirus infections that have not responded to a nucleoside analogue

such as **ganciclovir**. It is poorly absorbed from the GI tract and is given by slow intravenous injection. It causes a range of side-effects, including serum electrolyte changes, which in turn can cause neurological abnormalities including paraesthesia and seizures.

INHIBITORS OF VIRAL UNCOATING AND RELEASE

Examples: amantadine, zanamivir, oseltamivir

Amantadine was first developed in the 1960s as an antiviral agent effective against influenza virus, but its use is currently very limited because of widespread viral resistance, and it is used more frequently in Parkinson's disease. It disrupts a key viral protein essential for viral uncoating inside the host cell so that the influenza virus cannot release its nucleic acid. Because this protein is unique to the virus, amantadine usually causes few significant adverse effects. **Zanamivir** and **oseltamivir**, both active against influenza virus, inhibit a viral enzyme called neuraminidase, which frees new viral particles from the host cell. Inhibiting this enzyme means that even though viral replication has proceeded within the host cell, the new viruses cannot be released and so cannot infect adjacent healthy cells.

INHIBITORS OF VIRAL PROTEIN SYNTHESIS

Examples: darunavir, ombitasvir, ritonavir

Viral proteins produced on the host ribosome from the viral RNA are usually in the form of large polypeptides which contain the functional viral protein interspersed with nonfunctional sections. The functional proteins are snipped out of this larger chain by specific viral proteases (Fig. 11.19). These viral proteases are the targets for protease-inhibitor drugs. Because they are unique to virus biology, inhibiting these proteases does not affect host cell protease activity. Protease inhibitors are used mainly in hepatitis C and HIV treatment.

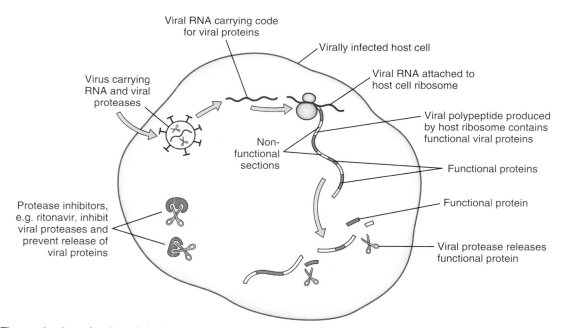

Fig. 11.19   The mechanism of action of viral protease inhibitors. Viral RNA is translated on the host cell ribosomes to make viral polypeptides. Viral proteases then cut the viral polypeptides up to release the functional proteins. Protease inhibitors bind to and block the viral proteases.

Focus on: Antiretroviral Drugs and HIV (Human Immunodeficiency Virus) Treatment

Acquired immunodeficiency syndrome (AIDS) first came to global attention in the early 1980s, when clusters of rare opportunistic infections and cancers in otherwise healthy, gay young men were identified in Los Angeles, California, and New York. These opportunistic conditions arose because affected individuals became seriously immunocompromised, and the causative agent, HIV, was identified in 1983. HIV is an RNA virus and is classified as a retrovirus because in order to replicate, once in its host cell it must convert its RNA into DNA. 'Retro-' in this context means 'going backwards', because in living cells DNA is always the template for RNA, and RNA is never converted into DNA. The DNA generated from the viral RNA is then inserted into the host cell's DNA and copies of viral nucleic acid and viral proteins are produced according to the mechanism described in Fig. 11.17. This process presents a useful selective drug target because retroviruses use an enzyme unique to viral biology and not present in human cells to catalyse the conversion of RNA to DNA. This enzyme is called reverse transcriptase, and the 'reverse' label here also reflects the fact that it catalyses a reaction that goes in the opposite direction to normal biological processes (Fig. 11.20). A range of drugs is now available to treat HIV infection and has transformed the condition from a rapidly and almost uniformly lethal disease to a chronic but controllable condition. No cure has yet been developed, although life expectancy with modern treatment is near normal.

Nucleoside HIV Reverse-Transcriptase Inhibitors

Examples: zidovudine, abacavir, lamivudine, stavudine

Zidovudine, which had been trialled unsuccessfully in the 1960s as an anticancer drug, became the first effective anti-HIV drug on the market and was licensed in the USA in March 1987. It initially showed great promise in HIV treatment, but interest waned when it became clear that when used alone, HIV rapidly developed resistance. However, in combination therapy, which greatly reduces the incidence of resistance, it is still widely used today. It works because it closely resembles the nucleotide containing the base thymine and is used in error by the viral reverse transcriptase when building new DNA from the viral RNA: it is therefore classed as a nucleoside analogue or false nucleoside. When the drug is incorporated into the growing nucleic-acid chain, it halts chain synthesis because it does not have a binding site for the next nucleotide to latch on to (Fig. 11.18). Zidovudine cuts transmission from an infected mother to child both through the placenta and in breast milk and delays the onset of HIV-related conditions, including HIV dementia.

Pharmacokinetics. Nucleoside HIV reverse-transcriptase inhibitors (NRTIs) are given orally. Zidovudine is a pro-drug and is activated in the infected cell. It is well absorbed and distributes widely, including across the placenta and into the CSF.

Adverse Effects. NRTIs as a group are very toxic and cause significant side-effects that can involve any body organ, probably by interfering with host cell energy pathways in the mitochondria. Adverse effects include reduced white blood cell counts, bone marrow disorders, and liver impairment. Regular full blood counts are needed, and care is needed in reduced renal function, because the drug may accumulate if renal excretion is impaired. The side-effects can be severe enough to require withdrawal of treatment.

Non-Nucleoside HIV Reverse-Transcriptase Inhibitors

Examples: efavirenz, etravirine, Rilpivirine

Non-NRTIs (NNRTIs), like NRTIs, inhibit HIV reverse transcriptase and prevent the conversion of viral RNA into DNA. Their mechanism of action is, however, different. They do not resemble normal nucleotides and are not assembled into new DNA strands; instead, they bind to the enzyme, changing the shape of its active site and deactivating it. The final result is the same: production of new DNA from viral RNA is halted, and without it the virus cannot replicate. NNRTIs are less toxic and more potent than NRTIs.

Pharmacokinetics. As a group, the NNRTIs have long half-lives of 2 days or more. **Efavirenz** is given orally despite unpredictable GI absorption, and distributes widely, including crossing the blood–brain barrier and causing central side-effects such as insomnia. **Etravirene** is well absorbed when given orally, although absorption is more effective following a meal, and is useful in treating HIV infections resistant to other NNRTIs.

Adverse Effects. NNRTIs can cause a range of adverse effects including hypersensitivity reactions and GI upsets. **Etravirine** increases the risk of myocardial infarction, likely because it interferes with glucose metabolism, can induce diabetes, and increases blood lipids.

HIV Protease Inhibitors

Examples: atazanavir, ritonavir, darunavir, saquinavir

The mechanism of action of protease inhibitors is described above (Fig. 11.19). **Saquinavir**, approved in 1995, was the first protease inhibitor licensed to treat HIV infection. It is given with **ritonavir** because ritonavir inhibits the liver enzyme CYP450, which breaks saquinavir down. In this way, ritonavir increases the half-life and plasma lev-

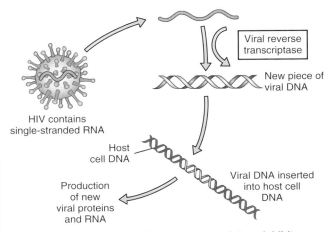

HIV contains single-stranded RNA

Viral reverse transcriptase

New piece of viral DNA

Host cell DNA

Viral DNA inserted into host cell DNA

Production of new viral proteins and RNA

Fig. 11.20   The action of reverse-transcriptase inhibitors.

Continued

els of saquinavir, and for the same reason is often used in low concentrations with other protease inhibitors.

Pharmacokinetics. Inhibiting metabolism of these agents with ritonavir extends their half-lives sufficiently that most require only once-daily dosing.

Adverse Effects. The protease inhibitors cause a range of adverse effects, including peripheral neuropathy, seizures, and hypersensitivity reactions including Stevens–Johnson syndrome (Fig. 3.13).

ANTIFUNGAL DRUGS

KEY DEFINITIONS

- Mycosis:
  an infection caused by a fungus
- Yeast:
  a fungus that grows as individual cells, often in colonies
- Mould:
  a fungus that grows as multicellular colonies in the form of long, thread-like hyphae

There may be as many as five million species of fungus on Earth, of which only a few hundred cause human disease. Most fungal infections are superficial, involving the skin, nails, or mucous membranes. Very few fungi are pathogenic enough to cause systemic infection in otherwise healthy people, and in general, those with functionally effective immune systems rarely develop systemic fungal infection, except in certain circumstances, for example following broad-spectrum antibiotic treatment. In the vulnerable, fungal infections can be life-threatening: for example, *Cryptococcus neoformans*, a very common yeast, causes no problems in healthy individuals but produces cryptococcal meningitis in immunocompromised people. In recent decades, the rate of invasive fungal infections is rising, because the numbers of immunocompromised people are rising: an ageing population, whose immunity is naturally declining, along with rising rates of certain chronic disorders, e.g. cancers and HIV infection, are significant contributors to this. Globally, the burden of fungal disease is disproportionately borne by resource-limited populations, with poor living conditions and limited diagnostic and treatment facilities.

The Biology of Fungi

Fungal cells are saprophytic, meaning they live on dead or decaying organic matter. They are more similar to human cells than are bacterial cells, making it challenging to find selective drug targets that damage the microbe but spare the host. As a result, many antifungal drugs are highly toxic in systemic use. Like human cells, fungal cells are eukaryotes, but unlike other eukaryotic cells, they possess a rigid outer cell wall to protect themselves from their external environment (Fig. 11.21). This cell wall contains substances not found in mammalian biology, including chitin and glucans. Echinocandins, e.g. **caspofungin**, inhibit glucan synthesis, disrupting cell wall integrity. Underlying the cell wall is the fungal cell membrane, which contains ergosterol, a substance related to cholesterol but not found in mammalian cell membranes. It offers a selective target for a range of antifungal drugs including

nystatin, amphotericin, terbinafine, and the azole antifungals, e.g. **iconazole.** Within the nucleus lies the cell's DNA, which must be copied prior to cell division. Each of the two copies then migrates to opposite ends of the cell, guided by a system of microtubules, in preparation for the cell to split into two daughter cells. **Griseofulvin** interrupts this process, halting cell division.

Pathology of Fungal Infections

Fungi frequently involved in superficial infections include *Trichophyton, Microsporum,* and *Epidermophyton* species, which may all cause ring-shaped, itchy, red skin lesions called tinea or ringworm (bear in mind this is a fungal infection and nothing to do with worms). Tinea infections are categorised according to location. The main groups are tinea pedis (athletes' foot, Fig. 11.22A), tinea cruris (jock itch, affecting the groin, Fig. 11.22B), tinea corporis affecting the body (Fig. 11.22C), tinea unguium affecting the nails (Fig. 11.22D), and tinea capitis affecting the scalp, eyebrows, and eyelashes (Fig. 11.22E). Tinea species are all dermatophytes (skin-loving) and feed on the keratin content of the upper epidermis. The other main organism causing superficial infection is *Candida*, the yeast responsible for thrush infections.

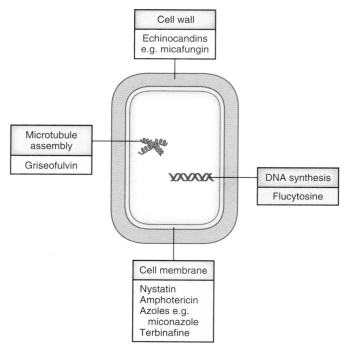

Fig. 11.21 The main features of fungal cell biology that provide useful drug targets. (Modified from Waller DG, Sampson A, and Hitchings A (2022) Medical pharmacology and therapeutics, 6th ed, Fig. 51.5. Oxford: Elsevier.)

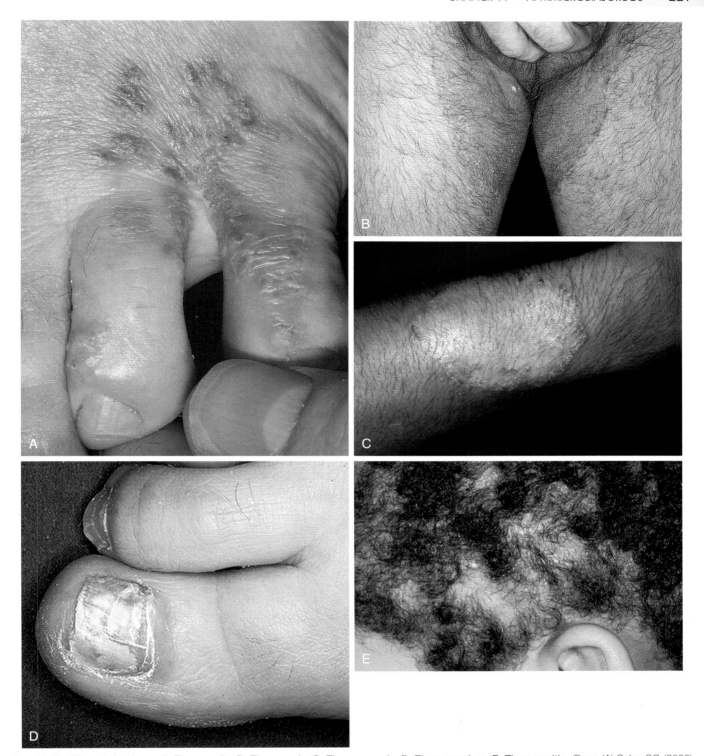

Fig. 11.22   Tinea infections. A. Tinea pedis. B. Tinea cruris. C. Tinea corporis. D. Tinea unguium. E. Tinea capitis. (From (A) Salvo SG (2009) Mosby's pathology for massage therapists, 2nd ed, Fig. 4.15B. St. Louis: Mosby; (B) Habif T (2016) Clinical dermatology: a color guide to diagnosis and therapy, 6th ed. St Louis: Elsevier; (C) Micheletti R, James W, Elston D, et al. (2023) Andrews' diseases of the skin clinical atlas, 2nd ed, Fig. 2.62. Oxford: Elsevier; (D) Terhorst-Molawi D (2020) BASICS dermatologie, 5th ed, Fig. 11.4. Munich: Elsevier Urban-Fischer Germany; and (E) Paller A and Mancini A. (2021) Hurwitz clinical pediatric dermatology, 6th ed, Fig. 17.4. St. Louis: Elsevier.)

A much wider range of fungi can cause systemic infections, which may establish in a range of body organs. Frequently affected is the respiratory system, because inhalation of fungal spores is a common route of infection. Fungi can also access the internal environment via wounds, or the GI or genitourinary tracts, and cause sepsis, endocarditis, meningitis, arthritis, osteomyelitis, peritonitis, and pyelonephritis. Many plant fungi produce toxins, which may be

ROSS & WILSON PHARMACOLOGY

stable to food processing and storage processes especially if not carried out to high-enough standards, and then consumed in contaminated foods. For example, aflatoxins produced by *Aspergillus* species contaminating cereals can cause hepatitis and liver cancer.

ANTIFUNGALS THAT INTERFERE WITH CELL WALL INTEGRITY

Without an intact cell wall, a fungal cell cannot resist the osmotic extremes of its external environment and disintegrates and dies.

ECHINOCANDINS

Examples: caspofungin, micafungin, anidulafungin

These are semi-synthetic agents, based on antimicrobial substances produced naturally by a range of fungi. The first of this family of drugs, **caspofungin**, was made available in 2001. Their target is an enzyme that produces glucans, essential components of fungal cell walls. Because glucans are not used in mammalian biology, this pathway provides a selective drug target. Echinocandins are only active against *Candida* and *Aspergillus* species.

Pharmacokinetics

As a group, the echinocandins have long half-lives: **caspofungin's** half-life is up to 50 hours. They are heavily plasma protein-bound and although they distribute well throughout tissues, very little enters the CSF. They are not absorbed across the wall of the GI tract and must be given intravenously.

Adverse Effects

These drugs cause a range of side-effects but are generally well tolerated, better so than other classes of systemic antifungals. They can trigger **histamine** release from mast cells, which can cause bronchospasm, bradycardia, hypotension, itch, and angioedema.

ANTIFUNGALS THAT INTERFERE WITH CELL MEMBRANE INTEGRITY

The cell membrane controls the entry and exit of substances in and out of the cell, and damage leads to microbial cell death.

NYSTATIN

Nystatin, one of the WHO's essential medicines, was isolated in 1950 from a soil-based bacterium. Although it is broad-spectrum, it is highly toxic in systemic use so is mainly used topically to clear *Candida* infections. It can be given orally to clear infections of the GI tract, including oral thrush, because its molecules are large, bulky, and highly ionised and so are not absorbed, avoiding systemic effects. Nystatin binds directly to ergosterol and generates damaging oxidising free radicals, which punch holes in the membrane. This immediately allows rapid and uncontrolled movement of fluid and other substances in and out of the fungal cell, killing it. Resistance to nystatin is very rare, because ergosterol is so fundamentally important to fungal cell membrane biology that it is preserved throughout generations. However, reports of resistant isolates are increasing.

AMPHOTERICIN

Amphotericin works like **nystatin**. It is however used systemically for a range of serious fungal infections, including invasive candidiasis, aspergillosis, and cryptococcus infections. It must be given intravenously and is very toxic because although its favoured target is fungal ergosterol, it also binds to cholesterol in host cell membranes, giving widespread adverse effects. Amphotericin is both nephrotoxic and hepatotoxic, and kidney and liver function should be monitored during treatment. The drug should be immediately stopped if liver function tests begin to show liver impairment.

TERBINAFINE

Terbinafine prevents ergosterol synthesis by inhibiting the enzyme that produces it. Without an adequate supply of ergosterol, the fungal cell cannot grow and divide because it cannot make a functionally intact cell membrane. Terbinafine is strongly keratinophilic and accumulates in skin and nails, which are rich in this protein, and is very useful in skin and nail infections. It is broad-spectrum and can be given orally or topically. It is highly lipophilic, so distributes very well throughout body tissues, and is generally well tolerated even in extended oral therapy for stubborn nail infections, which can be up to 6 months' duration. It can however cause severe hypersensitivity reactions including Stevens–Johnson syndrome (see Fig. 3.13) and hepatotoxicity, which requires discontinuation of the drug.

AZOLES

Triazoles: fluconazole, itraconazole, voriconazole
Imidazoles: ketoconazole, clotrimazole, econazole

The triazoles and imidazoles are closely related synthetic antifungals used in a wide range of infections. Clinically, the triazoles are all used systemically whereas the imidazoles are generally used topically. Although **ketoconazole** was the first antifungal azole licensed for oral use, it was withdrawn from systemic therapy in the UK 2013 because of hepatotoxicity and is rarely used systemically elsewhere because there are safer drugs available. As a group, the azoles act by blocking ergosterol synthesis. This prevents the fungal cell from producing new cell membrane, so that it cannot grow or divide.

Pharmacokinetics

Orally administered agents have long half-lives; for example, **fluconazole** has a half-life of 25 hours and **itraconazole's** half-life is 21 hours. **Fluconazole** is well absorbed with a bioavailability of over 90%, distributes into the CSF, and is one of the least toxic azoles. **Itraconazole** is erratically absorbed from the GI tract. Absorption of the liquid formulation is better than the capsules and is even better when gastric pH is low. It is therefore best taken on an empty stomach because food and drink in the stomach dilute the contents and increase pH. The azoles are metabolised in the liver and **itraconazole** is the only agent to have an active metabolite.

Adverse Effects

Systemic use can cause a range of potentially significant side-effects, including GI disturbances, blood disorders, and skin reactions. Azole antifungals are also associated with multiple drug interactions via a range of mechanisms. One important cause of interactions is azole-mediated inhibition of the important metabolising liver enzyme CYP3A4, which metabolises a wide range of drugs, including **anticonvulsants**, **non-steroidal anti-inflammatory drugs**, **immunosuppressants**, **benzodiazepines**, **antidepressants**, **antivirals**, **anticoagulants**, and many others. When co-administered with an azole antifungal, increased plasma levels of these drugs should be anticipated and managed appropriately. Even when applied topically, absorption through the skin can lead to plasma levels high enough to cause systemic side-effects, including these drug interactions. Because azoles are better absorbed when gastric pH is low, co-administration with drugs that reduce stomach pH, e.g. **proton-pump inhibitors** and **antacids**, reduces their absorption. **Itraconazole** should be used with caution in patients with heart disease because it has a direct, negative inotropic effect on the myocardium: that is, it reduces cardiac contractility, although the mechanism by which it does this is uncertain. **Posaconazole** can cause drowsiness and impair motor skills such as driving.

ANTIFUNGALS THAT INTERFERE WITH CELL DIVISION

Fungal cells divide much more slowly than bacteria, and because of this slow rate of proliferation and because, like human cells, they are eukaryotes, there are few available antifungals that target cell division.

GRISEOFULVIN

Griseofulvin is produced naturally by *Penicillium* species and is thought to interfere with the function of microtubules in the cell. Microtubules are hollow threads made of protein, used to give internal structure, to aid in motility in motile cells, and to guide and transport materials, granules, and organelles around within the cell. They form the mitotic spindle when a cell is dividing, which acts as tramlines to direct chromosome movement to each end of the cell. Disruption of these guiding pathways prevents mitosis and blocks fungal cell division. Griseofulvin is given orally, although its absorption is poor; fatty foods in the GI tract improve this. It has a high affinity for keratin and accumulates in hair, nails, and skin, and is used in tinea infections. Its half-life can be up to 21 hours and it should not be used in serious liver disease. It is teratogenic in animal studies, and effective contraception should be practiced if sexually active people are being treated with the drug. It is a potent inducer of liver cytochrome P450 enzymes and may therefore reduce the effect of a wide range of other drugs, including **oral contraceptives** and **warfarin**. It commonly causes GI side-effects and may cause serious skin reactions and peripheral neuropathy.

FLUCYTOSINE

Flucytosine is a synthetic agent mainly active against *Candida* and *Cryptococcus* species. Within the fungal cell, it is converted to 5-fluorouracil (5-FU, used in the treatment of some cancers, see also p. 236). 5-FU binds to and inhibits the enzyme thymidylate synthase, which builds RNA and DNA. Therefore, in the presence of the drug, the fungal cell can neither produce new proteins nor copy its DNA for cell division and does not survive. Resistance develops rapidly if it is used alone, and it is usually paired with **amphotericin** to prevent this. It is usually given intravenously and distributes well throughout body tissues, including into the CSF. Little is metabolised in the liver, so most is excreted unchanged by the

kidney and the dose must therefore be reduced in patients with poor renal function. Flucytosine can inhibit blood cell production, probably because it exerts its antiproliferative action in the rapidly dividing tissues of the bone marrow, and blood counts should be made weekly.

ANTIPARASITICAL DRUGS

All living creatures are susceptible to colonisation by parasites, organisms that establish themselves within the body of the host and survive and proliferate at the host's expense without providing any benefit in the relationship. Viruses by definition are therefore parasitic and are considered above. Parasites may enter the body via insect bites, contamination of wounds, via the GI tract in contaminated food or water, or from mother to child across the placenta. The main groups of organisms that parasitise humans and cause disease include protozoa, helminths (worms), and arthropods (insects).

PROTOZOAL INFECTIONS

Protozoa, a diverse group of single-celled organisms that vary hugely in size, preferred habitats, feeding habits, and methods of locomotion, include *Plasmodium*, *Leishmania*, and *Trichomonas* species.

ANTIMALARIAL DRUGS

Malaria is caused by five different species of *Plasmodium*, which spend part of their lifecycle in the *Anopheles* mosquito and part in their human host. The WHO estimated the total number of cases worldwide in 2019 was 219 million, 94% of which occurred in Africa.

Chloroquine
Chloroquine has been used to treat malaria since the 1940s and is still used today, although resistance is a growing problem. *Plasmodium* spends part of its life cycle in the infected person's erythrocytes, where they ingest haemoglobin, the haem portion of which is toxic to the parasite. Normally, the parasite converts haem to non-toxic metabolites, but chloroquine and the related agents, **quinine** and **mefloquine** inhibit this. Accumulation of toxic haem poisons and kills the parasite. **Mefloquine** is given orally, and **quinine** and **chloroquine** are given orally or intravenously. These drugs cause GI upsets, and a range of more significant problems: for example, at higher doses, **chloroquine** binds to melanin in the retina and damages the photoreceptors, leading to permanent loss of vision. They interfere with cardiac conduction and should be used with care in patients with known conduction disorders.

Primaquine
Although structurally related to **chloroquine**, primaquine interrupts the *Plasmodium* life cycle at a different point. Prior to entering host erythrocytes, the parasite spends time in the host liver, and while it is at this stage, primaquine poisons it by inhibiting its mitochondrial ATP production. It is given by mouth, is well absorbed, and is usually well tolerated although it can cause GI upsets. Care should be taken in patients who are deficient in glucose-6-phosphate dehydrogenase, and all patients should be tested prior to beginning

treatment. This enzyme is important for protecting the plasma membrane of red blood cells, and a degree of deficiency is relatively common in the general population. Primaquine worsens the effects of this deficiency and can cause serious haemolysis.

HELMINTHIC INFESTATION

Helminths (worms) may be transmitted orally, from contaminated food, water, or soil, or by invasion through the skin. Some helminths, e.g. tapeworms (Fig. 11.23) and roundworms, live in the host's GI tract, and others, e.g. *Schistosoma* species (flukes), invade other body tissues, e.g. the eye or the liver. Helminthic infections are of global importance: WHO 2020 data estimates that 24% of the world's population are infested with soil-transmitted helminths, most of which occur in tropical and sub-tropical areas.

ANTIHELMINTHIC DRUGS

Ivermectin
Ivermectin is given orally to treat a range of helminthic infestations and is also effective against the scabies mite *Sarcoptes scabei*. It interferes with calcium entry into the parasite's nervous and muscle tissue, paralysing it and causing death. It does not enter the CSF in humans, thought to be the main reason why it causes few side-effects.

Benzimidazoles
Examples: mebendazole, albendazole

These drugs inhibit motility in helminths by blocking their ability to take up glucose. Starved of their main source of energy, the helminth is paralysed and dies. **Mebendazole** is given orally, and little is absorbed across the wall of the GI tract. Most of what is absorbed is destroyed by first-pass metabolism in the liver, so this drug has little systemic toxicity in humans and is mainly used to treat infestations of the GI tract.

ARTHROPOD (INSECT) INFESTATIONS

These include fleas, mites, ticks, and lice. These parasites may themselves carry microbes that cause human disease,

e.g. tick bites can transmit Lyme disease. Common among these infections are head lice (*Pediculus capitis*), pubic lice (*Pthirus pubis*), body lice (*Pediculus corporis*), and scabies mite (*Sarcoptes scabei*) and are usually transmitted by direct person-to-person contact.

INSECTICIDES

The two main agents used to treat these infestations are **permethrin** and **malathion**, applied topically, usually as creams and lotions.

Permethrin
Permethrin is a neurotoxin, blocking nerve conduction in the insect's nervous system. It is poorly absorbed through the skin, so has no measurable effect on the host's neurological function, although it can cause local irritation at the site of application. Resistant variants in insect populations have been reported.

Malathion
Malathion is an organophosphate insecticide, a neurotoxin that blocks the enzyme acetylcholinesterase. This enzyme clears the neurotransmitter acetylcholine from nerve endings, including at the neuromuscular junction (the synapse of a motor nerve at skeletal muscle tissue). Acetylcholine therefore accumulates, and its action is significantly prolonged causing lethal interference with normal neurological function. When applied topically, some drug is absorbed across the skin, but it is rapidly metabolised, and does not cause measurable change in host nervous system function. Resistance has been reported, but less frequently than permethrin.

REFERENCES

Bhat, Z.S., Rather, M.A., Maqbol, M., et al., 2018. Drug targets exploited in *Mycobacterium tuberculosis*: pitfalls and promises on the horizon. Biomed. Pharmacother. 103, 1733–1747.

Dinos, G.P., 2017. The macrolide antibiotic renaissance. Br. J. Pharmacol. 174 (18), 2967–2983.

Gest, H., 2004. The discovery of microorganisms by Robert Hooke and Antoni van Leeuwenhoek, Fellows of the Royal Society. Notes Rec. R. Soc. 58 (2), 187–201.

Lobanovska, M., Pilla, G., 2017. Penicillin's discovery and antibiotic resistance: lessons for the future. Yale J. Biol. Med. 90 (1), 135–145.

Rehman, K., Kamran, S.H., Akash, M.S.H., 2020. Toxicity of antibiotics. In: Hashmi, M.Z. (Ed.), Antibiotics and Antimicrobial Resistance Genes in the Environment. Elsevier, Oxford.

Rubinstein, E., Lagace-Wiens, P., 2017. Quinolones. In: Cohen, J., Powderly, W.G., Opal, S.M. (Eds.), Infectious Diseases, fourth ed. Elsevier, Oxford.

Wanger, A., Chavez, V., Huang, R.S.P., et al., 2017. Antibiotics, antimicrobial resistance, antibiotic susceptibility testing and therapeutic drug monitoring for selected drugs. In: Wanger, A., Chavez, V., Huang, R.S.P., et al. (Eds.), Microbiology and Molecular Diagnosis in Pathology: A Comprehensive Review for Board Preparation, Certification and Clinical Practice. Elsevier, Oxford.

ONLINE RESOURCES

National Institute for Health and Care Excellence, 2015. Antimicrobial stewardship: systems and processes for effective antimicrobial medicine use: NICE guideline [NG15]. Available at: https://www.nice.org.uk/guidance/ng15.

Preston, S.L., Drusano, G.L., 2017. Penicillins. Antimicrobe. Available at: http://www.antimicrobe.org/d24.asp.

Very good review of the pharmacology of the penicillins.

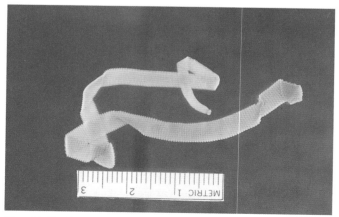

Fig. 11.23 Tapeworm. (From VanMeter K and Hubert R (2022) Microbiology for the healthcare professional, 3rd ed, Fig. 16.8. St. Louis: Elsevier.)

Reygart, W.C., 2018. An overview of the antimicrobial resistance mechanisms of bacteria. AIMS Microbiol. 4 (3), 482–501. Available at: https://www.ncbi.nlm.nih.gov/pmc/articles/PMC6604941/.

Uthayakumar, A., 2018. Cutaneous adverse reactions to antibiotics. DermNet. Available at: https://dermnetnz.org/topics/cutaneous-adverse-reactions-to-antibiotics/.

Clear and well-illustrated guide to skin reactions caused by antibiotics.

World Health Organisation, 2020. Global Tuberculosis Report: Executive Summary. Available at: https://www.who.int/docs/default-source/documents/tuberculosis/execsumm-11nov2020.pdf?s-fvrsn=e1d925f_4.

12 Cytotoxic Drugs

INTRODUCTION

The literal meaning of 'cytotoxic' refers to an agent which damages or kills a living cell, and in its widest sense includes adverse effects of drugs in physiological systems and antimicrobial agents used to kill or halt division of pathogenic micro-organisms. Its common use, however, has come to mean a drug used to treat cancer, and because cancer is such a common disease, the study and development of cytotoxic drugs is one of the most rapidly advancing areas in pharmaceutical research. Cancer is a disease that predates the history of our species. The oldest known case of cancer is an osteosarcoma in a toe bone of an earlier relative of *Homo sapiens* and is around 1.7 million years old (Fig. 12.1). Ancient Egyptian mummified remains show lesions indicative of bone cancer, and cases of what is clearly breast cancer are described in ancient Egyptian writings. The word 'cancer' is believed to have been first coined by Hippocrates (460–370 BC), the Greek physician sometimes also referred to as the father of medicine. It derives from the Greek word for 'crab', and likely originates because of the finger-like projections of abnormal tissue extending from a superficial breast tumour and which distort the surface of the breast. Chemotherapy, the treatment of cancer with cytotoxic agents, is the most recent of the three main therapeutic approaches, the others being radiotherapy and surgery.

The prospect of using drugs to treat cancer first emerged in the 1940s. Following the observation that the highly toxic chemical warfare agent sulphur mustard (mustard gas) caused a drastic fall in white blood cell counts, it was trialled in the treatment of lymphoma. In the 1950s, antifolates including **methotrexate** were used to treat leukaemia and other cancers. Since those early days, as understanding of the genetic, immunological, hormonal, and molecular basis of malignancy rapidly advanced, it has become clear that cancer is a collection of at least 200 different types. Based on this, a raft of new therapies has been developed, and the concept of targeted treatments has become a standard approach in many cancers. Cytotoxic drugs are amongst the most noxious therapeutic agents in clinical pharmacology because of their harmful actions on healthy tissues. However, our expanding understanding of the biochemistry, genetics, and molecular biology of cancer cells is driving the development of novel drugs which selectively target some aspect of malignant cell biology, reducing toxicity and improving the tolerability and efficacy of treatment regimens. Reflecting the ingenuity of the researchers engaged in this work, a bewildering and expanding array of drugs with a wide range of highly specific mechanisms of action is now available, many of which are only helpful in a small number of cancers because of their targeted action. This chapter does not aim to provide a comprehensive list of chemotherapeutic agents: indeed, with the speed with which the field is advancing, it is likely that any such list would be incomplete at publication anyway. However, it explains the scientific principles underpinning the pharmacology of the main groups of anticancer drugs and discusses important examples in more detail.

With improved diagnostics and treatment options, survival times and cure rates for many cancers have improved dramatically, but globally cancer remains the second leading cause of death.

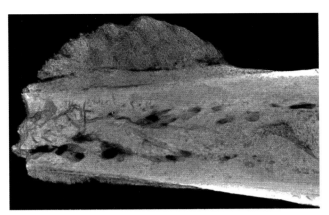

Fig. 12.1 The oldest known case of cancer. Osteosarcoma in the toe bone of an earlier relative of *Homo sapiens*: around 1.7 million years old. (Photo by P. Randolph-Quinney, Northumbria University; Weblink 1. Reprinted with permission.)

KEY POINTS

All tumours originate from a body cell whose DNA has suffered one or usually more mutations, the consequence of which is to release the cell from normal growth controls and allow it to replicate in a disorderly and unregulated fashion. The cell population produced from this malignant transformation becomes progressively more genetically unstable as the tumour expands, accumulating more and more mutations and becoming more and more abnormal. Cancers can be classified according to their tissue of origin:

- Carcinomas originate in epithelial tissues. Epithelial tissues cover and line body organs and surfaces, e.g. the skin and the lining of the gastrointestinal tract, and cell division rates are high. Multiple cell divisions increase the likelihood of copying errors occurring in the cell's DNA, leading to mutations appearing in the cell line. Eighty to ninety percent of cancers are carcinomas.
- Sarcomas originate in connective tissues like bone, cartilage, fat, and muscle.
- Blastomas originate in precursor cells (blasts). These cancers are most common in children.

DNA, THE CELL CYCLE, AND HEALTHY CELL DIVISION

Deoxyribonucleic acid (DNA) carries the genetic code that allows every nucleated cell to produce the structural and functional proteins it needs to fulfil its role. It is the largest molecule in the body: if all the DNA in a single typical body cell was extracted and laid out to its full length, it would be around 2 m long, an incredible feat of packaging given that most body cells are so tiny they can only be seen under a microscope. The cell's DNA is found in the cell nucleus but is only clearly visible in a cell preparing to divide, when it condenses into visible sausage-like structures called chromosomes. Nucleated body cells (except for sperm and ova) contain 46 chromosomes matched up into 23 pairs.

Ninety-eight percent of the DNA in a healthy human cell does not code for a protein and is referred to as 'non-coding'. Some of this DNA regulates gene expression, but most of it has no known function. The sections of DNA that do carry the code for a protein are called genes and are found at specific locations on a particular chromosome: for example, the gene that codes for insulin is found on chromosome 11. The human genome, the complete set of genes within the cell, contains between 20,000 and 25,000 genes.

DNA Structure

The DNA molecule is formed of two chains twisted around each other into a double helix like a twisted ladder (Fig. 12.2). The 'uprights' of the ladder are formed of alternating phosphate and sugar (deoxyribose) groups. Each sugar group has a base attached to it, and the bases on one chain are bound to the bases on the other chain with hydrogen bonds, stabilising the molecule and forming the 'rungs' of the ladder. Each sugar/base group is collectively called a nucleoside (see Fig. 11.18), and the sugar/base/phosphate unit is called a nucleotide (Fig. 12.2).

There are only four bases in DNA, thymine, adenine, guanine, and cytosine, and they display specific pairings. Thymine always binds to adenine and guanine to cytosine. Therefore, knowing the base sequence on one DNA strand accurately identifies the base sequence on the second strand. This is called complementary base pairing. The genetic code is written in the base sequences. Mutations in the base sequence of genes generate errors in the code and lead to the production of faulty, often non-functional protein.

Chemically speaking, adenine and guanine are purines, and thymine and cytosine are pyrimidines. Pyrimidine analogues, e.g. **fluorouracil** (FU), and purine analogues, e.g. **mercaptopurine**, are long-standing members of the

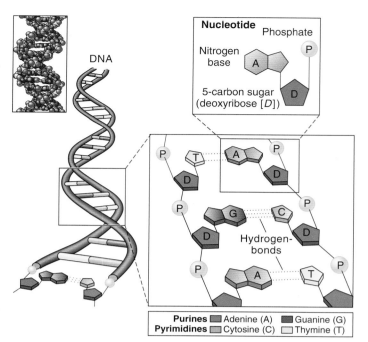

Fig. 12.2   The structure of DNA. DNA is formed from two chains of alternating sugar and phosphate groups, linked in a ladder-like structure by bases attached to the sugar units. The molecule is then twisted into a double helix. (From Thibodeau G and Patton K (2019) Anatomy and physiology, 10th ed. St. Louis: Mosby.)

chemotherapeutic drug armoury, and act by substituting for the true base when a cell is producing new nucleic acids. Nucleic acid containing the fake bases is non-functional.

DNA Replication

In body cells preparing for mitosis, the cell's DNA is duplicated, the fundamental event in the S phase of the cell cycle (Figs 12.3 and 12.5). DNA replication is a complex event involving several important enzymes, some of which are important targets for cytotoxic drugs. The DNA molecule is first uncoiled by DNA helicase, and the hydrogen bonds between the bases of the two strands are broken. This gives two complementary single strands of DNA, each of which is used to make a new double-stranded molecule: two identical daughter molecules are therefore produced from the original parent molecule. The enzyme which assembles the second strand on each original strand is called DNA polymerase. DNA topoisomerase stabilises and repairs DNA during DNA replication, and DNA ligase stitches newly synthesised segments of DNA together.

Because malignant cells usually divide more quickly than normal cells, DNA replication is an established chemotherapeutic target. Anticancer drugs can interfere with DNA synthesis in a number of ways. For example, cytotoxic anthracyclines such as **doxorubicin** and **idarubicin** insert themselves between the base 'rungs' of DNA (intercalation), damaging the molecule and preventing DNA replication.

mRNA and Protein Synthesis

To manufacture the protein product coded for by a gene, its code (the base sequence) is used to produce a single-stranded nucleic acid called messenger ribonucleic acid (mRNA). This is called transcription: the base sequence of the DNA is rewritten (transcribed) into the base sequence of the mRNA molecule, which travels from the nucleus into the cytosol and attaches to a ribosome, the organelle responsible for protein synthesis. The ribosome reads the mRNA code and assembles the new protein accordingly. This is called translation: the language of the base sequence code in DNA is translated into the correct sequence of amino acids making up the new protein (Fig. 12.4).

RNA is structurally different from DNA in three main ways: it is single-stranded instead of double-stranded, it contains the sugar ribose instead of the sugar deoxyribose, and it contains uracil instead of thymine. Like thymine and cytosine, uracil is a pyrimidine.

THE CELL CYCLE

A body cell undergoing cell division follows a tightly controlled series of steps called the cell cycle (Fig. 12.5). At key checkpoints, the cell and its genetic material are examined to ensure that they are healthy and that conditions are favourable before the cell can proceed to the next stage in the cycle: for example, cell division is inhibited if abnormalities are detected in the cell's DNA or if the nutrient supply is inadequate. These safeguards ensure that potentially dangerous mutations in DNA are not copied and passed to the next generation of cells. If damage is detected in a cell's DNA, pathways are activated to initiate repair if possible; if not, the cell's apoptosis (cell suicide, see below) genes are activated and the cell is eliminated.

The M (mitosis) phase comprises the process of cell division, producing two genetically identical daughter cells. During mitosis, the duplicated chromosomes separate, and a copy of each chromosome travels to opposite ends of the cell, attached to microtubules which direct chromosome movement. The vinca alkaloids, e.g. **vincristine**, and the taxanes, e.g. **paclitaxel**, inhibit microtubule formation and arrest the cancer cell in mitosis.

Following mitosis, the daughter cells enter G1 (the first gap phase), during which they grow and produce new proteins. Depending on the requirements of the tissue, the cell may now enter the S (synthesis) phase to prepare it to divide again, or it may be shunted into what is called the G0 phase,

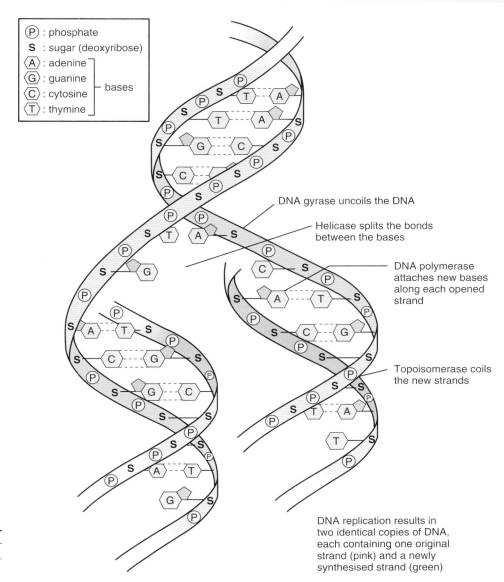

P : phosphate
S : sugar (deoxyribose)
A : adenine ⎤
G : guanine ⎥
C : cytosine ⎥ bases
T : thymine ⎦

DNA gyrase uncoils the DNA

Helicase splits the bonds
between the bases

DNA polymerase
attaches new bases
along each opened
strand

Topoisomerase coils
the new strands

DNA replication results in
two identical copies of DNA,
each containing one original
strand (pink) and a newly
synthesised strand (green)

Fig. 12.3 The steps in DNA replication. (Modified from HESI (2021) Admission assessment exam review, 5th ed, Fig. 5.11. St. Louis: Elsevier.)

in which it is fully functionally active but its ability to divide is disabled. If the cell is destined to divide again immediately, the health of its DNA is inspected at a checkpoint called the G1/S restriction point. If abnormalities are detected in the cell, its progress in the cell cycle is halted here. If the cell is found to be healthy, it passes into the S phase, during which the cell's chromosomes are duplicated in preparation for its next division. In the next stage, the G2 or second gap phase, the cell continues to grow and copies its organelles in preparation for mitosis. In addition, the microtubules, which will line the duplicated chromosomes up, separate them, and pull them to each end of the cell during mitosis, are assembled. Before progressing to the M phase, the cell's health and the integrity of its DNA is checked again at what is called the G2/M checkpoint. Damaged or abnormal cells are halted in their progression through the cell cycle here and are not permitted to undergo mitosis.

Cell cycle-checkpoint defects are characteristic of cancer cells, leading to repeated and uncontrolled cell division. Each time a damaged cell is allowed to proceed round the

cell cycle and divide, the number of mutated cells increases, and because one mutation predisposes the cell to developing others (genetic instability), it leads to an expanding population of cells accumulating multiple mutations and increasing risk of malignant transformation. Some of the most common genetic mutations leading to checkpoint failure are discussed below; they are an important target in anticancer drug research.

Key enzymes called cyclin-dependent kinases (CDKs) drive the cell cycle; CDKs need to bind to a regulatory protein called cyclin for activation. Both are potential targets in cancer drug development.

APOPTOSIS

Apoptosis is programmed cell death, sometimes referred to as cell suicide. It is an essential part of embryonic and fetal development, during which many more cells are produced than are actually needed, and the extra cells are eliminated by apoptosis to bring cell numbers down to within the desired range. Old, damaged, or mutated cells

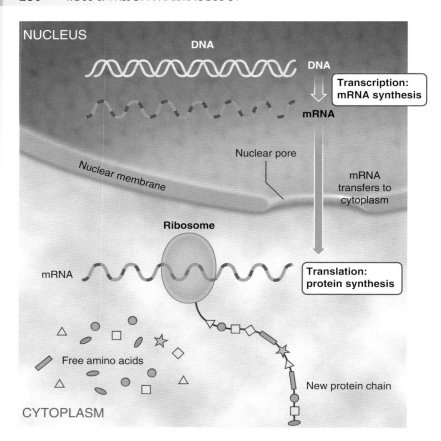

Fig. 12.4 Transcription and translation: the role of DNA, RNA, and ribosomes in protein synthesis. (From Waugh A and Grant A (2020) Ross & Wilson anatomy and physiology in health and illness, 14th ed, Fig. 17.5. Oxford: Elsevier.)

are also disposed of this way, as are cells that have arrested during mitosis, including as a result of chemotherapy. Apoptosis is therefore essential for growth and repair and in maintaining healthy function of cell populations in adult life. The key enzymes that drive apoptosis are called caspases. During apoptosis, the cell undergoes controlled but rapid disintegration: typically, half an hour is all that is needed for a cell to destroy itself. As the cell breaks up, macrophages rapidly scavenge the fragments to prevent the cellular contents from stimulating an inflammatory response. Identifying drugs that selectively stimulate apoptosis in cancer cells is an active area in anticancer drug development. Fig. 12.6 shows advancing stages of apoptosis in a malignant pig kidney cell exposed to the chemotherapeutic drug **etoposide**.

THE BIOLOGY OF CANCER

In health, cell proliferation, tissue growth, and the regulation of apoptosis are tightly controlled to safeguard against unrestrained, unwanted, or abnormal cell division. The fundamental pathological event in all cancers is one or more non-lethal mutations in the DNA of a body cell, which confer several important properties on the cell and allow it to escape the mechanisms normally governing the cell cycle and cell division. These properties give the cancer cell several survival advantages over its healthy counterparts.

PROPERTIES OF CANCER CELLS

Malignant transformation of a cell means that the cell has suffered one or more genetic mutations that have converted

it from a normal body cell to a cancer cell, with the acquisition of properties (Fig. 12.7) that allow it to move unchecked through the cell cycle, escaping the normal control points and dividing without restraint in a disorderly manner.

Loss of Differentiation Features

Differentiation is the process by which cells acquire their specialised (differentiated) characteristics, which allow them to carry out their particular function in the body. For example, muscle cells need to produce contractile proteins, and phagocytes need to produce quantities of degradative enzymes and other toxic substances to destroy their targets. A key feature of malignant cells is the loss of these specialised functions, and this is called dedifferentiation. Dedifferentiation correlates with malignancy; the more malignant a cell is, the more likely that it has lost its ability to carry out its specialised role. Drugs such as **retinoids** promote differentiation and are therefore anti-tumorigenic.

Immortality and Evasion of Apoptosis

Healthy cells are limited to between 50–60 divisions, after which the cell either has its ability to divide disabled, or its apoptosis pathways are activated. This ensures that old and potentially damaged cells do not continue to divide, reducing the chance that they develop malignant change. Malignant cells can continue replicating indefinitely and are resistant to apoptosis. Activating apoptosis is an attractive potential target for new chemotherapeutics. Although no agents have yet reached the market, some are in clinical trials, including turmeric derivatives such as **curcumin**.

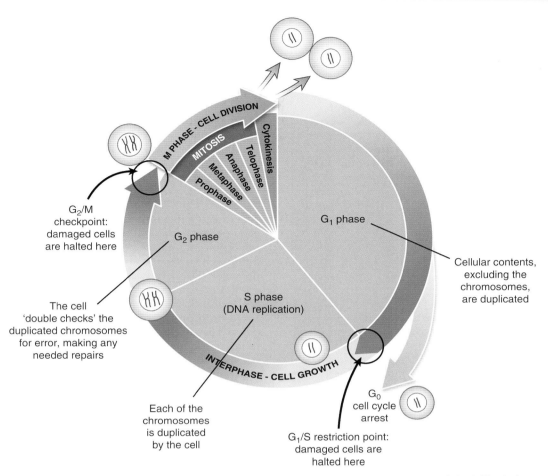

Fig. 12.5   The cell cycle. (From Grant A (2024) Ross & Wilson pathophysiology, Fig. 3.4. Oxford: Elsevier.)

Telomerase

At each end of a chromosome is a section of DNA which is there to protect the chromosome end and prevent it from damage, a bit like the short plastic sleeves protecting the ends of shoelaces. These protective caps are called telomeres. With each cell division, the telomere gets shorter. When it becomes too short to protect the chromosome end, cell division is arrested, and the cell may even have its apoptosis genes activated. This limits the number of divisions that a cell can undergo and ensures that older cells are shunted out of the cell cycle. Telomerase is the enzyme that builds telomere DNA onto the ends of chromosomes. Healthy body cells do not produce this enzyme, but cancer cells frequently do. This allows them to constantly repair the telomere caps on their chromosomes, theoretically allowing them to continue dividing indefinitely, producing expanding populations of malignant cells. Telomerase offers a selective target for cancer drugs; however, although telomerase inhibition strips the cancer cells of their immortality, it does not disrupt their ability to divide or exert direct cytotoxic effects. Although research in this area is ongoing, it has so far produced limited success and only one telomerase inhibitor, **imetelstat**, has so far reached the market.

Angiogenesis

When a tumour is very small, less than 2 mm in diameter, nutrients and oxygen can reach its centre by simple diffusion. As the tumour grows, diffusion is inadequate to supply its metabolic requirements, and it needs its own blood supply. Cancer cells produce growth factors like vascular endothelial growth factor (VEGF) that stimulate blood vessel growth (angiogenesis), developing a vascular network within the growing tumour and supporting its expansion. Several anticancer drugs, including **aflibercept** and **sorafenib**, inhibit angiogenesis.

Loss of Contact Inhibition

In health, cells dividing in a tissue observe social restrictions: once they have made contact with adjacent cells, their cell cycle is arrested and they stop dividing. This keeps the structure of the tissue orderly and cell numbers normal. Malignant cells lose this property and continue to divide even when in direct contact with their neighbours, producing excessive cell numbers and abnormal tissue architecture.

Motility

During periods of normal tissue growth, e.g. embryogenesis and wound healing, newly divided cells may be motile, allowing them to migrate along pre-determined pathways to their destination. This is a tightly regulated process, and once at its destination, the cell's motility is inhibited, and the cell takes up its position in the developing tissue. Cancer cells display increased and unhindered motility which allows them to invade locally and to cross basement membranes and other physiological barriers, permitting distant spread. Inhibition of cancer cell motility is a potential target in cancer therapeutics and several agents currently under investigation have shown promise in animal models.

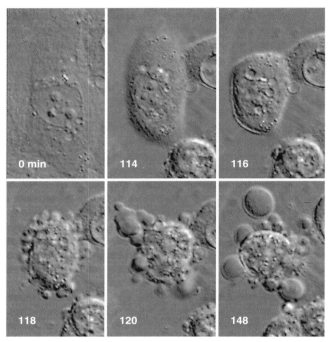

Fig. 12.6   The progression of apoptosis in a malignant pig kidney cell exposed to etoposide. (Courtesy L.M. Martins and K. Samejima, Wellcome Trust Institute for Cell Biology, University of Edinburgh, UK.)

Altered Nutrient Requirements

Because cancer cells generally divide faster than healthy cells, their nutrient requirements are high. Sometimes cancer cells can adapt their metabolism to use additional or alternative substances for energy. This is advantageous for the cancer cell in terms of improving its ability to grow and proliferate at the expense of non-cancerous cells, but it may also present potential drug targets: if a cancer cell has become dependent on a novel metabolic pathway not essential to healthy cells, it may be vulnerable to drugs which interrupt or interfere with that pathway, while minimising toxicity to normal tissues.

Genetic Instability

Genetic instability is the increased likelihood of further mutations when a mutated cell divides: that is, once one mutation is present, that cell will accumulate more and more mutations as it continues to divide. This is an important feature in cancer cells because cancer requires more than one, often multiple, mutations to be present. This can be exploited in chemotherapy because the more mutations accumulate, the likelier it is that the cell will be tripped into apoptosis and destroy itself. Poly-ADP ribose polymerase (PARP) inhibitors such as **niraparib** prevent a tumour cell from repairing DNA breaks and so push it towards cell suicide.

THE GENETICS OF CANCER

Two main groups of genes, proto-oncogenes and tumour-suppressor genes, are involved in the regulation of cell division, differentiation, and apoptosis, ensuring that cell proliferation is tightly controlled, halted when not required, and that old, defective, and worn-out cells are destroyed by apoptosis. Proto-oncogenes stimulate cell proliferation, and tumour-suppressor genes inhibit it. Mutations in one or

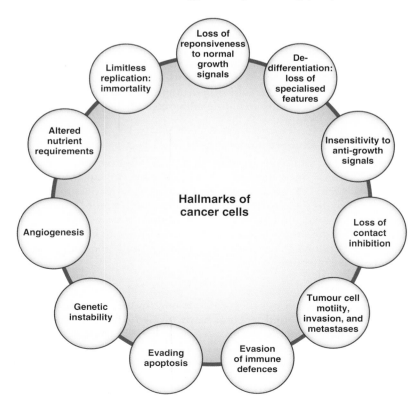

Fig. 12.7   Properties of malignant cells. (Modified from Craft J, Gordon C, Huether S, et al. (2023) Understanding pathophysiology ANZ, 4th ed, Fig. 37.3. Sydney: Elsevier Australia.)

more of these genes, leading to failure of their function, are found in all cancers, and an understanding of the genetic mechanisms underpinning specific cancers has allowed the development of an increasing pool of targeted therapies.

Proto-Oncogenes

Proto-oncogenes are healthy genes important in embryonic development, in growth, in healing and repair, and in replacement of cells that have reached the end of their useful life. They code for proteins which stimulate cell division and differentiation, and which inhibit apoptosis. Mutations in a healthy proto-oncogene can produce an abnormal oncogene (Fig. 12.8), which produces excessive quantities of a growth-stimulating protein, driving the cell through the cell cycle and allowing it to escape normal growth checks and halt signals. This is a common feature in cancer, and oncogenes are an important molecular target for the design of new cytotoxic drugs.

One example illustrating how understanding the molecular genetics of an oncogene has translated into clinical therapeutics is the story of **trastuzumab** (Herceptin), which came on the market in 1998. In the mid-1980s, researchers discovered an oncogene, called *HER2*, which produces a protein called human epidermal growth factor receptor (HER) 2. HER2 belongs to a family of cell-surface receptors called epidermal growth factor receptors (EGFRs). Epidermal growth factor (EGF) is a common growth factor which stimulates cell division in a range of cell types by binding to EGFRs. It was then shown that the *HER2* gene is overactive in a subset of women with breast cancer, increasing HER2 protein expression on the cell surface and

increasing the cells' responsiveness to growth stimuli and promoting tumour growth. This type of breast cancer was designated HER2-positive. Trastuzumab is a monoclonal antibody which binds to and blocks the HER2 protein at the cell surface, blocking the incoming growth stimuli and preventing the cell from dividing. Introduction of trastuzumab into the treatment regimes for HER2-positive primary and metastatic breast cancers significantly improves survival and reduces relapse rates: it has been a game-changing medical advance for this cohort of patients. It has also since been shown that the *HER2* oncogene is involved in other cancers including some stomach and oesophageal malignancies, and trastuzumab is now also used in these cases (Fig. 12.9).

Tumour-Suppressor Genes

Genes that produce proteins with anti-proliferative properties are called tumour-suppressor genes. These proteins act as brakes on the cell cycle, suppress cell division, and induce apoptosis in old and damaged cells. Mutations in one or more tumour-suppressor genes are commonly found in cancer cells. Important tumour-suppressor genes include *TP53*, which is mutated in over half of human cancers. The protein it codes for, p53, is essential for normal function of the G1/S restriction checkpoint in the cell cycle. Mutation of the *TP53* gene and loss of p53 allows damaged and abnormal cells to progress through this checkpoint, proceed through the cell cycle, and divide. Other tumour-suppressor genes directly linked to cancer include *BRCA1* and *BRCA2*. Mutations in the *BRCA* (**B**reast **Ca**ncer) genes increase the risk of a range of malignancies, including breast, prostate,

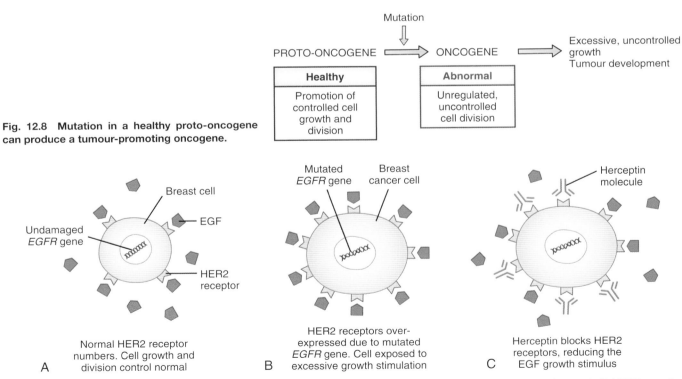

Fig. 12.8 Mutation in a healthy proto-oncogene can produce a tumour-promoting oncogene.

Fig. 12.9 The action of trastuzumab. A. Normal HER2 receptor numbers. Breast cell growth and division control normal. B. HER2 receptor over-expression due to mutated *EGFR* gene. Cell exposed to excessive growth stimulation. C. Trastuzumab blocks HER2 receptors, reducing the EGF growth stimulus. EGF, Epidermal growth factor; EGFR, epidermal growth factor receptor; HER2, human epidermal growth factor receptor 2. (From Grant A (2024) Ross & Wilson pathophysiology, Fig. 3.19. Oxford: Elsevier.)

pancreatic, and ovarian cancers. The proteins coded for by these genes are enzymes that ensure that damage to the cell's DNA is accurately repaired and so maintain DNA integrity. Loss of these enzymes leads to DNA instability, which predisposes the cell to malignant transformation. An understanding of the basic science underlying BRCA function led to the development of the PARP inhibitors, like **niraparib** (see below).

APPROACHES AND ISSUES IN CYTOTOXIC THERAPY

The perfect anticancer drug would kill cancer cells without causing toxicity to healthy body cells. In practice, cytotoxic drugs usually cause significant injury to healthy tissues, which often limits the dose that can be administered. Ideally, the drug should target some aspect of the malignant cell's metabolism or structure that is not present in normal body cells; but as all cancer cells originate from a body cell, finding such a target is a challenging proposition and requires a detailed understanding of the biology of the cancer cell in question. By definition, cancer cells have changed in some way compared to the healthy body cell from which they originated, and identifying these changes may expose vulnerabilities in the cancer cell which can be exploited by targeted drug design. For example, they are likely to divide more quickly, they may express different cell-surface markers, or respond differently to hormones or to growth factors. The progression from the basic research done at the lab bench to a clinically useful drug which extends and saves lives is the essential story in all areas of modern medical pharmacology, but perhaps the successes achieved in the development of novel, targeted anticancer agents is the most impressive illustration of this relationship.

Chemotherapy in cancer is often used in combination with other therapeutic approaches including surgery and radiotherapy, and drugs are often used in combination. In practice, because cancer treatment usually causes significant side-effects, the risk-benefit balance must be carefully considered when considering treatment options.

Staff administering cytotoxic agents must take steps to protect themselves. Pregnant women should not handle them.

COMMON ADVERSE EFFECTS OF CHEMOTHERAPY

A range of adverse effects are seen with many cytotoxic agents because of potential toxicity in multiple tissues and organs (Fig. 12.10). In addition, many are directly toxic to the liver and kidney, causing hepatic and renal impairment.

Teratogenicity

Women of childbearing age are always counselled to avoid pregnancy during chemotherapy because chemotherapeutic agents are almost always teratogenic in animal studies. The anti-proliferative and growth-suppressive activity of most chemotherapeutic agents confer significant risk of birth defects, especially in the first trimester.

Nausea and Vomiting

Along with anorexia, these are common and debilitating side-effects of many cytotoxic regimes. The physiology of vomiting is discussed in Chapter 10. Cytotoxic drugs in the bloodstream may stimulate the chemosensitive trigger zone and trigger vomiting, or they may stimulate the vomiting centre directly. Other agents may irritate sensory nerves in the GI tract and stimulate the vomiting centre via vagal afferents. Using anti-emetics to prevent or relieve these unpleasant symptoms is important.

Suppression of Rapidly Dividing Healthy Tissues

Healthy tissues with rapid cell turnover rates, including bone marrow, hair, skin, testis, and the epithelial lining of the gastrointestinal (GI) tract, are particularly susceptible to the anti-proliferative action of chemotherapy. Bone marrow suppression inhibits production of red blood cells, platelets, and some white blood cells. This causes anaemia, with tiredness, breathlessness, and palpitations. Thrombocytopenia (reduced platelet count) increases the risk of bleeding, and leukopenia (reduced white cell count) increases the risk of infection and suppresses healing. Cell renewal in the epithelial lining of the GI tract is affected,

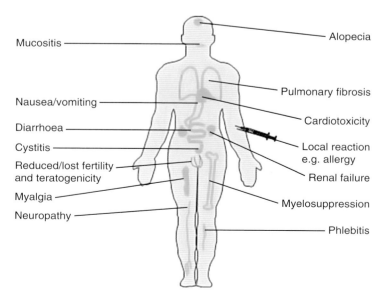

Mucositis
Nausea/vomiting
Diarrhoea
Cystitis
Reduced/lost fertility and teratogenicity
Myalgia
Neuropathy

Alopecia
Pulmonary fibrosis
Cardiotoxicity
Local reaction e.g. allergy
Renal failure
Myelosuppression
Phlebitis

Fig. 12.10   Common adverse effects of chemotherapy. (Modified from Herrmann J (2018) Clinical cardio-oncology, Fig. 1.5. St. Louis: Elsevier.)

leading to painful ulcerations, especially in the mouth, and diarrhoea. Rapidly dividing cells in hair follicles are suppressed, giving alopecia.

Future Malignancies

Many chemotherapy agents kill or eliminate cancer cells by damaging DNA so are themselves carcinogenic. Their action also extends to healthy tissues, and even if the cancer is cured, there is the likelihood that mutations in normal cells can persist and themselves cause secondary cancers, usually haematological, sometimes years down the line.

Reproductive Consequences

Cytotoxic drugs may eliminate or critically damage stem cells in the testes and permanently damage the oocytes of the ovary, leading to reduced or lost fertility. Freezing of sperm or ova in advance of chemotherapy may be an option in patients who may want to have a family in the future.

DRUG RESISTANCE IN CHEMOTHERAPY

Cancer cells, by definition, are genetically unstable. This means that the malignant cells within a tumour are not all genetically identical because of random mutations within the cancer cell population as they divide. Because of this, the sensitivity to cytotoxic drugs across the tumour-cell population is likely to vary, sometimes quite significantly. Treating the cancer with a particular drug may kill or irreversibly damage a significant proportion of the tumour cells, but cells which are less sensitive to the drug may survive and proliferate, producing a population of malignant cells resistant to the original treatment. This is fundamentally similar to the development of antimicrobial resistance in microbial populations (see Fig. 11.6). As with antimicrobial therapy, combination treatment, i.e. the use of two or more cytotoxic agents simultaneously, can help to reduce the emergence of drug-resistant cancer cells.

DRUGS THAT INTERFERE WITH ONE OR MORE STAGES OF THE CELL CYCLE

The increased rate and unrestrained manner of cancer cell division compared to healthy body cells makes cell division a useful target for anticancer drugs. However, many of these drugs are also highly toxic to healthy cells, particularly those with high proliferation rates, giving rise to some of the most common side-effects as described above.

SPINDLE POISONS

Examples of **vinca alkaloids:** vincristine, vinblastine, vindesine

Examples of **taxanes:** paclitaxel, docetaxel, cabazitaxel

Other agents: **eribulin**

The spindle is the network of fibres (also called microtubules) radiating out from each pole of the cell in a cell undergoing mitosis. Microtubules are built from proteins called tubulins (Fig. 12.11A). The spindle lines the chromosomes up in the correct alignment in the middle of the cell and then pulls the separating chromosomes to opposite ends of the cell, so that when the cell divides, each daughter cell has a full set of chromosomes. Spindle poisons arrest the cell cycle in the M phase and are used in a wide range of malignancies. They are usually given by injection or infusion because of poor oral absorption, although **vinorelbine** can be given orally. **Eribulin** is used in advanced breast cancer: it inhibits microtubule elongation and aggregates tubulin into non-functional masses in the cell. This disrupts the mitotic spindle, prevents mitosis, and triggers apoptosis.

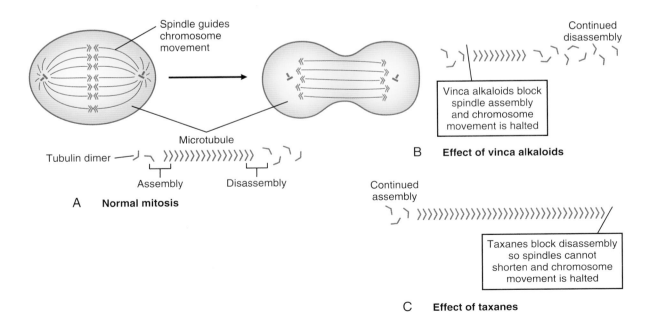

Fig. 12.11   Action of the spindle poisons. A. The mitotic spindle is formed from tubulin dimers. B. The vinca alkaloids prevent tubulin dimers from assembling into the linear microtubule fibres. C. Taxanes prevent disassembly of microtubules so that they cannot shorten to move chromosomes around the cell. (Modified from Stevens CW (2023) Brenner and Stevens' pharmacology, 6th ed, Fig. 45.5. St. Louis: Elsevier.)

The Vinca Alkaloids

Extracts of the periwinkle plant, *Catharanthus roseus*, had been used in traditional medicine for centuries for their hypoglycaemic effect, but in the 1950s two Canadian scientists isolated **vinblastine**, the first of the spindle poisons to be extracted from this plant. They prevent the assembly of tubulin proteins into the linear microtubule fibres (Fig 12.11B). Without an intact spindle, chromosome separation is not possible and cell division is arrested. The vinca alkaloids are mainly metabolised in the liver and have variable and potentially very long half-lives: for example, **vincristine's** half-life varies from 19–155 hours. The vinca alkaloids are neurotoxic and should not be given intrathecally. The main dose-limiting adverse effect of vincristine is dose-dependent peripheral neurotoxicity, affecting both sensory and motor function, although sensory manifestations, e.g. paraesthesias, dysaesthesias, and numbness, are more common. Some studies report up to 100% of patients developing some degree of neurological dysfunction. It is largely reversible on cessation of treatment, but some patients report persistent symptoms several years following chemotherapy.

Taxanes

The first taxane, **paclitaxel**, was derived from fungi living in the bark of the Pacific yew tree (*Taxus brevifolia*) and was first tested in cancer in the early 1970s. The newer taxanes are semi-synthetic taxane derivatives. These drugs prevent tubulin proteins from dissociating from each other (depolymerisation), which prevents the normal dynamic shortening and lengthening of spindle fibres essential for pulling chromosomes around within the cell (Fig. 12.11C). In addition to inhibiting mitosis, taxanes activate caspases, the enzymes that drive apoptosis, stimulating programmed cell death. The taxanes are metabolised in the liver. On infusion, they commonly cause mild to severe hypersensitivity reactions including urticaria, angioedema, and bronchoconstriction, and an antihistamine or corticosteroid is usually given in advance to reduce the risk or severity of this.

DRUGS THAT ACT ON DNA

Drugs that damage DNA, inhibit the enzymes needed for DNA synthesis, replication, or repair, or mimic the nucleoside (Fig. 11.18) building blocks of DNA are cytotoxic because they prevent cell division, and the DNA injury they produce may trigger apoptosis. They are discussed below under their main mechanism of action.

NUCLEOSIDE ANALOGUES (FALSE NUCLEOSIDES)

Examples of **pyrimidine analogues:** fluorouracil, azacitidine, decitabine, cytarabine

Examples of **purine analogues:** mercaptopurine, cladribine, gemcitabine, nelarabine, tioguanine

These drugs are structurally very similar to true nucleosides and compete with them during DNA and RNA synthesis, arresting DNA replication in the S phase of the cell cycle. Some bind to and inhibit one or more of the enzymes of the pathways producing nucleosides, halting nucleoside synthesis: examples include **fluorouracil** and **azacitidine**. Without a supply of nucleosides, DNA and RNA manufacture is not possible and the cancer cell cannot divide. Others are used by the polymerase enzymes building DNA or RNA instead of the true nucleoside, and newly synthesised nucleic acid contains both true and fake nucleosides. DNA/RNA containing fake nucleosides does not function normally and DNA cannot be replicated, thus preventing the cancer cell from dividing again. Examples include **gemcitabine** and **cladribine**. Whatever the mechanism of action of the fake nucleoside, the result is the same: the cancer cells' capacity to copy its DNA and produce proteins is impaired and the cell does not survive. Two representative examples are discussed here.

Fluorouracil

Fluorouracil is a pyrimidine analogue which is taken up more extensively in malignant cells than in healthy cells and binds to and blocks thymidylate synthetase (Fig. 12.12). Thymidylate synthetase converts 2-deoxyuridylate to 2-deoxythymidylate. This is a key step in the synthesis of DNA, and FU therefore blocks the cancer cell's ability to replicate its DNA and prevents it from dividing. It was first produced in 1957 and is still widely used today in a range of solid tumours, including some GI and breast cancers, and in pre-malignant and malignant skin conditions such as actinic keratosis. It has a short plasma half-life of 10–20 minutes and is metabolised mainly in the liver. Among others, it causes the standard range of cytotoxic adverse effects (see above) and may cause cardiotoxicity. **Capecitabine** and **tegafur** are pro-drugs which are converted in the tumour to FU.

Mercaptopurine

Mercaptopurine is used to treat leukaemia and is used for its immunosuppressant action in some autoimmune disorders including inflammatory bowel disease and severe psoriasis. It is an adenine analogue, is mistaken for a true adenine nucleoside, and is incorporated into DNA and RNA in cancer cells. It can cause the standard range of cytotoxic adverse effects and may cause significant hepatotoxicity: liver function should be monitored while the drug is being used.

TOPOISOMERASE INHIBITORS

Examples of **topoisomerase I inhibitors:** irinotecan, topotecan

Examples of **topoisomerase II inhibitors:** etoposide

Topoisomerase I and II are essential enzymes in DNA synthesis and repair. They cause the general cytotoxic adverse effects described above. Topoisomerase II inhibitors increase the risk of developing acute myeloid leukaemia later in life.

Topoisomerase I Inhibitors

Topoisomerase I stabilises and repairs DNA during transcription and replication, when the DNA strands are separated and vulnerable to damage. **Irinotecan** and **topotecan** are derived from camptothecin, which was first isolated from the bark of the Chinese tree *Camptotheca acuminata* and has been used in traditional Chinese medicine for thousands of years. They bind to and block topoisomerase I, causing double-strand breakages in the DNA molecule which are not repaired and lead to cell death. They are not absorbed when given orally and so are administered intravenously. Care should be taken in patients with hepatic or renal impairment. **Irinotecan** is used in advanced colorectal cancer and **topotecan** is used in ovarian, cervical, and small-cell lung cancer.

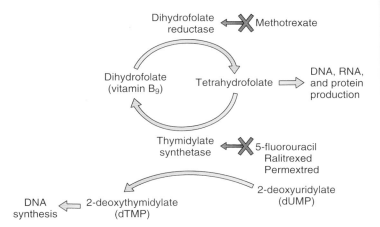

Fig. 12.12 The cytotoxic action of fluorouracil and methotrexate.

Topoisomerase II Inhibitors

Topoisomerase II stitches together (ligates) newly synthesised fragments of DNA in DNA synthesis. Topoisomerase II inhibition causes double-strand breaks in DNA, which are not repaired and cause cell death. **Etoposide** is derived from the mandrake root *Podophyllum paltatum*. It binds to and inhibits topoisomerase II, preventing DNA ligation and leaving the cell with non-survivable DNA damage. It is given orally, is partly metabolised in the liver and partly excreted unchanged, and has a plasma half-life of 4–11 hours. It is used in testicular cancer, in lymphoma, and in small-cell lung cancer.

FOLATE ANTAGONISTS

Examples: methotrexate, pemetrexed, raltitrexed, fluorouracil

Vitamins are co-factors, essential 'helper' substances without which an enzyme cannot function. Folic acid (vitamin B$_9$) is essential for several key enzymatic steps in the biochemical pathways that synthesise purine and pyrimidine nucleosides and some key amino acids, including methionine, serine, glycine, and histidine. Folic acid deficiency therefore inhibits DNA, RNA, and protein synthesis and so is particularly important in actively dividing cells. This makes folate metabolism a potential target in cancer therapy because cancer cells usually divide at a faster rate than normal cells.

Dietary folic acid is converted to dihydrofolate and then to tetrahydrofolate by the action of the enzyme dihydrofolate reductase (Fig. 12.12; see also Fig. 11.15). Dihydrofolate reductase is inhibited by **methotrexate**. Fig. 12.12 shows that tetrahydrofolate is a co-factor for the enzyme thymidylate synthetase, a key enzyme in the production of thymine nucleosides for DNA synthesis. This reaction converts tetrahydrofolate back to dihydrofolate, but dihydrofolate is then recycled back to tetrahydrofolate by dihydrofolate reductase, keeping tetrahydrofolate availability high. FU (see above), **raltitrexed**, and **pemetrexed** bind to and block thymidylate synthase, thus blocking the recycling of tetrahydrofolate and blocking DNA, RNA, and protein production.

Methotrexate

Methotrexate has been used as an anticancer drug since the 1950s and is still widely used in a range of malignant diseases including some leukaemias, non-Hodgkin's lymphoma, and some breast, lung, and ovarian cancers. It is also used as an anti-inflammatory and immunosuppressant agent in rheumatoid arthritis, inflammatory bowel disease, and psoriasis. Methotrexate inhibits several enzymes involved in folic acid metabolism, including dihydrofolate reductase and thymidylate synthase, preventing the tumour cell from manufacturing DNA, RNA, and key proteins and leading eventually to apoptosis of the cancer cell (Fig. 12.12). It is given orally or by injection and causes the standard range of cytotoxic side-effects (see above) and others, including neurotoxicity, confusion, respiratory problems, and hepatotoxicity. It is poorly metabolised and is mainly excreted unchanged in the urine, so great care is needed in people with impaired renal function. It is given once weekly and the half-life is dose-dependent: it is shorter (3–10 hours) in low-dose treatment, which extends to up to 15 hours in higher-dose treatment and even longer in renal impairment. Clearance varies significantly between patients.

Folinic acid (also called **leucovorin**) is used as a rescue medication and is given 24 hours after high-dose methotrexate to help reverse methotrexate-induced myelosuppression.

DNA ALKYLATING AGENTS

Alkylating agents possess one or two active groups (usually two) which damage DNA by attaching reactive alkyl groups to its guanine and/or adenine bases. Because most of these agents have two reactive groups, each group can react with a different base which cross-links the two bases (Fig. 12.13). Alkylated DNA cannot be replicated because the cross-links prevent the strands from separating, and it is subject to mutations and breakages, leading to cell death. These agents damage cellular DNA at all stages of the cell cycle and are among the most toxic of the chemotherapeutic medications. They cause the general cytotoxic side-effects described above, often with particularly severe bone marrow toxicity, and increase the risk of leukaemia in later life in a dose-dependent fashion. Although they are very toxic, they are used in a range of malignancies. They fall into a few chemically diverse groups.

Nitrogen Mustard Derivatives

Examples: chlorambucil, cyclophosphamide, melphalan, thiotepa

These drugs are derived from or chemically related to nitrogen mustards, which are related to the sulphur mustards used in World War I as chemical warfare agents and since

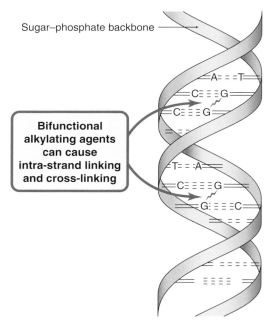

Sugar–phosphate backbone

Bifunctional alkylating agents can cause intra-strand linking and cross-linking

Fig. 12.13 Cross-linking of bases in DNA by alkylating agents.
(From Ritter JM, Flower RJ, Henderson G, et al. (2020) Rang & Dale's pharmacology, 8th ed, Fig. 56.3. Oxford: Elsevier.)

banned under the 1925 Geneva Convention. Their chemical structures have been modified to make them more stable.

Cyclophosphamide

Cyclophosphamide is used to treat a wide range of cancers in addition to severe rheumatoid arthritis with systemic complications. Its plasma half-life is between 3 and 12 hours. It is given orally and is a pro-drug activated in the liver and body tissues to the cytotoxic substances **acrolein** and **phosphoramide**. Phosphoramide is thought to be mainly responsible for alkylation and cross-linking, and acrolein is responsible for most of cyclophosphamide's toxicity; it produces large quantities of reactive oxygen species, which injure cell organelles including the cell membrane, damage DNA, and impair enzyme function. **Acrolein** is particularly toxic to the bladder, causing haemorrhagic cystitis especially at higher doses of cyclophosphamide.

Nitrosoureas

Examples: carmustine, lomustine, streptozocin

Unlike most other alkylating agents, carmustine and lomustine cross the blood–brain barrier and are used to treat central nervous system tumours. In addition, they are used in Hodgkin's lymphoma, and **lomustine** is used in melanoma and some lung cancers. They have short plasma half-lives of usually less than 30 minutes, but both are metabolised in the liver to active metabolites which extend their biological activity. Intravenous **carmustine** can cause delayed pulmonary toxicity, which is dose-related and may be fatal. **Streptozocin** is not absorbed orally and is given by infusion. It does not cross the blood–brain barrier; its plasma half-life is usually less than 15 minutes and it is metabolised mainly in the liver. It has an affinity for pancreatic islet cells and so is used to treat pancreatic tumours and is particularly renotoxic.

Platinum Compounds (Platins)

Examples: cisplatin, carboplatin, oxaliplatin

The anti-proliferative effects of platinum were discovered by accident in the 1960s when researchers observed that electrical fields inhibited *Escherichia coli* division. It was eventually realised that it was not the electrical field blocking the bacterial cells' ability to divide, but a platinum compound released from the platinum electrodes used to generate it. This compound, **cisplatin**, was trialled in the 1970s in a range of cancers and platinum compounds have established themselves as important therapies in a range of cancers, particularly testicular and ovarian cancer. **Oxaliplatin** is only used in advanced colorectal cancer.

Cisplatin is particularly renotoxic and a good fluid intake is very important during courses of therapy. It is also ototoxic, and hearing should be monitored.

Miscellaneous Agents

Examples: busulfan, mitomycin C

Busulfan is rapidly metabolised in the liver and has a plasma half-life of less than 3 hours. It is given orally, is well absorbed, and crosses the blood–brain barrier. In 6–8% of patients, chronic inflammatory and fibrotic pulmonary changes can occur, often after the drug has been withdrawn; the risk increases with dose. It is sometimes used in leukaemia, but its main use is in conditioning treatment before stem cell or bone marrow transplantations.

Mitomycin C is an old cytotoxic antibiotic derived from *Streptomyces caespitosus*. It is mainly metabolised in the liver and can cause chronic lung inflammation and pulmonary fibrosis.

OTHER AGENTS THAT DIRECTLY DAMAGE DNA

These drugs usually have more than one mechanism of action, but the end result is damaged, broken, or deformed DNA which cannot be translated into mRNA for protein production or copied for cell division.

Anthracyclines

Examples: daunorubicin, doxorubicin, epirubicin, idarubicin, mitoxantrone

The anthracyclines are intercalating agents which have a range of cytotoxic actions. They bind (intercalate) between base pairs, distorting the normal shape of the DNA molecule, preventing DNA replication and the action of RNA transcriptase, the enzyme which reads the DNA code and produces the mRNA needed for protein synthesis. Additionally, they produce toxic free radicals when metabolised, which breaks DNA and damages the cell membrane and cellular proteins. They are used in a range of haematological malignancies and solid tumours and are given intravenously because their oral absorption is poor.

Doxorubicin

Doxorubicin is produced by *Streptomyces peucetius*. Its mechanisms of action include those described above. Additionally, by inserting itself between the DNA strands, it prevents topoisomerase II (see above) from stitching together newly synthesised strands of DNA, and so halts cell division. Its half-life is 20–40 hours and it does not cross the blood–brain barrier. It should be avoided if possible in those with a current or past history of heart disease because it is cardiotoxic.

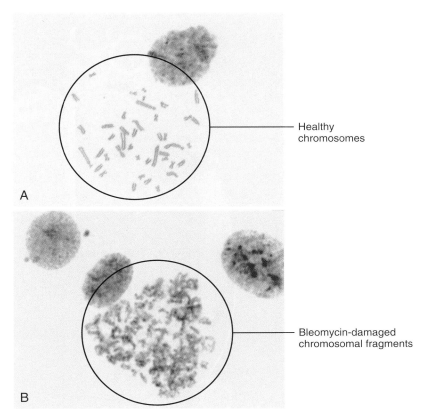

Fig. 12.14 Bleomycin-induced chromosomal damage. A. Healthy chromosomes isolated from rat cells. B. Fragmentation of chromosomes induced by bleomycin. (From Caporossi D, Ciafrè SA, Pittaluga M, et al. (2003) Cellular responses to H_2O_2 and bleomycin-induced oxidative stress in L6C5 rat myoblasts. *Free Radical Biology and Medicine*, 35 (11), pp. 1355-1364.)

Cytotoxic Antibiotics

Examples: bleomycin, dactinomycin

Bleomycin

Bleomycin is a mix of antibiotics from *Streptomyces verticillus*. It binds metal ions into a complex on the DNA strand, which generates reactive oxygen free radicals and produces both single- and double-strand breaks. The damage bleomycin inflicts on DNA is visible under the light microscope as abnormal and fragmented chromosomes (Fig. 12.14). Bleomycin is not given orally because it is not absorbed and is given by injection or infusion. Its plasma half-life is around 2 hours, and it is metabolised mainly in the liver. It should be avoided in people with pre-existing lung disease because it is highly toxic to the lungs, causing potentially fatal pulmonary fibrosis (Fig. 8.2). Incidence of bleomycin-induced lung toxicity may be as high as 1 in 10 patients. Other adverse effects include hypersensitivity-type reactions, fever, and skin toxicity including hyperpigmentation.

DRUGS THAT INHIBIT CYCLIN-DEPENDENT KINASE

Examples: abemaciclib, palbociclib, ribociclib

CDKs, in conjunction with cyclin proteins, are the enzymes that catalyse the co-ordinated sequence of events that drives a cell through the cell cycle. CDK activity and cyclin levels are frequently increased in cancer cells. Inhibiting CDK activity therefore reduces cancer cell progress through the cell cycle, reducing their proliferation and increasing apoptosis. There are at least 20 known CDKs, offering multiple potential drug targets. This is one of the newest areas of drug development and, at the time of writing, several potentially useful agents including **alvocidib** and **seliciclib** were in clinical and pre-clinical trials.

Abemaciclib was first approved in 2017. It is currently used to treat some advanced breast cancers but is being trialled in other malignancies. It inhibits CDK4 and CDK6 and prevents cancer cells from progressing from G1 to the S phase of the cell cycle. It is given orally, and its side-effects include increased risk of clotting, neutropenia, and anaemia. **Palbociclib** and **ribociclib** are similar.

PARP INHIBITORS

Examples: niraparib, olaparib, rucaparib

The enzyme poly-ADP ribose polymerase (PARP) binds to and repairs single-strand breaks in DNA. Inhibition of this enzyme means that strand breaks are not re-joined; this destabilises the DNA, makes it more susceptible to damage by DNA mutagenic agents such as radiation, and increases the risk of further damage including double-strand breaks. This normally triggers apoptosis and cell death. The first PARP inhibitor to reach the market, **olaparib**, was approved in 2015, and these drugs are mainly used in breast and ovarian cancer.

PARP inhibitors have been found to be up to 1000 times more effective in their anticancer activity in cancers associated with *BRCA* mutations than those with normal *BRCA* function. The *BRCA* genes are tumour-suppressor genes (see above) that produce proteins important for DNA repair. When these genes are mutated and non-functional, the cell is more reliant than normal on DNA repair carried out by PARP. Therefore, inhibiting PARP in cancer cells without functional *BRCA* genes means that DNA break repair either cannot proceed at all or, if a repair is made, it is prone to

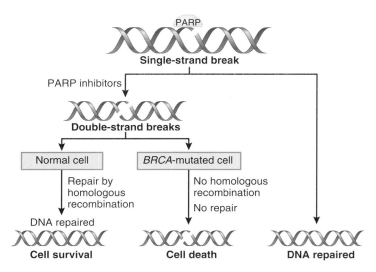

Fig. 12.15 **PARP (poly-ADP ribose polymerase) inhibitors are particularly effective in cells with mutated, non-functional *BRCA* genes.** PARP normally repairs single-strand breaks. In cells with *BRCA* mutations, the normal repair function of BRCA protein is lost. In the presence of a PARP inhibitor, DNA damage cannot be repaired, and the cell undergoes apoptosis. (From Sonnenblick A, de Azambuja E, Azim Jr HA, et al. (2015) An update on PARP inhibitors—moving to the adjuvant setting. *Nature Reviews Clinical Oncology*, 12 (1), pp. 27-41.)

error. Either way, the cell experiences genetic instability, predisposing it to further DNA damage and eventual cell death (Fig. 12.15). PARP inhibitors are therefore used to treat BRCA-associated tumours not only of the breast and ovary but also, for example, of the prostate, uterine tube, and peritoneum.

PARP inhibitors are well absorbed following oral administration and mainly metabolised in the liver. Their half-lives are variable (**olaparib,** 6 hours; **rucaparib,** 26 hours) and they cause general cytotoxic side-effects. They increase the risk of developing secondary myelodysplastic syndrome and acute myeloid leukaemia, usually within 8 months to 2.5 years.

CELL SIGNALLING PATHWAY INHIBITORS

Cell signalling is the umbrella term used to mean all the metabolic pathways in the cell which allows the cell to detect and respond to signals from hormones, growth factors, neurotransmitters, cytokines, and other chemicals in its environment. Identifying pathways that are unique to or over-expressed in cancer cells can lead to the design of specific inhibitors.

PROTEIN KINASE INHIBITORS

Examples: gefitinib, imatinib, lapatinib, sorafenib

Protein kinases are a large family of enzymes that activate proteins by adding a phosphate group to them. They have a wide range of functions in the cell and regulate the activity of proteins important in cell growth and proliferation and in immune responses. They have become important targets in cancer because protein kinases are dysregulated in malignant disease and contribute to the abnormal behaviours and properties of cancer cells, and a wide range of protein kinase inhibitors is now available, most for specialist use only in a very limited range of malignancies. Some of these drugs block more than one protein kinase, and others are much more selective and block very specific protein kinases in very specific roles. For example, the CDK inhibitors (see above) specifically target CDKs involved in the cell cycle. **Lapatinib** blocks protein kinases associated

with HER1, HER2, and EGFRs, and is used in HER2-positive breast cancers.

HEDGEHOG PATHWAY INHIBITORS

Examples: glasdegib, vismodegib, taladegib

The charmingly named Hedgehog (Hh) signalling pathway is essential for embryonic development and cell differentiation. In mature tissues, the Hh pathway is only selectively activated, e.g. in healing, repair and epithelial regeneration: in most tissues the pathway is switched off. When an Hh protein binds to its receptor on the cell surface, it activates a pathway which drives the cell through the cell cycle and promotes its division. Hh pathway abnormalities are associated with around one-third of all malignant tumours. With the Hh pathway erroneously activated, cell proliferation and other characteristics of tumour cell biology such as angiogenesis and increased growth factor activity are promoted.

The Hh signalling pathway is complex, linking the Hh cell-surface receptors to the nucleus and to other intracellular structures. There are therefore several potential drug targets for anti-Hh drugs and currently many potentially useful substances are under investigation. **Glasdegib** and **vismodegib** bind to cell-surface Hh receptors and block the Hh pathway, suppressing its ability to divide. They are given orally. Vismodegib is mainly excreted unchanged and is used mainly in advanced basal cell carcinoma; glasdegib is mainly metabolised in the liver and is used in acute myeloid leukaemia.

HORMONE-RESPONSIVE CANCERS

Cancers developing in sex-hormone-responsive tissues such as breast and prostate may be hormone-dependent, and so drugs that block the hormone have anti-tumour activity. Breast cancers that express oestrogen receptors are designated oestrogen (ER)-positive and those that express progesterone receptors are designated PR-positive. Tumours may have both (ER/PR-positive), either, or neither (ER/PR-negative). Most breast cancers are hormone-sensitive, so determining the receptor status of a tumour is an early standard part of breast cancer management because it dictates treatment decisions.

ANTIOESTROGENS

Oestrogen has a range of proliferative actions on breast tissue, and lifetime exposure to oestrogen is a recognised risk factor for breast cancer. About 75% of breast cancers are ER-positive, and drugs that block oestrogen receptors are therefore an important treatment option.

Tamoxifen

Tamoxifen was first developed in the search for oral contraceptives, and although it has no contraceptive activity in humans, it was trialled in the 1970s as chemotherapeutic agent in breast cancer. It competes with oestrogen for the ER and blocks its proliferative effect. It is taken orally, and its plasma half-life is between 5 and 7 days, but it produces active metabolites with much longer half-lives. It increases the coagulability of the blood, predisposing to clots, and should not be used in women with a history of thromboembolism. It can cause endometrial changes including malignant change. Patients should be advised to report vaginal bleeding or discharge, menstrual irregularities, or pelvic pain or pressure for prompt investigation. In pre-menopausal women, it causes menopausal side-effects such as hot flushes.

Tamoxifen may also be used prophylactically in women who have a strong family history of breast cancer.

AROMATASE INHIBITORS

Oestrogens are synthesised from testosterone by the action of the enzyme aromatase (see Fig. 5.14). Aromatase inhibitors therefore block the conversion of testosterone to oestrogen and reduce oestrogen levels, which inhibits growth of an oestrogen-dependent tumour. In addition, some breast cancers express elevated aromatase levels and so are particularly sensitive to the effect of aromatase inhibition.

Anastrozole

Anastrozole is an aromatase inhibitor, and it may be preferred to tamoxifen in ER-positive breast cancer because it has fewer side-effects. Common side-effects include osteoporosis, hair loss, vaginal dryness, and hot flushes. **Letrozole** is a similar agent; neither should be used in pre-menopausal women.

ANTIANDROGENS

Examples: abiraterone acetate, darolutamide, flutamide

Eighty to ninety percent of prostate cancers express androgen receptors (ARs) and are testosterone-dependent in the earlier stages of their development. Androgen-deprivation treatment using antiandrogens is therefore an important treatment; these drugs bind to the AR and block testosterone binding, depriving the tumour cell of this important growth signal. They are given orally.

GLUCOCORTICOIDS

Glucocorticoids have profound anti-inflammatory and immunosuppressant effects (see also Ch. 6) and are sometimes used as adjuvant treatment in cancer. Agents such as **prednisolone** and **dexamethasone** are used for their immunosuppressant effect in lymphomas, myelomas, and some leukaemias: they suppress the proliferation and activity of the malignant white blood cells and enhance cell death. In many cancers, however, glucocorticoids are not used as cytotoxic agents, but as supportive drugs to take the edge off the side-effects of chemotherapy and make the treatments more tolerable. For example, they may be given to reduce the severity of hypersensitivity reactions common with agents such as **pemetrexed** and **cisplatin**. Their anti-inflammatory action can help reduce the swelling and inflammation around a tumour, especially important when an expanding mass is compressing adjacent normal tissues, i.e. in the confined space of the skull. In this situation, **dexamethasone** is preferred because it has no fluid-retaining activity. Glucocorticoids are anti-emetic and stimulate appetite, so are useful in countering chemotherapy-induced nausea and vomiting and encouraging food intake. They can have a positive effect on mood and induce feelings of well-being and contentment, always a beneficial contribution in what is likely to be a difficult set of life circumstances for anyone dealing with cancer.

MONOCLONAL ANTIBODY THERAPIES

Antibodies are defensive proteins specific to a single target and are generated by B-lymphocytes (B-cells) in response to an immunological challenge, e.g. infection. Because of their genetic abnormalities, cancer cells express abnormal proteins (antigens) on their cell membranes, which may offer a good selective target for tumour-specific antibodies (Fig. 12.16).

Monoclonal antibodies (mAbs) used in cancer treatments are produced in the laboratory by a population of B-cells all derived from a single B-cell, which are therefore selective for a single protein. The explosion of knowledge in cancer cell biology in the last decade has enabled the development of mAbs directed specifically against tumour-specific proteins, offering an increasingly important contribution to targeted cancer treatment. The rapidly expanding list of therapeutic mAbs, all with long and complex names, may seem confusing at first sight, but mAb nomenclature does actually follow a set of rules; for example, the generic names end in '-mab', indicating that it is a monoclonal antibody. The one or two letters preceding 'mab' indicate the source of the antibody: for example, 'zu' means the source is mainly human but partly from another source, usually mouse. The one or two letters preceding that indicate the general

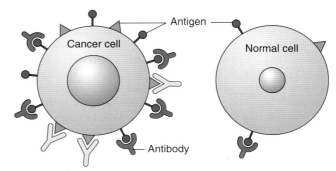

Fig. 12.16 The expression of abnormal antigens on tumour-cell membranes offer selective targets for monoclonal antibody treatments. (Modified from Craft J, Gordon C, Huether S, et al. (2023) Understanding pathophysiology ANZ, 4th ed, Fig. 37.31. Sydney: Elsevier Australia.)

target: for example, 'tu' means tumour and indicates the mAb is directed against a malignancy of some sort. Hence, **trastuzumab** is a monoclonal antibody derived from mainly human sources which targets cancer cells. mAbs are usually used in combination with other treatments and are always given by infusion or injection, because they are degraded by proteolytic enzymes in the GI tract and are poorly absorbed.

ADVERSE EFFECTS

In general, mAbs are less toxic than older chemotherapeutic agents, but they can induce severe allergic-type reactions, including skin eruptions, hypotension, fever, chills, and GI upsets. Some can cause target-specific adverse side-effects; for example, drugs which interfere with VEGF, an agent important in blood-vessel growth and development, can cause thromboembolism, bleeding, poor wound healing, and hypertension (see also **bevacizumab** below).

MECHANISMS OF ACTION OF mAbs

Monoclonal antibodies have a range of mechanisms of action in cancer treatment. In each case, the mAb binds to its target protein but there are a variety of effector mechanisms accounting for their cytotoxic action.

STIMULATION OF DEFENSIVE/IMMUNOLOGICAL MECHANISMS

Direct binding of the mAb to the cancer cell may stimulate a range of defensive and immunological mechanisms which lead to its destruction. Coating a target cell with antibodies activates complement, which causes cell lysis and attracts and activates cells of the immune system, including macrophages and T-cells, which destroy the target cell. Additionally, antibody binding may trigger apoptosis pathways, leading to cell suicide (Fig. 12.17).

Rituximab

Rituximab binds to a protein called **CD20** which is found on healthy B-cell membranes, but which is expressed in higher-than-normal quantities by B-cells in chronic lymphocytic leukaemia and some forms of non-Hodgkin's lymphoma, making it a relatively selective target. Binding of the antibody to the B-cell activates complement and triggers cell lysis, causing a rapid and sustained reduction in B-cell counts. It is also sometimes used in severe rheumatoid arthritis and other autoimmune disorders in which B-cells are thought to contribute to the disease pathology. It has a long half-life, which extends with repeated dosing and can exceed 30 days. Side-effects are numerous and can be severe. Severe infusion reactions, which can be fatal, have been reported: widespread cytokine release causes hypotension, cardiac arrhythmias, pulmonary infiltration, and acute respiratory distress syndrome and shock. Another serious and potentially fatal reaction is acute renal failure due to the sudden release of B-cell breakdown products into the bloodstream. Other agents with similar mechanisms of action to rituximab include **ofatumumab** and **alemtuzumab.**

BLOCKING CELL-SURFACE RECEPTORS FOR GROWTH FACTORS

Cancer cells are dependent on a range of growth factors to stimulate growth and survival. Monoclonal antibodies which

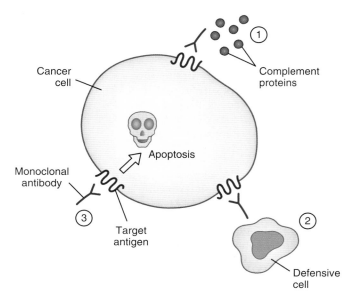

Fig. 12.17   Cytotoxic monoclonal antibodies may trigger cancer cell death by activating immune or defence mechanisms. Antibody binding: 1. Activates complement. 2. Attract and activates defence cells e.g. macrophages. 3. Triggers apoptosis and cell death.

target the cell's receptors for these growth factors block the cell's ability to respond. Examples include **ramucirumab**, which targets VEGF receptors, preventing the tumour from developing its own network of blood vessels.

Trastuzumab

Trastuzumab blocks EGFRs on some types of cancer cells and so silences this growth-stimulating signal. Its mechanism of action is described in more detail above. It is used mainly in HER2-positive breast cancer but also in other cancers that over-express the HER2 receptor, including some gastric cancers. Only about 15%–25% of breast cancers are HER2-positive and therefore respond to trastuzumab, but these tumours tend to be faster growing and more aggressive than HER2-negative disease, and this drug has significantly improved prognosis and survival in HER2-positive cases. Its most significant side-effect is cardiotoxicity, and it can cause arrhythmias, heart failure, and coronary artery disease, which are usually reversible when treatment stops. The reason behind this is not completely clear, but it is known that healthy cardiac myocytes express HER2, and that blocking this receptor may inhibit the myocardial cells' capacity to detoxify harmful products of cellular metabolism, including reactive oxygen species, which then accumulate and damage the cell. Cardiac function should be monitored during and after treatment. Other HER2 receptor inhibitors include **pertuzumab.** Because trastuzumab and pertuzumab block different sites on the HER2 receptor, they have a synergistic action and can usefully be combined.

BINDING TO CHEMICAL FACTORS ESSENTIAL FOR CANCER CELL GROWTH AND SURVIVAL

Monoclonal antibodies may be targeted against growth factors or other cytokines on which the cancer cell is dependent. When the mAb binds to the growth factor, it can no longer bind to its receptor.

Bevacizumab

As a solid tumour expands, it needs its own network of blood vessels to ensure an adequate supply of oxygen and nutrients, and most tumours produce increased levels of vascular endothelial growth factor (VEGF) to promote blood vessel growth and survival. Bevacizumab is a mAb directed against VEGF; it binds to and neutralises the VEGF molecule, depriving the tumour of this key mediator and inhibiting tumour angiogenesis. It is used in several cancers including breast, colon, and reproductive tract tumours and is currently also being trialled in the treatment of severe post–COVID-19 respiratory complications including acute lung injury, in which VEGF seems to contribute to the disease process. It has an average half-life of 20 days, although this can be more than doubled in some patients. It is associated with a wide range of side-effects, including the consequences of blocking VEGF in normal tissues (see above).

TARGETED DELIVERY OF OTHER CYTOTOXIC TREATMENTS

Monoclonal antibodies can be bound to a cytotoxic drug to form an antibody–drug conjugate. Because the conjugates bind directly to cancer cells via the mAb component, the cytotoxic effect of the conjugated drug is increased and its toxicity to healthy tissues is reduced. Once the mAb binds to its target receptor on the cancer cell, the conjugate is internalised, and the conjugate is degraded by intracellular enzymes to release the cytotoxic drug inside the cell (Fig. 12.18). For example, **trastuzumab deruxtecan** is a conjugate of trastuzumab and deruxtecan used in advanced HER2-positive breast cancer. Deruxtecan inhibits topoisomerase and so inhibits the cancer cell's ability to repair its DNA during cell division. **Trastuzumab emtansine** is a conjugate of trastuzumab with emtansine which is used in advanced breast cancer. Emtansine interferes with assembly of the microtubule spindle that directs chromosome separation

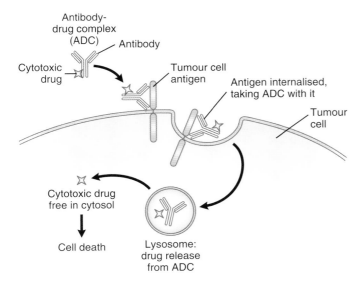

Fig. 12.18 The action of antibody–drug conjugates. The antibody gives the conjugate specificity for the target cell. After it binds, the conjugate is internalised, where the drug is released and exerts its cytotoxic action. (Modified from Senter PD and Sievers EL (2012) The discovery and development of brentuximab vedotin for use in relapsed Hodgkin's lymphoma and systemic anaplastic large cell lymphoma. *Nature Biotechnology*, 30 (7), 631–637.)

during mitosis. This arrests the cell cycle, and the tumour cell is killed by apoptosis. **Gemtuzumab ozogamicin** is a conjugate of gemtuzumab and ozogamicin. Gemtuzumab is directed against a cell-surface protein called CD33, which is found in elevated quantities on the surface of leukaemic myeloblasts in most patients with acute myeloid leukaemia. CD33 stimulates cell division, so blockade of these receptors inhibits leukaemic cell proliferation. Once internalised, ozogamicin, which is a cytotoxic antibiotic, binds to and damages the leukaemic cell's DNA, activating apoptosis and inducing cell death.

IMMUNOTHERAPY

The most familiar role of the immune system is in the prevention and control of infection, but part of its role is the constant surveillance of tissues to identify and destroy mutated or abnormal cells. Cancer cells develop ways to conceal and protect themselves from the unwanted attentions of T-cells and other body defences, including producing tumour-derived immunosuppressant factors which dampen down normal immune activity. Immunotherapy is an umbrella term meaning any treatment which in some way enhances the immune system's capacity to destroy tumour cells, and these are among the newest available cancer therapies. The mAbs which coat cancer cells and stimulate complement (e.g. **rituximab**, see above) are one example of immunotherapy. Other examples of immunotherapy include:

IMMUNE CHECKPOINT INHIBITORS

Immune checkpoint proteins are found on the surface of immune cells, and when activated they inhibit immune responses and promote immune tolerance. In health, this is an important regulator of immune cell function, putting the brakes on potentially damaging or inappropriate immune responses. One strategy used by malignant cells to evade immune killing is to up-regulate the immune checkpoint proteins on T-cells in the tumour environment. This suppresses T-cell function and reduces their ability to attack and destroy the cancer cells.

Work on three different immune checkpoint proteins has yielded useful anticancer drugs in recent years: the PD (programmed cell death)-1 protein, the cytotoxic T-lymphocyte-associated protein-4 (CTLA-4) and the lymphocyte activation gene-3 (LAG-3). Monoclonal antibodies that target these checkpoint proteins block them, releasing the brake on T-cells and increasing their capacity to attack and destroy tumour cells. **Nivolumab** and **pembrolizumab** are examples of PD-1 checkpoint inhibitors and are used in a range of advanced cancers including metastatic melanoma. **Opdualag** was licensed in the US in 2022 for the treatment of advanced malignant melanoma. It is a combination of two mAbs: nivolumab, which as described above blocks PD-1, and **relatlimab**, which blocks LAG-3. **Ipilimumab** is a CTLA-4 inhibitor licensed in 2011 for the treatment of melanoma.

IMMUNE SYSTEM MODULATORS

These drugs enhance the body's immune response to cancer. Interleukins (ILs) and interferons are cytokines produced naturally by white blood cells that stimulate lymphocyte numbers and activity. Used therapeutically, their

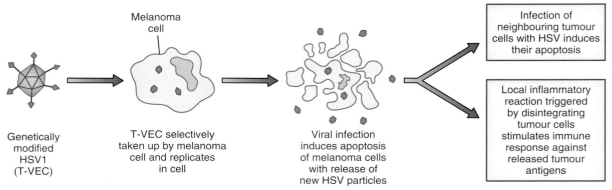

Fig. 12.19   **The mechanism of action of talimogene laherparepvec (T-VEC).** HSV, Herpes simplex virus

immunostimulant action increases immune responses to tumour cells. For example, **aldesleukin** is synthetic IL-2 used in some renal cancers. **Thalidomide** has a dark history because following its introduction in the 1960s to prevent pregnancy-related sickness, it proved to be a potent teratogen responsible for tens of thousands of babies born with significant birth defects. However, along with the related agents **pomalidomide** and **lenalidomide**, it is now used in multiple myeloma. These drugs stimulate the release of pro-inflammatory cytokines including IL-6 and tumour necrosis factor alpha, promoting inflammatory and immune function and enhancing malignant cell detection and destruction. There is also evidence that they inhibit the action of growth factors including VEGF, impairing the ability of the tumour to develop its own blood supply. This latter action probably accounts for their teratogenicity.

TREATMENT VACCINES

Although research in this area is still at a very early stage, it offers the exciting prospect of personally tailored cancer treatment. Unlike vaccination to prevent infection, cancer vaccines are not intended as prophylactic therapies. The principle here is that identification of tumour-specific proteins expressed on the surface of an individual's cancer cells can be used to make a vaccine specific to those cancer cells. Administration of the vaccine to that individual then stimulates an immune response specific to the cancer cells with resultant destruction of the tumour.

Virus Vaccines

Viruses are intracellular parasites. They enter a cell and hijack the cell's organelles to produce new viral proteins and nucleic acids, which are then assembled into new viral particles (see Fig. 11.17). Depending on the virus, these new viral particles may accumulate in the host cell until the host cell literally bursts (lysis), releasing the viral particles into the local vicinity to infect neighbouring cells. One novel approach to cancer therapy is to use viruses to infect and destroy cancer cells.

Talimogene Laherparepvec

This therapy is a genetically modified preparation of herpes simplex virus type 1. It is used in malignant melanoma and injected directly into the tumour. The virus is genetically engineered to selectively enter and replicate within tumour cells, causing the cell to lyse and release large quantities of melanoma-tumour antigens into the local environment. This activates defence and immune cells, which multiply and produce a local and systemic immune response directed against the tumour. The released viral particles infect neighbouring cancer cells, and the process is repeated (Fig. 12.19). Care is needed in immunosuppressed patients, for example those on steroid treatment, because although the pathogenicity of the genetically engineered virus has been substantially reduced, it may still cause systemic herpes infections in people whose immune function is impaired.

MISCELLANEOUS CHEMOTHERAPY DRUGS

Some drugs do not fall tidily into the categories used above.

PROTEASOME INHIBITORS

Examples: bortezomib, carfilzomib, ixazomib

The proteasome is a complex of proteolytic enzymes responsible for destroying unwanted, abnormal, or misfolded proteins inside the cell. Proteasomes are found in cells throughout the body, ensure that potentially harmful proteins do not accumulate, and allow the cell to maintain levels of key regulatory proteins within normal ranges. Proteasome inhibitors bind to one or more of the enzymatic sites within the proteasome and block them. This leads to the accumulation of a range of unwanted and abnormal proteins in the cell, interfering with the cell's ability to regulate its internal pathways and triggering apoptosis. These drugs are used in multiple myeloma and can cause a wide range of side-effects, including cardiovascular events and reactivation of latent viral infections including herpes zoster and hepatitis B.

ASPARAGINASE

The enzyme asparaginase breaks down the amino acid asparagine. Therapeutically, it is available in different formulations derived from different sources: for example, **crisantaspase** is the asparaginase produced by *Erwinia chrysanthemi* and there are formulations prepared from *Escherichia coli* asparaginase. **Pegaspargase** is a PEGylated formulation. Asparagine is needed for DNA and protein synthesis, and asparagine depletion inhibits the proliferation of tumour cells. Asparaginase is used in acute lymphoblastic leukaemia.

RETINOIC ACID AND ITS DERIVATIVES

Retinoic acid is a metabolite of vitamin A; it enters cells and acts on receptors in the nucleus to regulate genes that suppress cell proliferation, promote cell differentiation, and induce apoptosis. Retinoic acid and its derivatives therefore have an anti-tumour action, although they are highly toxic to healthy cells and in therapeutic use have significant side-effects including teratogenicity and neuropsychiatric reactions. **Bexarotene** is a synthetic retinoid used in T-cell lymphoma, and **tretinoin** is used in acute promyelocytic leukaemia. Because of their anti-proliferative activity, tretinoin and **isotretinoin** are also used in severe acne.

REFERENCES

Drew, Y., 2015. The development of PARP inhibitors in ovarian cancer: from bench to bedside. Br. J. Cancer 113 (Suppl. 1), S3–S9.

Pufall, M.A., 2015. Glucocorticoids and cancer. Adv. Exp. Med. Biol. 872, 315–333.

Tadesse, S., Caldon, E.C., Tilley, W., et al., 2019. Cyclin-dependent kinase 2 inhibitors in cancer therapy: an update. J. Med. Chem. 62 (9), 4233–4251.

Wang, J., Fang, Y., Fan, R.A., et al., 2021. Proteasome inhibitors and their pharmacokinetics, pharmacodynamics and metabolism. Int. J. Mol. Sci. 22 (21), 11595.

ONLINE RESOURCES

Chial, H., 2008. Proto-oncogenes to oncogenes to cancer. Nat. Educ. 1 (1), 33. Available at: https://www.nature.com/scitable/topicpage/proto-oncogenes-to-oncogenes-to-cancer-883/#:~:text=Often%2C%20pro-to%2Doncogenes%20encode%20proteins,maintenance%20of%20tissues%20and%20organs.

Emory Winship Cancer Institute, 2024. Cancer biology. Available at: https://www.cancerquest.org/cancer-biology.

Sun, Y., Liu, Y., Ma, X., et al., 2021. The influence of cell cycle regulation on chemotherapy. Int. J. Mol. Sci. 22 (13), 6923. Available at: https://www.ncbi.nlm.nih.gov/pmc/articles/PMC8267727/.

Zahavi, D., Weiner, L., 2020. Monoclonal antibodies in cancer therapy. Antibodies 9 (3), 34. Available at: https://www.mdpi.com/2073-4468/9/3/34/htm.

Index

Page numbers followed by "*f*" indicate figures, "*b*" indicate boxes, and "*t*" indicate tables.

246